Providing Health Care in the Context of Language Barriers

Full details of all our publications can be found on http://www.multilingual-matters.com, or by writing to Multilingual Matters, St Nicholas House, 31–34 High Street, Bristol BS1 2AW, UK.

Providing Health Care in the Context of Language Barriers

International Perspectives

Edited by
Elizabeth A. Jacobs and Lisa C. Diamond

MULTILINGUAL MATTERS
Bristol • Blue Ridge Summit

DOI 10.21832/JACOBS7760
Library of Congress Cataloging in Publication Data
Names: Jacobs, Elizabeth A., editor. | Diamond, Lisa (Physician), editor.
Title: Providing Health Care in the Context of Language Barriers: International Perspectives/ Edited by Elizabeth A. Jacobs and Lisa Diamond.
Description: Bristol, UK; Blue Ridge Summit, PA : Multilingual Matters, [2017] | Includes bibliographical references and index.
Identifiers: LCCN 2016053229| ISBN 9781783097760 (hbk : alk. paper) | ISBN 9781783097753 (pbk : alk. paper) | ISBN 9781783097791 (kindle)
Subjects: LCSH: Medicine—Translating. | Health facilities—Translating services. | Communication in medicine. | Transcultural medical care. | Linguistic minorities—Medical care. | Translating and interpreting.
Classification: LCC R119.5 .P76 2017 | DDC 610--dc23 LC record available at https://lccn.loc.gov/2016053229

British Library Cataloguing in Publication Data
A catalogue entry for this book is available from the British Library.

ISBN-13: 978-1-78309-776-0 (hbk)
ISBN-13: 978-1-78309-775-3 (pbk)

Multilingual Matters
UK: St Nicholas House, 31-34 High Street, Bristol BS1 2AW, UK.
USA: NBN, Blue Ridge Summit, PA, USA.

Website: www.multilingual-matters.com
Twitter: Multi_Ling_Mat
Facebook: https://www.facebook.com/multilingualmatters
Blog: www.channelviewpublications.wordpress.com

Copyright © 2017 Elizabeth A. Jacobs, Lisa C. Diamond and the authors of individual chapters.

All rights reserved. No part of this work may be reproduced in any form or by any means without permission in writing from the publisher.

The policy of Multilingual Matters/Channel View Publications is to use papers that are natural, renewable and recyclable products, made from wood grown in sustainable forests. In the manufacturing process of our books, and to further support our policy, preference is given to printers that have FSC and PEFC Chain of Custody certification. The FSC and/or PEFC logos will appear on those books where full certification has been granted to the printer concerned.

Typeset by Nova Techset Private Limited, Bengaluru and Chennai, India.
Printed and bound in the UK by Short Run Press Ltd.
Printed and bound in the US by Edwards Brothers Malloy, Inc.

Contents

	Contributors	vii
	Introduction	xv
1	The Drivers of Demand for Language Services in Health Care *Allison Squires*	1
2	Three Critical Steps to Enhance Delivery of Language Services in Health Care *Leah S. Karliner*	20
3	Conceptualizing Bilingual Health Communication: A Theory-based Approach to Interpreter-mediated Medical Encounters *Elaine Hsieh*	35
4	Challenges to and Recommendations for Working with a Community Interpreter in Mental Health: A Canadian Perspective *Yvan Leanza, Camille Brisset, Rhéa Rocque and Alexandra Boilard*	56
5	Toward a Theoretical Framework of Informal Interpreting in Health Care: Explaining the Effects of Role Conflict on Control, Power and Trust in Interpreter-mediated Encounters *Barbara Schouten*	71
6	Understanding the Advantages and Disadvantages of the Diversity of Approaches to Overcoming Language Barriers in Medical Encounters *Rebecca Schwei, Mary Rhodes and Elizabeth A. Jacobs*	93
7	Language Concordance Between Limited English Proficient Patients and Their Clinicians *Dana Canfield and Lisa C. Diamond*	102

8   Breaking the Silence: Identifying the Needs of Bilingual
    Speakers in Health Care   116
    Gwerfyl Roberts

9   Engaging the Community to Develop Solutions for Languages of
    Lesser Diffusion   149
    *Francesca Gany, C. Javier González, E. Zoe Schutzman
    and Debra J. Pelto*

10 Chinese Voices: Improving Access to Health Care   170
    Fiona Irvine, Martin Partridge and Echo Yeung

11 A New Zealand Perspective on Providing Health Care for
    Patients with Limited English Proficiency   190
    *Ben Gray, Jo Hilder, Lindsay Macdonald, Rachel Tester,
    Anthony Dowell and Maria Stubbe*

12 Toward a New Approach for Culturally and Linguistically
    Responsive Health Care: A Case Study of Developments
    in Victoria, Australia   211
    Lidia Horvat

    Epilogue   235
    Glossary   236
    Index   239

Contributors

Alexandra Boilard has completed her Bachelor of Arts and doctoral studies in Psychology at Laval University (Québec, Canada). During her studies she worked as a research assistant in the Psychology and Cultures Laboratory. Her PhD research focused on representations of Colombian and Quebecer parents on parental practices, maltreatment and youth protection. She is now working as a clinician in an inpatient child psychiatry department.

Camille Brisset after a post-doctoral fellowship at Laval University in the Psychology and Cultures Laboratory, became an associate professor in developmental psychology and cross-cultural psychology at the University of Bordeaux in France. She is specialized in the study of human development in context. As such, she is interested in psychosocial adaptation in terms of developmental and cultural transition (representation of attachment, emotional regulation and transition to university), but also in the roles practitioners play in this process (interpreting in mental health, professional development of future psychologists in the context of cultural diversity).

Dana Canfield is a medical student at Case Western Reserve University School of Medicine in the class of 2018. Throughout college and medical school her passion for social justice and healthcare policy has instigated her involvement in various research projects and student organizations aimed at eliminating healthcare inequality. As a medical student researcher in the Memorial Sloan Kettering Summer Research Fellowship program, she was given the opportunity to work with physician researchers in MSK's Immigrant Health and Cancer Disparities Service, where she met Dr Lisa Diamond and was introduced to the additional obstacles faced by patients with limited English proficiency (LEP). This work has broadened her understanding of medically underserved populations and alerted her to the many specific areas of care where the needs of LEP patients are not being met. She plans to continue advocating for all underserved groups through research and involvement in healthcare policy organizations throughout her career.

Lisa C. Diamond, MD, MPH, FACP is an Assistant Attending Physician at Memorial Sloan Kettering Cancer Center and an Assistant Professor of Healthcare Policy and Research at Weill Cornell Medical College. She attended the George Washington University School of Medicine and Health Sciences and received a Master of Public Health degree from the Johns Hopkins Bloomberg School of Public Health. She trained as a general internist at New York Presbyterian Hospital/Columbia University Medical Center in New York, followed by a Robert Wood Johnson Clinical Scholars Program Fellowship at Yale University. After noticing during medical school and residency that patients with limited English proficiency (LEP) received worse care than English-speaking patients, she began pursuing a research career to eliminate these disparities. Her research focuses on understanding how clinician non-English language proficiency affects the quality of care delivered to patients with LEP. Ultimately, she plans to use the results of her research to establish standards for the appropriate use of non-fluent non-English language skills by clinicians and to identify process and outcome measures that capture the quality of cancer care being delivered to LEP patients. Her research has been supported by grants from the National Institutes of Health and The California Endowment. She has published several peer-reviewed journal articles and book chapters. She also works clinically as a hospitalist physician, supervising medical interns and residents at Memorial Sloan Kettering.

Anthony Dowell is Professor of Primary Health Care and General Practice and Head of the Department of Obstetrics and Gynaecology at the University of Otago in Wellington. He is a General Practitioner at Island Bay Medical Centre. He has worked in primary care in New Zealand, the UK and Central Africa. His research interests include communication between patients and health professionals and mental health problems in primary care. He is a Co-Director of the Applied Research in Communication on Health research group.

Francesca Gany, MD, MS was the founder and Director of the Center for Immigrant Health, New York University School of Medicine, of the New York University Cancer Institute CORE Center (Cancer Outreach, Outcomes and Research for Equity), and of the Health Promotion, Disease Prevention and Human Migration concentration in the New York University Global Masters of Public Health program. Dr Gany is now the founding Chief of the Immigrant Health and Cancer Disparities Service and the Center for Immigrant Health and Cancer Disparities at Memorial Sloan Kettering Cancer Center. She has served as the Principal Investigator on a number of pioneering immigrant health studies and programs in the areas of cancer treatment adherence and quality of life, health disparities, language access and cultural responsiveness, technology and immigrant health, and healthcare access. Her translational community-engaged work has led to the development of long-term policy and programmatic changes.

C. Javier González, MFA is Director of Language Initiatives at the Immigrant Health and Cancer Disparities Service of Memorial Sloan Kettering Cancer Center in New York City. He has worked to develop standards and curricula in interpreting and translation in health care. He co-directed the Remote Simultaneous Medical Interpretation project and developed its curriculum and Quality Control program. He has created nationally recognized educational videos and distance-learning modules for interpreters, patients and providers. He is an item writer and advisor to the Certification Commission for Healthcare Interpreters. He has participated in groundbreaking research that has translated into policies for language access to health care.

Ben Gray is a senior lecturer at the University of Otago Wellington in the Department of Primary Health Care and General Practice. He convenes the undergraduate course in Professional Skills Attitudes and Ethics. He works half-time in General Practice at Newtown Union Health Service, a multi-ethnic multilingual high-needs practice. His research interests focus on cross-cultural care, working with interpreters and bioethics.

Jo Hilder is a Research Fellow at the University of Otago Wellington, based in the Department of Primary Health Care and General Practice. She has a background in applied linguistics, and her research interests include communication in health care, particularly with patients with limited English proficiency.

Lidia Horvat works in in the Victorian Department of Health and Human Services. Her main focus is to support the Victorian health sector in the systematic improvement of health care quality and safety. This work includes policy development and research in consumer participation, cultural responsiveness, equity, person- and family-centered care, health literacy and communication. Lidia is currently leading the development of a new partnering in healthcare policy. She is lead author of a Cochrane Systematic Review, entitled 'Cultural competence education for health professionals' investigating the effects of cultural competence education interventions for health professionals on patient-related outcomes.

Dr Elaine Hsieh has been involved in research on cross-cultural care and health communication for over a decade. She has conducted ethnographic studies, in-depth interviews, focus groups, surveys and multi-phases studies that examine the interactions between providers and patients who do not share the same language. She has received funding from the National Institutes of Health to further expand her Bilingual Health Communication model. The results have been published in *Journal of General Internal Medicine, Social Science and Medicine, Patient Education and Counseling, Health Communication, Qualitative Health Research*, among others. Her model of bilingual health communication has received several national and international top paper awards for its theoretical advancement and practical implications.

Fiona Irvine is the Jenny Jones Chair of Nursing and Head of Nursing. Her research is primarily focused on the organization and delivery of health and nursing services and she has published widely in this area. She has secured major research funding from the National Institute of Health Research, the Welsh Government and other prestigious bodies to support her work in this area. Irvine is a referee for numerous journals and grant giving bodies such as NIHR and NISCHR. She has a clinical background in District Nursing and End of Life Care and maintains her clinical activity by working closely with health service partners to undertake research in these areas and to apply the findings in nursing practice

Elizabeth A. Jacobs, MD MAPP FACP is Associate Vice Chair for Health Services Research in the Department of Medicine and Associate Professor of Medicine and Population Health Sciences at the University of Wisconsin School of Medicine and Public Health. She attended medical school at University of California at San Francisco, trained as a general internist at Brigham and Women's Hospital in Boston, and completed a Robert Wood Johnson Clinical Scholars Fellowship at the University of Chicago. After struggling to care for limited English-speaking patients during medical school and residency, she decided to pursue a research career investigating how to reduce disparities in health care. She has done research documenting that provision of adequate interpreter services positively impacts the delivery of health care provided to patients with limited English proficiency and that the provision of these services are cost-beneficial. Her research interests also include access to, and cultural specificity of, medical care delivered to minority patients, health literacy, measurement of trust across cultures, and the role that trust in health care plays in African American and Latino patients health care decisions. Her research has been supported by grants from the National Institutes of Health, The Robert Wood Johnson Foundation, The California Endowment, The Russell Sage Foundation, the Office of Minority Health, and the Patient Centered Outcomes Research Institute (PCORI). She is recognized as an expert on the provision of linguistically accessible and culturally competent care nationally and internationally and has served on Office of Minority Health, JCAHO, AHRQ, and PCORI expert panels. She has published numerous peer-reviewed journal articles and authored three book chapters. In addition, she works with other investigators to design culturally specific research, and teaches residents and medical students about practicing culturally sensitive medicine.

Dr Leah S. Karliner, MD MAS is Associate Professor in Residence in the Division of General Internal Medicine, Department of Medicine at the

University of California, San Francisco. She is also a member of the Medical Effectiveness Research Center for Diverse Communities at UCSF as well as the UCSF Helen Diller Family Comprehensive Cancer Center. She is both a practicing general internist and a health services researcher. She completed her training – including her MD degree, a residency in primary care internal medicine, a general internal medicine research fellowship and a Master's of Advanced Studies in Clinical Research – at UCSF. Dr Karliner's scholarly work centers on improving quality of care for limited English-speaking patients. Her research particularly focuses on language access and outcomes after hospitalization as well as communication during breast cancer diagnosis and treatment

Yvan Leanza, PhD After many migratory movements between Switzerland and Canada, is now full professor in the School of Psychology, Laval University (Québec City) where he teaches cross-cultural psychology and intervention and leads the 'Psychology and Cultures' laboratory (www.labo-psychologie-cultures.ca). His researches focus on working with interpreters and relations to the (culturally different) other in healthcare settings and on sleep in a cross-cultural perspective. He is a founding member and the actual director of *Alterstice – International Journal of Intercultural Research* (www.alterstice.org). He has edited or authored several books on migrant and minority integration processes and on the relation to the (culturally different) other in pediatrics. He is one of the authors of the only systematic review of interpreting qualitative studies (published in *Patient Education and Counselling* 91, 2013) and of a chapter on working with interpreters in mental health settings (in L. Kirmayer *et al.*, 2014, *Cultural Consultation*, Springer, New York).

Lindsay Macdonald is a Research Fellow at the University of Otago, Wellington. She is a Registered Nurse with a postgraduate degree in linguistics and nursing. Her postgraduate studies in linguistics and nursing led to an ongoing interest in health communication, particularly in how clinicians and patients talk with each other. She is a member of the Applied Communication in Health (ARCH) research group based in the Department of Primary Health Care and General Practice. Ms MacDonald's research focuses on communication in clinical practice, and using video-recordings of actual consultations and day-to-day health practice activity. Wherever possible, participants (clinicians and patients) are partners in the research process. Her other current research interests include interprofessional practice and approaches to weight management.

Martin Partridge, PhD has worked professionally for many years with people with intellectual disabilities, disabled people and older adults in many different roles, in both statutory and third sector organisations in the UK. He has conducted research in China and involvement in Chinese culture has enabled him to spend time in Beijing in developing contacts with disability services. With a PhD in disability studies from the University of Bristol, Dr Patridge's research has been centred on transcultural groups, health and social care and policy development. He is particularly interested in Chinese people outside of China, Chinese culture, social care, social work, cultural competence, dual-heritage and identity, disability, learning disability, diversity and social policy. In his academic and research role, he uses a variety of mixed and qualitative research methods in gaining in-depth understandings of participant's experiences. From his research recommendations, he now leads in partnership with local Chinese community welfare organisations an accessible, multilingual website (Chinese Social Care and Health). This website acts as a hub of information on welfare and social care issues for Chinese people in England who have little or no access to services.

Debra J. Pelto, MPH, PhD is a health disparities researcher whose work centers on access to health care and health information among underserved immigrant and minority populations. She is a Postdoctoral Research Fellow in the Immigrant Health and Cancer Disparities Service, Psychiatry and Behavioral Sciences, of Memorial Sloan Kettering Cancer Center in New York City, where her work addresses cancer and chronic disease prevention among the Mexican immigrant population. Her previous projects include patient and community health interventions addressing cancer, chronic and infectious disease and sexual and reproductive health, and an ethnography of family planning and access to care among Mexican immigrants in New York City. She has been a Health Disparities Scholar sponsored by the National Institute of Minority Health and Health Disparities.

Mary Rhodes, MD is an Assistant Professor of Medicine in the Division of Hematology and Oncology, Palliative Care Section at the Medical College of Wisconsin. She graduated from the University of Wisconsin School of Medicine and Public Health, completed an Internal Medicine residency at Montefiore Medical Center in Bronx, NY, and a fellowship in Hospice and Palliative Medicine at the University of Wisconsin Hospital and Clinics. She is enrolled in a masters program in Clinical and Translational Sciences at the Medical College of Wisconsin. Her research interests arose from observing the impact of communication and cultural barriers on patient decision-making. Her long-term research goals are to alleviate these disparities and her current focus is on the experience of medical interpreters in mediating discussions at end of life.

Mrs Gwerfyl Roberts's research focuses on enhancing and implementing the evidence base for language appropriate practice in health and social care. She works collaboratively with stakeholders through international engagement around the bilingual contexts of health care; leading government policy; improving health research in Wales; enhancing the healthcare workforce; and creating an evidence base for organizational support for language competence. Gwerfyl leads LLAIS, the Welsh language awareness methodology support hub, and is an active member of the Welsh Government Task Group for Welsh Language Services in Health and Social Care, and academic board of the Coleg Cymraeg Cenedlaethol.

Rhéa Rocque has completed her Bachelor of Arts Honours in Psychology at the University of Manitoba (Winnipeg, Canada). Her Honours thesis aimed to explore African immigrants' and refugees' representations of mental illness. She is now completing her doctoral studies in Psychology at Laval University (Quebec, Canada). As part of her PhD research, she is exploring patients' experiences of communicating with physicians. Intercultural issues in health remains her primary research interest.

Barbara Schouten, PhD works as an assistant professor at the University of Amsterdam. Her research focuses on intercultural health communication, in particular on cultural differences in patients' information and participation preferences and communicative behavior, interpreter-mediated communication processes, patient-provider interaction and health intervention evaluations.

E. Zoe Schutzman, MA New York State Certified Court Interpreter and Nationally Certified Healthcare Interpreter (CHI™) is Specialist, Educator and Staff Development II in the Interpreter Language Services Department at The University of New Mexico Health Science Center's UNM Hospitals in Albuquerque, New Mexico. As a linguist, she has taught at institutions of higher education and been a leader in training individuals to become professionally qualified medical interpreters. She has developed and enhanced curricula, assessment and quality assurance protocols, as well as provided linguistic and culturally appropriate expertise to myriad research endeavors. Her contributions have extended to meaningful access to healthcare services for immigrant communities with limited English proficiency; sociolinguistic, language acquisition and language documentation projects, including methodology creation and implementation; analysis of internal and national regulatory policies; and development, translation and trans-creation of research, outreach and educational materials.

Rebecca J Schwei received her MPH in Global Health from Emory University and is currently an Assistant Researcher at the University of Wisconsin Madison School of Medicine and Public Health. Her research interests include health equity, provision of linguistically appropriate health care, healthcare decision making and the social determinants of health.

Allison Squires, PhD, RN, FAAN is a global health workforce researcher with a special interest in improving immigrant health outcomes. She is an internationally recognized expert in cross-language research methods and a board member of the National Council for Interpreting in Health Care. With research experience in 30 countries, she has consulted with the Migration Policy Institute in Washington, DC and The World Bank on health workforce and immigrant health issues. She joined New York University after completing her PhD in Nursing and Global Health Policy at Yale University and a post-doctoral fellowship in health outcomes research at the University of Pennsylvania.

Maria Stubbe is an interactional sociolinguist working in the Department of Primary Health Care and General Practice, University of Otago (Wellington), New Zealand. She is co-director of the Applied Research on Communication in Health Group, which investigates communication issues in clinical practice using video-recordings of authentic interactions between health professionals and patients. She has published widely in the fields of pragmatics, workplace language and health communication.

Rachel Tester is a Research Fellow at the University of Otago Wellington, based in the Department of Primary Health Care and General Practice. She has a background in psychology, and her research interests include communication in health care on sensitive subjects such as addiction and mental health.

Echo Yeung, Echo qualified as a social worker in 1989, having studied at the University of Hong Kong. She worked in Hong Kong as a social worker for two years and as a Chinese social worker for in Liverpool for 10 years. Currently she is a senior lecturer teaching on social work programmes at Liverpool John Moores University. Echo's research interests lie in the field of health and social care of minority ethnic groups. Her PhD study was to examine the pathway to mental health care of Chinese people with mental health problems in England. She was also involved in a study, funded by NIHR, to look at the experience of social care of Chinese people with physical disabilities. She also conducted a number of studies to explore different ways to involve service users and carers from minority ethnic communities in the training of social work students.

Introduction

As immigration continues and grows across the globe, linguistic diversity grows in parallel. As a result, many patients and their healthcare providers have to communicate across a language barrier. This occurs when a patient and/or their family is most proficient in a language other than that of their healthcare provider and communication is hampered. In this situation, patients' needs may not be understood or met because of lack of adequate communication. The nature and complexity of language barriers in health care vary within and across nations owing to the culture and political nature of the nation and/or the culture and political nature of the linguistic groups residing in and seeking health care in those countries. With this diversity of contexts comes a need for diverse approaches to overcoming language barriers in health care. The aim of this book to provide a collection of chapters describing these different approaches, their advantages and disadvantages, and special issues which need to be considered in particular contexts or linguistic groups. The chapters proceed from general topics to more focused topics, including examples from several international settings. As such, there is variability of terminology used. Several terms which may be unfamiliar to a reader are defined in the glossary provided. Some issues arise in multiple chapters. We have elected to leave these areas of overlap in each chapter so that each may stand on its own in the event that one chapter is used for teaching a specific topic.

In the first chapter, Dr Allison Squires examines how domestic and international migration, driven by the forces of globalization, is changing how health systems need to respond to indigenous and immigrant healthcare needs. It provides a 360° view of the global phenomenon and provide suggestions for macro-level policy strategies that can facilitate research and strengthen health system's capabilities to respond to the phenomenon in a way that promotes optimal health outcomes.

While healthcare systems often struggle to deliver quality care across a language barrier, in fact the fundamentals of providing linguistic access are simple. The first is to identify who needs the service and in which language; The second is to identify the human resources to provide the service; and the third is to deliver the service in-person or remotely (via telephone or video-conferencing). The second chapter, by Dr Leah Karliner, discusses each of these fundamentals in detail, including the challenges and opportunities presented by the ever-changing landscape of technologic advances.

Although interpreter-mediated medical encounters have been gaining interdisciplinary attention, its research focus traditionally has been on interpreters' linguistic performances. In Dr Elaine Hsieh's chapter, she presents a conceptual framework for bilingual health care, highlighting the quality and equality of care as the guiding principle in resolving interactional dilemmas in medical encounters and in evaluating the success of interpreter-mediated interactions. By recognizing that the communicative process, meanings of an illness event and even the quality and equality of care are socially constructed, Dr Hsieh's Model of Bilingual Health Communication provides multiple opportunities and entry points for theory development and practice implications.

In mental health care, language holds a particular place not only as a vehicle of information, but also as the main way of expressing inner states and feelings and it is the major tool for therapy. This chapter, by Dr Yvan Leanza and colleagues, explores the issues in working with interpreters in psychological assessment and in psychotherapy. Interpreters' extent of involvement in the therapeutic process is one of the central questions clinicians need to answer. Clinician therapeutic orientation, institutional choices about linguistic issues and larger social issues (like language politics) also influence how interpreters are integrated in mental health clinical teams.

Migrant patients with limited language proficiency in the dominant language often bring along informal interpreters to medical consultations. In this chapter, Dr Barbara Schouten discusses the perspectives of patients, informal interpreters and healthcare providers on informal interpreting by reviewing the empirical and theoretical literature. The analysis focuses on discrepancies and commonalities between the perspectives of the three parties involved, as well as on actual communication discourses in consultations with informal interpreters. Dr Schouten provides a discussion of the notion of trust, for example, which demonstrates the conflicting research findings in this area and the need to operationalize abstract constructs with care and precision. Based on the results, practical recommendations for working with informal interpreters in health care are given and a future research agenda is proposed.

The number of healthcare encounters in which patients and their provider do not speak the same language is increasing worldwide. Approaches to address these language barriers in health care vary internationally from providing professional, trained interpreters within healthcare systems to utilizing friends and family to help communicate with patients. Each of these approaches has strengths and weaknesses and the best approach may vary across nations and cultural groups. In this chapter, Rebecca Schwei and Dr Elizabeth Jacobs summarize the international literature about overcoming language barriers in health care and provide some guidance, with caveats, as to how to effectively reduce language barriers in health care internationally.

Patients with limited English proficiency (LEP) are at risk of impaired communication with their clinicians and thus disparities in care. As noted in other chapters, professional interpreters and truly bilingual clinicians can reduce disparities for LEP patients. Despite knowledge that the use of professional interpreters improves patient care for LEP patients, research has shown that clinicians underuse language services in favor of their own, often limited, non-English skills. This fact, combined with the rapid growth of the US LEP population and the complex discussions that take place in clinical care, highlights a compelling unmet need for standards to guide the use of non-fluent language skills by clinicians with LEP patients. Dana Canfield and Dr Lisa Diamond's chapter reviews the literature on language concordance and the relationship between clinician language proficiency and quality of care.

Despite the growing commitment in health care to establish communicative competence with service users, the language needs of bilingual speakers often remain invisible, leading to the marginalization of vulnerable groups and compromising the quality of their care. Nevertheless, with the revitalization of many of the world's indigenous minority languages, healthcare systems must adapt to legislative change and advances in language policy. Dr Gwerfyl Roberts's chapter reviews the research evidence from bilingual Wales, UK, and beyond that contributes to our understanding of the dynamics of bilingual healthcare communication and examines the implications for implementing the evidence from an individual and organizational perspective.

Languages of lesser diffusion – languages spoken by relatively small populations in a given area – pose a unique challenge to healthcare systems around the world. Drs Francesca Gany, Debra Pelto and colleagues focus their chapter on how to track the emergence of such languages and how to engage communities who speak languages of lesser diffusion, using community-based participatory methods to create culturally responsive solutions to language barriers faced by those accessing health care. This chapter lays out the particular problems faced with regard to less widely spoken languages in the US and provides concrete information about how various communities of speakers have worked to confront and deal with those challenges. It also helps readers understand those challenges and the strengths and weaknesses of possible solutions. Techniques described include the establishment of partnerships with community-based organizations, integrating normally excluded community affiliates and developing robust resolutions to promote health equity.

The provision of culturally and linguistically sensitive services for minority ethnic communities is a constant challenge to the UK health service, particularly when the diversity of a particular ethnic group is not fully acknowledged. One such diverse group is the Chinese population of the UK, who originate from a number of countries and use several languages (and dialects) including Mandarin, Cantonese and Hakka. Drawing on recent research studies, Dr Fiona Irvine and colleagues consider some of the challenges faced by different Chinese-speaking people in understanding, accessing and using health services, and present examples of good practice that can be implemented within the current confines of limited financial resources.

Outside of the US and UK, other countries have made unique contributions to improving language access for speakers of non-dominant languages. New Zealand has made the transition from an almost monolingual country to a country with many languages in a relatively short space of time. This chapter, by Ben Gray and colleagues, provides a background to New Zealand's cultural diversity with particular emphasis on the important place of Maori, and the more recent influx of migrants from non-English speaking countries. It then describes the context of the health system (predominantly state funded) and the regulatory approach that has been taken. The resulting approach to the issue of increasing language diversity is compared with their neighbor Australia and the US. They describe the pragmatic response that has developed with more of a focus on cost efficacy and patient safety than on rights. They report on the research they have done studying the complexity of video-recorded interpreted consultations and describe how this could inform language policy. The information in this chapter is the sort of information necessary to begin cross-national comparisons.

Victoria, Australia has one of the most culturally and linguistically diverse populations in the world and a strong history of policy, programmatic and legislative initiatives in building accessible and equitable health care. Approaches to building a more responsive healthcare system for all consumers, patients and communities are numerous and diverse in foci. However, identifying what works best, where, for whom and how to improve care and health outcomes in culturally and linguistically diverse patient groups remains a challenge. Dr Lidia Horvat's chapter focuses on policy development initiatives in Victoria, Australia and examines how a strategy around standards for culturally responsive care is evolving toward a coherent framework. Such a framework may bring together key interrelated approaches with common underlying principles. These principles include equity, person- and family-centered care, health literacy, consumer participation, human rights, cultural responsiveness, intersectionality and quality and safety in health care. From the perspective of sociolinguistics and applied linguistics, this is a model of how to analyze and implement a plan to deal with linguistic and cultural diversity.

Taken together, these chapters describe the landscape of how best to provide linguistically appropriate care to speakers of non-dominant languages. This book provides a collection from several countries and research traditions to provide the collective wisdom of healthcare professionals working together across national and disciplinary boundaries.

1 The Drivers of Demand for Language Services in Health Care

Allison Squires

> *Societies with a rich diversity of skills and experiences are better placed to stimulate growth through their human resources, and migration is one of the ways in which the exchange of talent, services, and skills can be fostered. Yet migration remains highly politicized and often negatively perceived, despite the obvious need for diversification in today's rapidly evolving societies and economies.*
> (Appave & Laczko, 2011: 15)

Figure 1.1 illustrates the current complexity of global migration. Geographically, individuals tend to migrate first within their country, usually from rural to urban areas. Reasons for domestic migration may include changes in local conditions that force migration owing to economic (job seeking or employment changes), political (conflict or war), educational (degree or training seeking) or ecological reasons. If international migration occurs, this may happen first within the local region (e.g. South Asia) and then internationally. The most common pattern is from a low or middle income country to a high income country. Additionally, an individual's education level will often dictate how migration occurs, whether it is voluntary and driven by a confirmed opportunity, voluntary and driven by potential opportunity, or involuntary driven by a variety of reasons.

More than ever before, individuals migrate to other countries primarily for work opportunities when career advancement opportunities arise, their local economies do not produce enough opportunities for paid employment or when underemployment prevails. War and conflict zones may also drive workers from their country temporarily or permanently and transferring the skills of these migrants can prove challenging (The International Bank for Reconstruction and Development 2011; Appave & Laczko, 2011; Docquier *et al.*, 2009). Nonetheless, migration for work often benefits many workers as they develop new technical, social and linguistic skills that may make them more competitive in their originating country labor markets and act as buffers

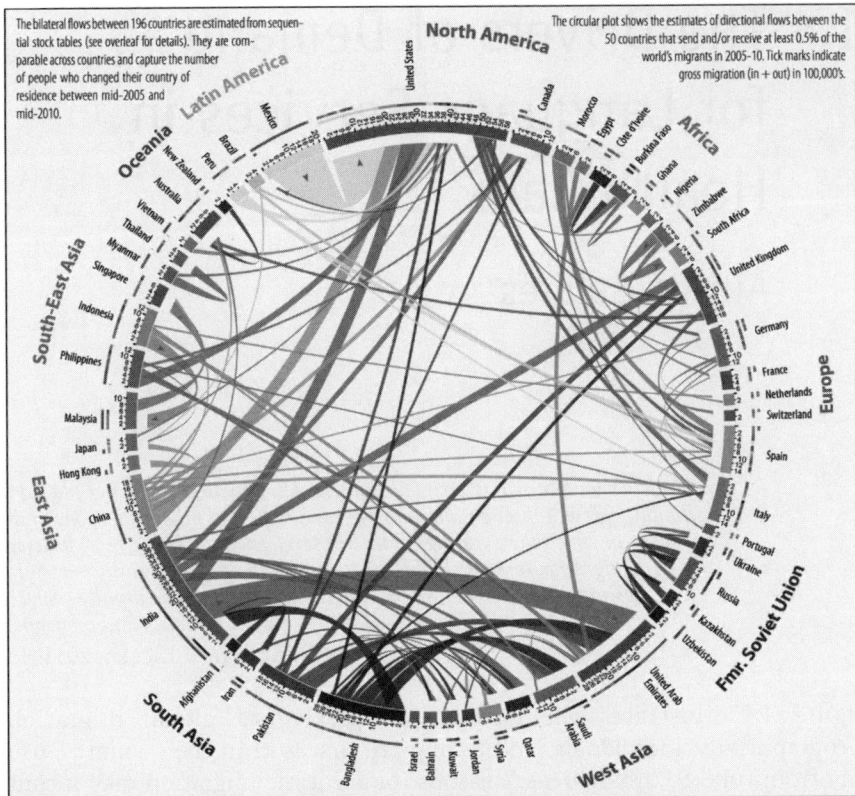

Figure 1.1 Global migration flows 2005–10 Adapted from http://www.global-migration.info/VID_Global_Migration_Datasheet_web.pdf Team at the Wittgenstein Centre for Demography and Global Human Capital (IIASA,VID/ÖAW,WU): Nikola Sander, Guy J. Abel and Ramon Bauer. Circular plots created with Circos (Krzywinski, M. *et al*. Circos: an Information Aesthetic for Comparative Genomics. *Genome Res*, 2009, 19:1639–1645).

against economic shocks (Durand & Massey, 2010; Siqueira *et al.*, 2013; Walani, 2013; Shihadeh & Barranco, 2010; Bartram, 2010; Hagan *et al.*, 2011; Tilly, 2011; Docquier *et al.*, 2009). Migrating workers are also major contributors to the global economy through remittances: earnings sent back to the home country to the migrant's family often to pay for housing and healthcare costs (Carling, 2009). In 2014, the World Bank estimated that remittances sent home by migrating workers contributed US$400 billion to the global economy and would increase by 7–9% annually through 2020 (The World Bank, 2016). With international travel easier than at any other point in history, the 21st-century worker has a high probability of migrating permanently or temporarily for work at some point in their lifetime.

Yet as a global phenomenon, 21st century global migration patterns are changing health services delivery in countries around the world. For some healthcare systems, this presents new demands on service delivery while others see increased challenges on already stretched ones. Changing countries is stressful in good and bad ways and often impacts individual and family health. Legacies of origin country health system strengths and deficiencies will travel with the migrant in terms of their health profile. Whether they are an investment banker who has moved from New York to London or an internationally educated nurse from the Philippines who moves to the Middle East to staff healthcare systems or a Central American migrant fleeing stagnant economies and drug violence, newly arrived migrant workers undergo a transition period, often known as culture shock. The stress of the transition often affects their mental health as some individuals adapt more readily than others to new cultures, contexts and stressors while others may develop depression, anxiety and other mental health sequelae that affect their physical health, all as a direct result of their migration experiences and sudden absence of traditional support systems (Rudmin, 2010; Bauer et al., 2010; Riggs et al., 2012; Viruell-Fuentes et al., 2012; Teruya & Bazargan-Hejazi, 2013; Lassetter & Callister, 2008). Even though the cumulative causation of migration may increase social networks and support systems abroad (Fussell, 2010; Sanderson & Kentor, 2008) that may lessen the effects of migration experiences on health, the phenomenon's effects on health are complex.

Consequently, migrants may or may not access the healthcare system in their destination country when needed. Several factors influence these behaviors. First, insurance schemes play a large role in whether or not the migrant accesses the local healthcare system simply owing to whether or not they can get coverage in their new country. Even countries with universal health coverage do not necessarily provide coverage to new immigrants (Biswas et al., 2011; Docquier et al., 2009; Reyes & Hardy, 2015; Siddiqi et al., 2013). The second major factor is a language barrier. Even if a migrant comes from a country, for example, where English is an or the official language and has migrated to another English-speaking country, the language of healthcare systems and illness descriptors can be different enough to affect how and when the migrant accesses the healthcare system (Squires et al., 2013). When the migrant has little to no language skill in the official language(s) of a country, it becomes a major barrier to accessing and utilizing healthcare services. Even countries with long histories of receiving immigrants can be unprepared for the reality of individuals who cannot communicate effectively with a healthcare provider.

Migrant Identity and Health

Regardless of the reason for migration, researchers categorize migrants as documented, undocumented and refugee. The latter two situations have the greatest likelihood of affecting the health of individuals and their families because of the nature of the migration experience. *Documented* individuals who migrate generally have no greater risk for health issues when living and working in high-income countries than in their home country. Health risks associated with living and working in a low- or middle-income country are related to the disease burden inherent to the country and the ability of the local health system to respond to their needs or transfer the individual to another country for treatment.

Undocumented individuals migrate to a country without legal citizenship or work papers. Many may arrive in the country via a tourist visa and remain after it expires. Others arrive through human traffickers and may have been subject to emotional, physical or sexual abuse during the process. Nonetheless, once they arrive they contribute economically to countries by providing inexpensive labor, primarily in the service, agricultural and construction sectors. Health issues in this population can result from the migration experience, the success or failure of their integration into the new community or occupationally related injuries which may or may not receive timely treatment.

Refugees have fled their home country for political reasons. The United Nations (UN) defines them as:

> Any person who, owing to a well-founded fear of being persecuted for reasons of race, religion, nationality, membership of a particular social group or political opinion, is outside the country of his nationality and is unable or, owing to such fear, is unwilling to avail himself of the protection of that country; or who, not having a nationality and being outside of the country of his former habitual residence as a result of such events, is unable or, owing to such fear, unwilling to return [to it]. (Source: UN Convention Related to the Status of Refugees and the 1967 Protocol)

The skills of these individuals and their education levels vary widely. Translating their skills into equivalent positions in the receiving country is often a challenge. Proof of education documents may be lost or unobtainable and training curricula may be sufficiently different that they do not meet the competency or credentialing standards of the receiving country. This means this population is at risk for underemployment or may need to repeat their education. These individuals are also at high risk for post-traumatic stress disorder and may manifest these symptoms physically. Asylum seekers may face similar challenges.

Conclusion

Language often cannot be separated from migrant status, which also impacts health, so healthcare organizations must also be knowledgeable about the particular health risks that result from the migration experience. In consideration of the aforementioned factors, this chapter focuses on how migration dynamics influence demand for language services in healthcare systems and the subsequent implications for policy (both organizational and national) and research. It will examine how these experiences start to create demand for language services in healthcare systems and conclude with recommendations to better account for the demands that language services place on healthcare organizations and systems.

Language Services: Definition, Outcomes Impact and Implementation Factors

Regardless of how the individual migrates, their ability to access the system through insurance schemes and bridging language barriers is what creates the demand for language services in health systems. It is widely reported in anecdotal evidence sources that when it becomes known in an immigrant community that a provider speaks their language, more patients seek care through that person. Organizations that provide good-quality language services also attract more clients. Increasingly, research shows that facilities with good-quality language services reduce 30 day readmissions and other costly complications of hospitalization (Lindholm *et al.*, 2012; Betancourt *et al.*, 2012; Tuot *et al.*, 2012).

Language services, for the purposes of this chapter, are defined as the services or personnel an organization provides to bridge a client's language barrier. These services are essential for optimizing patient outcomes (Hacker *et al.*, 2012; Jacobs *et al.*, 2007, 2011a; Kosmider *et al.*, 2010; Karliner *et al.*, 2007; Eamranond *et al.*, 2009; Fernandez *et al.*, 2011; Ipsiroglu *et al.*, 2005; Levas, 2011), even when controlling for potential confounders, and reducing differences in patient satisfaction with care (Jacobs *et al.*, 2001, 2007, 2011b; Green *et al.*, 2005; Grover *et al.*, 2012; Ngo-Metzger *et al.*, 2007; Karliner *et al.*, 2007; Bagchi *et al.*, 2011; Kanter *et al.*, 2009; Ayanian *et al.*, 2005). Language services can include language-concordant personnel who are not certified to conduct medical interpretation, language-concordant personnel who are certified to conduct medical interpretation, volunteer interpreters, paid interpreters, telephone interpreters and increasingly language interpretation technology available on smartphones and computers. It is well known that family members often provide interpretation for their relatives despite strong recommendations that they do not (Regenstein *et al.*, 2008; Betancourt *et al.*, 2012), but they are contributors to demand for language services because providers need to include them, as appropriate, in care planning. Interpreter use with limited English Proficient (LEP) patients, therefore, is essential for delivering patient-centered care (Green *et al.*, 2005; Jacobs, 2000; Karliner *et al.*, 2011; Nápoles *et al.*, 2009; Radwin *et al.*, 2013; Ngo-Metzger *et al.*, 2009; Charlton *et al.*, 2008).

Therefore, how these services are deployed in the healthcare delivery setting drives service demand and influences outcomes. Hsieh (2006) categorizes interpreters in the following ways: chance interpreter, untrained interpreter, bilingual healthcare provider, on-site interpreter and telephone interpreter. Chance and untrained interpreters have no formal training in interpretation, a bilingual healthcare provider may or may not, and the latter two have training.

Trained human interpreters are the most common ways that providers bridge a language barrier with a patient. Trained human interpreters view themselves as an integral part of the healthcare encounter, serving as communication brokers (Hsieh & Kramer, 2012; Hsieh, 2008), patient advocates for social justice (Hilfinger Messias et al., 2009; McDowell et al., 2011) and system brokers (El Ansari et al., 2009; Brisset et al., 2013). Policies that mandate or provide decision tools for interpreter service use have mixed results regarding their efficacy (Ginde et al., 2010).

Yet when demand for an interpreter arises, providers typically conduct a situational analysis that helps them determine when to use an interpreter, with situational acuity dictating interpreter need and not patient preference (Bischoff & Hudelson, 2010b; Rosenberg et al., 2007; Andres et al., 2013). When convenient for staff, telephone or computer-based interpreters are effective for bridging communication barriers with LEP patients (Tuot et al., 2012). Team-based strategies for interpretation are effective when there is a high volume of LEP patients (Schapira et al., 2008). It is more common, however, that providers use the most easily available interpreter, including other staff members and family, even when policies advise against this practice (Hsieh, 2006).

Generally, however, a lack of interpreter services causes most healthcare workers to alter their work patterns, thereby decreasing efficiency, increasing stress and increasing the threats to patient safety (Johnson et al., 1999; Cioffi, 2003; Jones, 2008; Elderkin-Thompson et al., 2001; Bernard et al., 2006). Interruptions to professional role execution increase threats to patient safety and underdiagnosis (Hadziabdic et al., 2011; Leng et al., 2010; Gany et al., 2007). Changes can result in increased provider stress owing to work reorganization (Bernard et al., 2005, 2006; Gany et al., 2007; Hadziabdic et al., 2011; Leng et al., 2010). Despite these risks, providers of all kinds tend to underutilize interpreter services and, therefore, affect both perceived and actual demand for language services (Gill et al., 2011; Bischoff & Hudelson, 2010a; Diamond et al., 2009, 2012).

Implementing language services

Language services are a critical component for meeting the goals of the Quadruple Aim – an international project to improve the quality, costs, and experiences of individuals accessing the health care system. The Quadruple Aim first emerged from the Institute for Healthcare Improvement as the Triple Aim and seeks to 'apply integrated approaches to simultaneously improve care, improve population health, and reduce costs per capita'

(Whittington *et al.*, 2015). The newest fourth part of the aim focuses on improving the health worker experience. It was added to the goals of the project because poor health worker job satisfaction and retention has consistently been found to adversely affect the patient experience and system costs.

The Quadruple Aim has evolved into a global movement with more than 50 countries now actively applying these goals to their healthcare systems. A main focal point of the effort centers on improving the experience of care. For patients with a language barrier and their providers, that means systematically addressing how language services are implemented so that communication improves between all parties.

To begin with, demand for language services will be driven by the local immigrant population. For healthcare organizations large and small, how many interpreters, how many languages, and the amount of service coverage for a 24 hour, 7 days a week operation will be driven by local demographics and utilization patterns. In the US, for example, the American Community Survey derived from the US Census data will provide information about the local immigrant population. While studies have yet to determine when it becomes cost effective for a facility to hire interpreters full time as opposed to alternatives, these decisions are largely driven by feedback provided from staff about their language services needs. Per-patient estimates of interpreter service costs in hospitals are around $234 but may be cost neutral for the organization because they can decrease readmissions (Jacobs *et al.*, 2007; Tuot *et al.*, 2012; Karliner *et al.*, 2010; Kripalani *et al.*, 2010; Lindholm *et al.*, 2012; Anderson *et al.*, 2005). Furthermore, research suggests that, in some instances, bilingual nurses may get as much as a 7% increase in salary for their bilingual skills (Coomer, 2011; Kalist, 2005); however, the cost offset of a higher salary for hiring a bilingual nurse has yet to be determined.

There are a few things to consider when planning language services in the absence of technical skills for forecasting demand. First, when implementing language services to meet demand, it is important to consider both 'planned' – something that would happen in primary care or same day surgery – and 'unplanned' – as would happen in acute care – encounters. In a planned encounter, the provider has access to organizational resources that allow them to plan ahead and organize interpreter services in advance of the patient encounter. This happens in primary care most often. In an unplanned encounter, the provider must organize resources to respond to 'spontaneous' interactions with the patient related to the nature of the encounter. Acute care services fit this category best since providers may not always have access to adequate interpreter services at the moment they are needed. Even with a nurse caring for hospitalized patients over a period of days, for example, it seems that the situation would be 'planned', but the moment-to-moment interactions of the nurse caring for the hospitalized patient may not always allow for planned encounters. Home care or community-based services could fall into either category because of the nature of the service referral process.

Overall, the quality of management behind care coordination between facilities (e.g. hospital to home care, long-term care to home care) will dictate if the encounter qualifies as planned or unplanned. That dynamic also has the potential to affect patient outcomes and drive demand for language services, even though it remains understudied.

For 'big picture' approaches, *language planning theory* can offer healthcare organizations a way to systematically structure the scaling up or new implementation of language services. Language Planning Theory (LPT) posits that the identification of language problems at the interactional level (i.e. between patients and providers) leads to the adoption of language planning efforts at the institutional level (Thomas & Lee, 2010). A core assumption of LPT is that the 'language function' serves as a vehicle between transmitter and receiver. It occurs in a specific sociolinguistic context to meet a basic communicative need. In said context, one language may effectively dominate another as the sole form of communication, as English does in the US healthcare system. Language dominance often leads to inadequate patient medical histories or poor health teaching (Cobarrubias & Fishman, 1983; Thomas & Lee, 2010; NACHC, 2008). Organizational level solutions then result to address the key interactional problem(s).

LPT developed as a unique area of study in the mid-20th century as a subfield of political science. It examined how colonial states viewed linguistic diversity as a resource (or not). Early researchers viewed language as an organizational resource or service delivery issue that was valuable and required careful management because it could block access to resources and information (Thomas & Lee, 2010). More recently, Cooper proposed a model for evaluating language planning initiatives (LPI) by organizations (Cooper, 1989). Cooper's model is composed of the following components for evaluation:

(1) *Implementation Actors* – who is involved in implementation of LPI?
(2) *Behaviors targeted* – what behaviors have been identified as constituting a 'problem' or a reason for shift?
(3) *Stakeholders* – who are the stakeholders (both direct and indirect)?
(4) *Goals* – what are the goals of the LPI effort?
(5) *Structural conditions* – what are the social, economic, and structural conditions that affect LPI efforts or outcomes?
(6) *Means of implementation* – by what means are changes implemented?
(7) *Decision process structures* – how are decision processes structured? How are they made?
(8) *Results or outcomes* – how are the results of LPI initiatives determined?

Cooper's model assumes that all of these factors could contribute equally to the organizational response(s), but will vary based on language services demand and organizational culture. Research can capture the extent to which each component contributes to the outcome under study.

Conclusion

This section illustrated the complex nature of language services and how their organization and implementation can affect patient outcomes and drive demand. Even though the evidence is present to show the drivers of demand through increased migration, there are still significant gaps in knowledge that need answers.

The Need for More Evidence About the Outcomes Impact of Language Services and Their Organization

In general, there is a lack of research about most other healthcare contexts besides the hospital and primary care setting. Aside from physicians, researchers have produced few studies examining nurses and allied health personnel and how an increased demand for language services impacts their roles. Even fewer studies have examined the impact on patient outcomes in any setting, although the US Agency for Health Care Research and Quality has funded several outcomes studies that confirm that poor management of language barriers by organizations increases length of stay by 15–20% and increases risk for 30 day readmission (Lindholm et al., 2012; Karliner et al., 2010; Jacobs et al., 2007). Combine that with the current deficiencies in language barriers research, and the dearth of evidence is significant.

For example, even with its extensive and nationally standardized patient database, the homecare setting remains understudied. What few publications in this area exist are descriptive and anecdotal at best, identifying resources for practitioners or providing guidelines for culturally competent practice. The evidence in the long-term care setting, from a demand for language services perspective, offers an angle on the topic not commonly seen in other contexts. Because of the historically extensive use of internationally educated registered nursing personnel to staff long-term care, literature for that context focuses on language issues of the staff and not the patients, even when language barriers in patients are acknowledged as a significant issue in care transitions between healthcare organizations (Naylor et al., 2009; Bourgeault et al., 2010; Ku & Flores, 2005; White et al., 2012; Ulmer et al., 2009). In contrast, non-physician-led studies in rehabilitation services on this topic are few simply because health services studies in allied health occupations are a new and emerging area of research. For that same reason, there are few studies about demand for language services that include physical therapists, occupational therapists, and speech and communication professionals. Understanding the demand for language services in a way that is sensitive to role implementation of these providers is an important component of ensuring patient access to their services.

Another profession specific example comes from nursing. Nurses have not conducted a lot of research on this topic despite how frequently nurses encounter language-barrier patients in their work. Only seven studies about how language barriers impact registered nurse or nurse practitioner role execution in any setting exist (Beckstrand *et al.*, 2010; Gerrish *et al.*, 2004; Whitman *et al.*, 2010; Tuot *et al.*, 2012; Diamond *et al.*, 2012; Taylor & Alfred, 2010; Bernard *et al.*, 2006). While we could hypothesize that the primary care literature applies to nurse practitioners working in those settings, the fact that nurse practitioners tend to work in more underserved areas and also have higher patient satisfaction scores (Charlton *et al.*, 2008; Buchan & Dal Poz, 2002; Desborough *et al.*, 2012; Institute of Medicine 2011) suggests that more specific research about nurse practitioners and the relationship to patient outcomes in limited-English-proficiency individuals is needed.

Several factors explain this gap in the research within nursing. First, in the US, the global leader in nursing research, few nurses are bilingual, and those who are often do not pursue research careers. This may change in future generations as the demographics of the profession change in the country to better reflect the demographics of the clientele. In other countries, both nursing research and the demand for language services are new, so at a national level, it becomes an emerging area of research that is dependent on funding mechanisms for further study.

A second reason is that, in the hospital setting, where the majority of nurses still work around the world, it is very difficult to monitor language-concordant encounters and thus study the impact of either nurses' use of interpreters or language-concordant nurses on patient outcomes. The unit-level interactions between patients and nurses, even with the advent of electronic medical records, remain difficult to track and analyze. Nonetheless, several studies have identified admission, discharge and patient teaching as key points in the hospital encounter that make a difference in outcomes of patients with a language barrier (Lindholm *et al.*, 2012; Jacobs *et al.*, 2007; Garrett *et al.*, 2008; Karliner *et al.*, 2010; Grover *et al.*, 2012; Levas, 2011). Nurses are key actors in these patient experience encounter points, so their use of interpreters during those periods may explain variations in related outcomes.

Regardless of which healthcare professional is studied, diversifying the healthcare human resources studied in language-barriers research will help enhance the understanding of how demand for language services is specific to and similar across the professions. Organizations that clearly designate the language skills of providers not only on identification badges, but also in the electronic health record will help make it possible to study how language concordance influences outcomes at the encounter or unit level, thereby enhancing the existing understanding of drivers of demand for language services (Bahl et al., 2008). With these changes, researchers can then better understand how much language concordance contributes to improving patient outcomes in the affected populations or how much language discordance contributes to health disparities.

Conclusion

Demand for language services is complex and specific to the immigration patterns in different regions and countries. The 21st-century workers' global mobility will only continue to influence the demand for language services in health systems as the century moves forward. The healthcare needs of these individuals will change as the reasons for migration and its associated experiences evolve in the natural course of human history. This means that accounting for language services should become part of any strategic development plan of any healthcare organization. Meeting the demand for language services driven by the dynamics of global migration will also be an important component of providing universal health coverage. Organizations with a long history of working effectively with LEP individuals can serve as critical resources for organizations located in areas where the demand for language services is growing rapidly.

Whatever approach key stakeholders choose to implement language services, above all else, the end product should result in improved patient experiences in the healthcare system. Patients with language barriers should be able to communicate in their preferred language whenever possible. When they can do that, it results in better health for populations and improved patient experiences.

References

Anderson, M.A., Clarke, M.M., Helms, L.B. and Foreman, M.D. (2005) Hospital readmission from home health care before and after prospective payment. *Journal of Nursing Scholarship* 37 (1), 73–79; doi: 10.1111/j.1547-5069.2005.00001.x. http://doi.wiley.com/10.1111/j.1547-5069.2005.00001.x.

Andres, E., Wynia, M., Regenstein, M. and Maul, L. (2013) Should I call an interpreter? – How do physicians with second language skills decide? *Journal of Health Care for the Poor and Underserved* 24 (2), 525–539; doi: 10.1353/hpu.2013.0060. http://www.ncbi.nlm.nih.gov/pubmed/23728026.

Appave, G. and Laczko, F. (2011) World Migration Report 2011: Communicating Effectively About Migration. International Organization for Migration (IOM).

Ayanian, J.Z., Zaslavsky, A.M., Guadagnoli, E., Fuchs, C.S., Yost, K.J., Creech, C.M., Cress, R.D., O'Connor, L.C., West, D.W. and Wright, W.E. (2005) Patients' perceptions of quality of care for colorectal cancer by race, ethnicity, and language. *Journal of Clinical Oncology: Official Journal of the American Society of Clinical Oncology* 23 (27), 6576–6586; doi: 10.1200/JCO.2005.06.102. http://www.ncbi.nlm.nih.gov/pubmed/16116149.

Bagchi, A.D., Dale, S., Verbitsky-Savitz, N., Andrecheck, S., Zavotsky, K. and Eisenstein, R. (2011) Examining effectiveness of medical interpreters in emergency departments for Spanish-speaking patients with limited English proficiency: Results of a randomized controlled trial. *Annals of Emergency Medicine* 57 (3), 248–256.e1–4; doi: 10.1016/j.annemergmed.2010.05.032. http://www.ncbi.nlm.nih.gov/pubmed/20678825.

Bahl, V., Thompson, M.A., Kau, T.-Y., Hu, H.M. and Campbell, D.A. (2008) Do the AHRQ patient safety indicators flag conditions that are present at the time of hospital admission? *Medical Care* 46 (5), 516–522; doi: 10.1097/MLR.0b013e31815f537f. http://www.ncbi.nlm.nih.gov/pubmed/18438200.

Bartram, D. (2010) The normative foundations of 'policy implications': Reflections on international labour migration. *Work, Employment & Society* 24 (2), 355–365; doi: 10.1177/0950017010362156. http://wes.sagepub.com/cgi/doi/10.1177/0950017010362156.

Bauer, A.M., Chen, C.-N. and Alegría, M. (2010) English language proficiency and mental health service use among Latino and Asian Americans with mental disorders. *Medical Care* 48 (12), 1097–1104; doi: 10.1097/MLR.0b013e3181f80749. http://www.pubmedcentral.nih.gov/articlerender.fcgi?artid=3135417&tool=pmcentrez&rendertype=abstract.

Beckstrand, R.L., Rawle, N.L., Callister, L. and Mandleco, B.L. (2010) Pediatric nurses' perceptions of obstacles and supportive behaviors in end-of-life care. *American Journal of Critical Care: An Official Publication, American Association of Critical-Care Nurses* 19 (6), 543–552; doi: 10.4037/ajcc2009497. http://www.ncbi.nlm.nih.gov/pubmed/20026650.

Bernard, A.C., Summers, A., Thomas, J., Ray, M., Rockich, A., Boulanger, B., Kearney, P., Barnes, S., Boulanger, B. and Kearney, P. (2005) Novel Spanish translators for acute care nurses and physicians: Usefulness and effect on practitioner stress. *American Journal of Critical Care* 14, 545–550.

Bernard, A., Whitaker, M., Ray, M., Rockich, A., Barton-Baxter, M., Barnes, S.-L., Boulanger, B., Tsuei, B. and Kearney, P. (2006) Impact of language barrier on acute care medical professionals is dependent upon role. *Journal of Professional Nursing: Official Journal of the American Association of Colleges of Nursing* 22 (6), 355–358; doi: 10.1016/j.profnurs.2006.09.001. http://www.ncbi.nlm.nih.gov/pubmed/17141719.

Betancourt, J.R., Renfrew, M.R., Green, A.R., Lopez, L. and Wasserman, M. (2012) Improving patient safety systems for patients with limited English proficiency: A guide for hospitals. Washington, DC.

Bischoff, A. and Hudelson, P. (2010a) Communicating with foreign language-speaking patients: Is access to professional interpreters enough? *Journal of Travel Medicine* 17 (1), 15–20; doi: 10.1111/j.1708-8305.2009.00314.x. http://www.ncbi.nlm.nih.gov/pubmed/20074097.

Bischoff, A. and Hudelson, P. (2010b) Access to healthcare interpreter services: Where are we and where do we need to go? *International Journal of Environmental Research and Public Health* 7 (7), 2838–2844; doi: 10.3390/ijerph7072838. http://www.pubmedcentral.nih.gov/articlerender.fcgi?artid=2922730&tool=pmcentrez&rendertype=abstract.

Biswas, D., Kristiansen, M., Krasnik, A. and Norredam, M. (2011) Access to healthcare and alternative health-seeking strategies among undocumented migrants in Denmark. *BMC Public Health* 11 (1), 560; doi: 10.1186/1471-2458-11-560. http://www.pubmedcentral.nih.gov/articlerender.fcgi?artid=3163547&tool=pmcentrez&rendertype=abstract.

Bourgeault, I.L., Atanackovic, J., Rashid, A. and Parpia, R. (2010) Relations between immigrant care workers and older persons in home and long-term care. *Canadian Journal on Aging/La Revue Canadienne Du Vieillissement* 29 (1), 109–118; doi: 10.1017/S0714980809990407. http://www.ncbi.nlm.nih.gov/pubmed/20202269.

Brisset, C., Leanza, Y. and Laforest, K. (2013) Working with interpreters in health care: A systematic review and meta-ethnography of qualitative studies. *Patient Education and Counseling* 91 (2), 131–140; doi: 10.1016/j.pec.2012.11.008. http://www.ncbi.nlm.nih.gov/pubmed/23246426.

Buchan, J. and Dal Poz, M.R. (2002) Skill mix in the health care workforce: Reviewing the evidence. *Bulletin of the World Health Organization* 80 (7), 575–580; http://www.pubmedcentral.nih.gov/articlerender.fcgi?artid=2567564&tool=pmcentrez&rendertype=abstract.

Carling, J. (2009) The determinants of migrant remittances. *Oxford Review of Economic Policy* 24 (3), 581–598; doi: 10.1093/oxrep/grn022. http://oxrep.oxfordjournals.org/cgi/doi/10.1093/oxrep/grn022.

Charlton, C.R., Dearing, K.S., Berry, J.A. and Johnson, M.J. (2008) Nurse practitioners' communication styles and their impact on patient outcomes: An integrated literature review. *Journal of the American Academy of Nurse Practitioners* 20 (7), 382–388; doi: 10.1111/j.1745-7599.2008.00336.x. http://www.ncbi.nlm.nih.gov/pubmed/18638178.

Cioffi, R.N.J. (2003) Communicating with culturally and linguistically diverse patients in an acute care setting: Nurses' experiences. *International Journal of Nursing Studies* 40 (3), 299–306; http://www.ncbi.nlm.nih.gov/pubmed/16295344.

Cobarrubias, J. and Fishman, J.A. (1983) *Progress in Language Planning: International Perspectives*, edited by Cobarrubias, J. and Fishman, J.A., 1st edn. Berlin: Walter de Gruyter.

Coomer, N.M. (2011) Returns to bilingualism in the nursing labor market – Demand or ability? *The Journal of Socio-Economics* 40 (3), 274–284; doi: 10.1016/j.socec.2010.10.001. http://linkinghub.elsevier.com/retrieve/pii/S1053535710001344.

Cooper, R.J. (1989) *Language Planning and Social Change*. New York: Cambridge University Press.

DEC (2016) Migration and Remittances Team of the Development Prospects Group from the Development Economics. Migration and Development Brief. Washington, DC; http://siteresources.worldbank.org/INTPROSPECTS/Resources/334934-1288990760745/MigrationandDevelopmentBrief22.pdf.

Desborough, J., Forrest, L. and Parker, R. (2012) Nurse-led primary healthcare walk-in centres: An integrative literature review. *Journal of Advanced Nursing* 68 (2), 248–263; doi: 10.1111/j.1365-2648.2011.05798.x. http://www.ncbi.nlm.nih.gov/pubmed/21834837.

Diamond, L.C., Schenker, Y., Curry, L., Bradley, E.H. and Fernandez, A. (2009) Getting by: Underuse of interpreters by resident physicians. *Journal of General Internal Medicine* 24 (2), 256–262; doi: 10.1007/s11606-008-0875-7. http://www.pubmedcentral.nih.gov/articlerender.fcgi?artid=2628994&tool=pmcentrez&rendertype=abstract.

Diamond, L.C., Tuot, D.S. and Karliner, L.S. (2012) The use of Spanish language skills by physicians and nurses: Policy implications for teaching and testing. *Journal of General Internal Medicine* 27 (1), 117–123; doi: 10.1007/s11606-011-1779-5. http://www.pubmedcentral.nih.gov/articlerender.fcgi?artid=3250531&tool=pmcentrez&rendertype=abstract.

Docquier, F., Lowell, B.L. and Marfouk, A. (2009) A gendered assessment of highly skilled emigration. *Population and Development Review* 35 (2), 297–321.

Durand, J. and Massey, D.S. (2010) New World Orders: Continuities and changes in Latin American migration. *The Annals of the American Academy of Political and Social Science* 630 (1), 20–52; doi: 10.1177/0002716210368102. http://www.pubmedcentral.nih.gov/articlerender.fcgi?artid=2931359&tool=pmcentrez&rendertype=abstract.

Eamranond, P.P., Davis, R.B., Phillips, R.S. and Wee, C.C. (2009) Patient–physician language concordance and lifestyle counseling among Spanish-speaking patients. *Journal of Immigrant and Minority Health/Center for Minority Public Health* 11 (6), 494–498; doi: 10.1007/s10903-008-9222-7. http://www.ncbi.nlm.nih.gov/pubmed/19152110.

El Ansari, W., Newbigging, K., Roth, C. and Malik, F. (2009) The role of advocacy and interpretation services in the delivery of quality healthcare to diverse minority communities in London, United Kingdom. *Health & Social Care in the Community* 17 (6), 636–646; doi: 10.1111/j.1365-2524.2009.00867.x. http://www.ncbi.nlm.nih.gov/pubmed/19486185.

Elderkin-Thompson, V., Silver, R.S. and Waitzkin, H. (2001) When nurses double as interpreters: A study of Spanish-speaking patients in a US primary care setting. *Social Science and Medicine (1982)* 52 (9), 1343–1358; http://www.ncbi.nlm.nih.gov/pubmed/11286360.

Fernandez, A., Schillinger, D., Warton, E.M., Adler, N., Moffet, N.H., Schenker, Y., Salgado, N.V., Ahmed, A. and Karter, A.J. (2011) Language barriers, physician–patient language concordance, and glycemic control among insured latinos with diabetes: The Diabetes Study of Northern California (DISTANCE). *Journal of General Internal Medicine* 26 (2), 170–176; doi: 10.1007/s11606-010-1507-6. http://www.pubmedcentral.nih.gov/articlerender.fcgi?artid=3019330&tool=pmcentrez&rendertype=abstract.

Fussell, E. (2010) The cumulative causation of international migration in Latin America. *The ANNALS of the American Academy of Political and Social Science* 630 (1), 162–177; doi: 10.1177/0002716210368108. http://ann.sagepub.com/cgi/doi/10.1177/0002716210368108.

Gany, F., Kapelusznik, L., Prakash, K., Gonzalez, J., Orta, L.Y., Tseng, C.-H. and Changrani, J. (2007) The impact of medical interpretation method on time and errors. *Journal of General Internal Medicine* 22 (Suppl 2), 319–323; doi: 10.1007/s11606-007-0361-7. http://www.pubmedcentral.nih.gov/articlerender.fcgi?artid=2078536&tool=pmcentrez&rendertype=abstract.

Garrett, P.W., Dickson, H.G. and Klinken Whelan H. (2008) Communication and healthcare complexity in people with little or no English: The communication complexity score. *Ethnicity & Health* 13 (3), 203–317; doi: 10.1080/13557850701837328. http://www.ncbi.nlm.nih.gov/pubmed/18568973.

Gerrish, K., Chau, R., Sobowale, A. and Birks, E. (2004) Bridging the language barrier: The use of interpreters in primary care nursing. *Health & Social Care in the Community* 12 (5), 407–413; doi: 10.1111/j.1365-2524.2004.00510.x. http://www.ncbi.nlm.nih.gov/pubmed/15373819.

Gill, P.S., Beavan, J., Calvert, M. and Freemantle, N. (2011) The unmet need for interpreting provision in UK primary Care. *PloS One* 6 (6), e20837; doi: 10.1371/journal.pone.0020837. http://www.pubmedcentral.nih.gov/articlerender.fcgi?artid=3113854&tool=pmcentrez&rendertype=abstract.

Ginde, A.A., Sullivan, A.F., Corel, B., Caceres, J.A. and Camargo, C.A. (2010) Reevaluation of the effect of mandatory interpreter legislation on use of professional interpreters for ED patients with language barriers. *Patient Education and Counseling* 81 (2), 204–6; doi: 10.1016/j.pec.2010.01.023. http://www.ncbi.nlm.nih.gov/pubmed/20193999.

Green, A.R., Ngo-Metzger, Q., Legedza, A.T.R., Massagli, M.P., Phillips, R.S. and Iezzoni, L.I. (2005) Interpreter services, language concordance, and health care quality. Experiences of Asian Americans with Limited English Proficiency. *Journal of General Internal Medicine* 20 (11), 1050–1056; doi: 10.1111/j.1525-1497.2005.0223.x. http://www.pubmedcentral.nih.gov/articlerender.fcgi?artid=1490255&tool=pmcentrez&rendertype=abstract.

Grover, A., Deakyne, S., Bajaj, L. and Roosevelt, G.E. (2012) Comparison of throughput times for limited English proficiency patient visits in the emergency department between different interpreter modalities. *Journal of Immigrant and Minority Health/Center for Minority Public Health* 14 (4), 602–607; doi: 10.1007/s10903-011-9532-z. http://www.ncbi.nlm.nih.gov/pubmed/21947693.

Hacker, K., Choi, Y.S., Trebino, L., Hicks, L., Friedman, E., Blanchfield, B. and Gazelle, G.S. (2012) Exploring the impact of language services on utilization and clinical outcomes for diabetics. *PloS One* 7 (6), e38507; doi: 10.1371/journal.pone.0038507. http://www.pubmedcentral.nih.gov/articlerender.fcgi?artid=3366945&tool=pmcentrez&rendertype=abstract.

Hadziabdic, E., Heikkilä, K., Albin, B. and Hjelm, K. (2011) Problems and consequences in the use of professional interpreters: Qualitative analysis of incidents from primary healthcare. *Nursing Inquiry* 18 (3), 253–261; doi: 10.1111/j.1440-1800.2011.00542.x. http://www.ncbi.nlm.nih.gov/pubmed/21790876.

Hagan, J., Lowe, N. and Quingla, C. (2011) Skills on the move: Rethinking the relationship between human capital and immigrant economic mobility. *Work and Occupations* 38 (2), 149–178; doi: 10.1177/0730888410397918. http://wox.sagepub.com/cgi/doi/10.1177/0730888410397918.

Hilfinger Messias, D.K., McDowell, L. and Estrada, R.D. (2009) Language interpreting as social justice work. *Advances in Nursing Science* 32 (2), 128–143.

Hsieh, E. (2006) Understanding medical interpreters: Reconceptualizing bilingual health communication. *Health Communication* 20 (2), 177–186; doi: 10.1207/s15327027hc2002_9. http://www.ncbi.nlm.nih.gov/pubmed/16965255.

Hsieh, E. (2008) 'I am not a robot!' Interpreters' views of their roles in health care settings. *Qualitative Health Research* 18 (10), 1367–1383; doi: 10.1177/1049732308323840. http://www.ncbi.nlm.nih.gov/pubmed/18832768.

Hsieh, E. and Kramer, E.M. (2012) Medical interpreters as tools: Dangers and challenges in the utilitarian approach to interpreters' roles and functions. *Patient Education and Counseling* 89 (1) (October), 158–162; doi: 10.1016/j.pec.2012.07.001. http://www.ncbi.nlm.nih.gov/pubmed/22857777.

Institute of Medicine (2011) *The Future of Nursing: Leading Change, Advancing Health Committee on the Robert Wood Johnson Foundation Initiative on the Future of Nursing, at the Institute of Medicine; Institute of Medicine*, 1st ed. Washington, DC: Institute of Medicine.

Ipsiroglu, O.S., Herle, M., Spoula, E., Möslinger, D., Wimmer, B., Burgard, P., Bode, H. and Stöckler-Ipsiroglu, S. (2005) Transcultural pediatrics: Compliance and outcome of phenylketonuria patients from families with an immigration background. *Wiener Klinische Wochenschrift* 117 (15–16), 541–547; doi: 10.1007/s00508-005-0327-x. http://www.ncbi.nlm.nih.gov/pubmed/16158204.

Jacobs, E.A. (2000) Patient centeredness in medical encounters requiring an interpreter. *The American Journal of Medicine* 109 (6), 515; doi: 10.1016/S0002-9343(00)00536-2. http://www.ncbi.nlm.nih.gov/pubmed/11184776.

Jacobs, E.A., Lauderdale, D.S., Meltzer, D., Shorey, J.M., Levinson, W. and Thisted, R.A. (2001) Impact of interpreter services on delivery of health care to limited-English-proficient patients. *Journal of General Internal Medicine* 16 (7), 468–474; doi: 10.1046/j.1525-1497.2001.016007468.x. http://www.ncbi.nlm.nih.gov/pubmed/11520385.

Jacobs, E.A., Sadowski, L.S. and Rathouz, P.J. (2007) The impact of an enhanced interpreter service intervention on hospital costs and patient satisfaction. *Journal of General Internal Medicine* 22 (Suppl 2), 306–311; doi: 10.1007/s11606-007-0357-3. http://www.pubmedcentral.nih.gov/articlerender.fcgi?artid=2078550&tool=pmcentrez&rendertype=abstract.

Jacobs, E.A., Sanchez Leos, G., Rathouz, P.J. and Fu, P. (2011a) Shared networks of interpreter services, at relatively low cost, can help providers serve patients with limited English skills. *Health Affairs (Project Hope)* 30 (10), 1930–1938; doi: 10.1377/hlthaff.2011.0667. http://www.ncbi.nlm.nih.gov/pubmed/21976337.

Jacobs, E.A., Mendenhall, E., Scheck Mcalearney, A., Rolle, I., Whitaker, E.E., Warnecke, R. and Estwing Ferrans, C. (2011b) An exploratory study of how trust in health care institutions varies across African American, Hispanic and White populations. *Communication and Medicine* 8 (1), 89–98. http://www.ncbi.nlm.nih.gov/pubmed/22616359.

Johnson, M., Noble, C., Matthews, C. and Aguilar, N. (1999) Bilingual communicators within the health care setting. *Qualitative Health Research* 9 (3), 329–343; doi: 10.1177/104973299129121893. http://qhr.sagepub.com/cgi/doi/10.1177/104973299129121893.

Jones, S.M. (2008) Emergency nurses' caring experiences with Mexican American patients. *Journal of Emergency Nursing: JEN: Official Publication of the Emergency Department Nurses Association* 34 (3), 199–204; doi: 10.1016/j.jen.2007.05.009. http://www.ncbi.nlm.nih.gov/pubmed/18558248.

Kalist, D. (2005) Registered nurses and the value of bilingualism. *Industrial and Labor Relations Review* 59 (1), 101–118. http://digitalcommons.ilr.cornell.edu/ilrreview/vol59/iss1/6.

Kanter, M.H., Abrams, K.M., Carrasco, M.R., Spiegel, N.H., Vogel, R.S. and Coleman, K.J. (2009) Patient–physician language concordance: A strategy for meeting the needs of Spanish-speaking patients in primary care. *The Permanente Journal* 13 (4), 79–84. http://www.pubmedcentral.nih.gov/articlerender.fcgi?artid=2911827&tool=pmcentrez&rendertype=abstract.

Karliner, L.S., Jacobs, EA. Chen, A.H. and Mutha, S. (2007) Do professional interpreters improve clinical care for patients with limited English proficiency? A systematic review of the literature. *Health Services Research* 42 (2), 727–54; doi: 10.1111/j.1475-6773.2006.00629.x. http://www.pubmedcentral.nih.gov/articlerender.fcgi?artid=1955368&tool=pmcentrez&rendertype=abstract.

Karliner, L.S., Kim, S.E., Meltzer, D.O. and Auerbach, A.D. (2010) Influence of language barriers on outcomes of hospital care for general medicine inpatients. *Journal of Hospital Medicine: An Official Publication of the Society of Hospital Medicine* 5 (5), 276–282; doi: 10.1002/jhm.658. http://www.ncbi.nlm.nih.gov/pubmed/20533573.

Karliner, L.S., Hwang, E.S., Nickleach, D. and Kaplan, C.P. (2011) Language barriers and patient-centered breast cancer care. *Patient Education and Counseling* 84 (2), 223–8; doi: 10.1016/j.pec.2010.07.009. http://www.ncbi.nlm.nih.gov/pubmed/20685068.

Kosmider, S., Shedda, S., Jones, I.T., McLaughlin, S. and Gibbs, P. (2010) Predictors of clinic non-attendance: Opportunities to improve patient outcomes in colorectal cancer. *Internal Medicine Journal* 40 (11), 757–763; doi: 10.1111/j.1445-5994.2009.01986.x. http://www.ncbi.nlm.nih.gov/pubmed/19460064.

Kripalani, S., Jacobson, T.A., Mugalla, I.C., Cawthon, C.R., Niesner, K.J. and Vaccarino, V. (2010) Health literacy and the quality of physician–patient communication during hospitalization. *Journal of Hospital Medicine: An Official Publication of the Society of Hospital Medicine* 5 (5), 269–275; doi: 10.1002/jhm.667. http://www.pubmedcentral.nih.gov/articlerender.fcgi?artid=3468649&tool=pmcentrez&rendertype=abstract.

Ku, L. and Flores, G. (2005) Pay now or pay later: Providing interpreter services in health care. *Health Affairs (Project Hope)* 24 (2), 435–444; doi: 10.1377/hlthaff.24.2.435. http://content.healthaffairs.org/content/24/2/435.abstract.

Lassetter, J.H. and Callister, L.C. (2008) The impact of migration on the health of voluntary migrants in Western societies: A review of the literature. *Journal of Transcultural Nursing* 20 (1), 93–104; doi: 10.1177/1043659608325841. http://tcn.sagepub.com/cgi/doi/10.1177/1043659608325841.

Leng, J.C.F., Changrani, J., Tseng, C.H. and Gany, F. (2010) Detection of depression with different interpreting methods among Chinese and Latino primary care patients: A randomized controlled trial. *Journal of Immigrant and Minority Health/Center for Minority Public Health* 12 (2), 234–241; doi: 10.1007/s10903-009-9254-7. http://www.ncbi.nlm.nih.gov/pubmed/19408119.

Levas, M.N. (2011) Effects of the limited English proficiency of parents on hospital length of stay and home health care referral for their home health care – Eligible children with infections. *Archives of Pediatrics & Adolescent Medicine* 165 (9), 831; doi: 10.1001/archpediatrics.2011.61. http://www.ncbi.nlm.nih.gov/pubmed/215 36949.

Lindholm, M., Hargraves, J.L., Ferguson, W.J. and Reed, G. (2012) Professional language interpretation and inpatient length of stay and readmission rates. *Journal of General Internal Medicine* 27 (10), 1294–1299; doi: 10.1007/s11606-012-2041-5. http://www.pubmedcentral.nih.gov/articlerender.fcgi?artid=3445680&tool=pmcentrez&rendertype=abstract.

McDowell, L., Hilfinger Messias, D.A.K. and Dawson Estrada, R. (2011) The work of language interpretation in health care: Complex, challenging, exhausting, and often invisible. *Journal of Transcultural Nursing: Official Journal of the Transcultural Nursing Society/Transcultural Nursing Society* 22 (2), 137–47; doi: 10.1177/1043659610395773. http://www.ncbi.nlm.nih.gov/pubmed/21317402.

NACHC (2008) Serving Patients with Limited Serving Patients with Limited English Proficiency: Results of A Community Health Cetner Survey. Bethesda, MD.

Nápoles, A.M., Gregorich, S.E., Santoyo-Olsson, J., O'Brien, H. and Stewart, A.L. (2009) Interpersonal processes of care and patient satisfaction: Do associations differ by race, ethnicity, and language? *Health Services Research* 44 (4), 1326–1344; doi: 10.1111/j.1475-6773.2009.00965.x. http://www.pubmedcentral.nih.gov/articlerender.fcgi?artid=2714869&tool=pmcentrez&rendertype=abstract.

Naylor, M.D., Kurtzman, E.T. and Pauly, M.V. (2009) Transitions of elders between long-term care and hospitals. *Policy, Politics and Nursing Practice* 10 (3), 187–94; doi: 10.1177/1527154409355710. http://www.ncbi.nlm.nih.gov/pubmed/20026453.

Ngo-Metzger, Q., Sorkin, D.H., Phillips, R.S., Greenfield, S., Massagli, M.P., Clarridge, B. and Kaplan, S.H. (2007) Providing high-quality care for limited english proficient patients: The importance of language concordance and interpreter use. *Journal of General Internal Medicine* 22 (Suppl 2), 324–30; doi: 10.1007/s11606-007-0340-z. http://www.pubmedcentral.nih.gov/articlerender.fcgi?artid=2078537&tool=pmcentrez&rendertype=abstract.

Ngo-Metzger, Q., Sorkin, D.H. and Phillips, R. (2009) Healthcare experiences of limited English-proficient Asian American patients. *Patient* 2 (2), 113–120.

Radwin, L.E., Cabral, H.J. and Siu Woodworth, T. (2013) Effects of race and language on patient-centered cancer nursing care and patient outcomes. *Journal of Health Care for the Poor and Underserved* 24 (2), 619–632; doi: 10.1353/hpu.2013.0058. http://www.ncbi.nlm.nih.gov/pubmed/23728032.

Regenstein, M., Huang, J., West, C., Mead, H., Trott, J. and Stegun, M. (2008) Hospital Language Services: Quality Improvement and Performance Measures. http://www.ahrq.gov/professionals/quality-patient-safety/patient-safety-resources/resources/advances-in-patient-safety-2/vol2/Advances-Regenstein_54.pdf.

Reyes, A.M. and Hardy, M. (2015) Health insurance instability among older immigrants: Region of origin disparities in coverage. *The Journals of Gerontology. Series B, Psychological Sciences and Social Sciences* 70 (2), gbu218; doi: 10.1093/geronb/gbu218. http://psychsocgerontology.oxfordjournals.org/content/70/2/303.abstract?maxtoshow=&HITS=10&hits=70&RESULTFORMAT=1&andorexacttitle=and&andorexacttitleabs=and&fulltext=Mexico&andorexactfulltext=and&searchid=1&FIRSTINDEX=0&sortspec=match&fdate=//&resourcetyp.

Riggs, E., Davis, E., Gibbs, L., Block, K., Szwarc, J., Casey, S., Duell-Piening, P. and Waters, E. (2012) Accessing maternal and child health services in Melbourne, Australia: Reflections from refugee families and service providers. *BMC Health Services Research*; doi: 10.1186/1472-6963-12-117. http://www.pubmedcentral.nih.gov/articlerender.fcgi?artid=3424108&tool=pmcentrez&rendertype=abstract.

Rosenberg, E., Leanza, Y. and Seller, R. (2007) Doctor–patient communication in primary care with an interpreter: Physician perceptions of professional and family interpreters. *Patient Education and Counseling* 67 (3), 286–292; doi: 10.1016/j.pec.2007.03.011. http://www.ncbi.nlm.nih.gov/pubmed/17448622.

Rudmin, F.W. (2010) Phenomenology of acculturation: Retrospective reports from the Philippines, Japan, Quebec, and Norway. *Culture & Psychology* 16 (3) (August 23), 313–332; doi: 10.1177/1354067X10371139. http://cap.sagepub.com/cgi/doi/10.1177/1354067X10371139.

Sanderson, M.R. and Kentor, J. (2008) Foreign direct investment and international migration: A cross-national analysis of less-developed countries, 1985–2000. *International Sociology* 23 (4), 514–539; doi: 10.1177/0268580908090726. http://iss.sagepub.com/cgi/doi/10.1177/0268580908090726.

Schapira, L., Vargas, E., Hidalgo, R., Brier, M., Sanchez, L., Hobrecker, K., Lynch, T. and Chabner, B. (2008) Lost in translation: Integrating medical interpreters into the multidisciplinary team. *The Oncologist* 13 (5), 586–592; doi: 10.1634/theoncologist.2008-0042. http://www.ncbi.nlm.nih.gov/pubmed/18515743.

Shihadeh, E.S. and Barranco, R.E. (2010) Latino immigration, economic deprivation, and violence: Regional Differences in the effect of linguistic isolation. *Homicide Studies* 14 (3), 336–355; doi: 10.1177/1088767910371190. http://hsx.sagepub.com/cgi/doi/10.1177/1088767910371190.

Siddiqi, A., Ornelas, I.J., Quinn, K., Zuberi, D. and Nguyen, Q.C. (2013) Societal context and the production of immigrant status-based health inequalities: A comparative study of the United States and Canada. *Journal of Public Health Policy* 34 (2), 330–344; doi: 10.1057/jphp.2013.7. http://www.ncbi.nlm.nih.gov/pubmed/23447028.

Siqueira, C.E., Gaydos, A.M., Monforton, C., Slatin, C., Borkowski, L., Dooley, P., Liebman, A., Rosenberg, E., Shor, G. and Keifer, M. (2013) Effects of social, economic, and labor policies on occupational health disparities. *American Journal of Industrial Medicine* 57 (5), 557–572; doi: 10.1002/ajim.22186.

Squires, A., Aiken, L.H., van den Heede, K., Sermeus, W., Bruyneel, L., Lindqvist, R., Schoonhoven, L. *et al.* (2013) A systematic survey instrument translation process for multi-country, comparative health workforce studies. *International Journal of Nursing Studies* 50 (2), 264–73; doi: 10.1016/j.ijnurstu.2012.02.015. http://www.ncbi.nlm.nih.gov/pubmed/22445444.

Taylor, R.A. and Alfred, M.A. (2010) Nurses' perceptions of the organizational supports needed for the delivery of culturally competent care. *Western Journal of Nursing Research* 32 (5), 591–609; doi: 10.1177/0193945909354999. http://www.ncbi.nlm.nih.gov/pubmed/20693336.

Teruya, S.A. and Bazargan-Hejazi, S. (2013) The immigrant and Hispanic paradoxes: A systematic review of their predictions and effects. *Hispanic Journal of Behavioral Sciences* 35 (4), 486–509; doi: 10.1177/0739986313499004. http://hjb.sagepub.com/cgi/doi/10.1177/0739986313499004.

The International Bank for Reconstruction and Development (2011) World Development Report 2012: Gender Equality and Development. Washington, DC; doi: 10.1787/9789264179370-6-en.

The World Bank (2016) Migration and Remittances Factbook 2016, 3rd edn. http://siteresources.worldbank.org/INTPROSPECTS/Resources/334934-1199807908806/4549025-1450455807487/Factbookpart1.pdf.

Thomas, C.A. and Lee, B. (2010) Language liaisons: Language planning leadership in health care. *Language Problems and Language Planning* 34 (2), 95–119; doi: 10.1075/lplp.34.2.01tho. http://openurl.ingenta.com/content/xref?genre=article&issn=0272-2690&volume=34&issue=2&spage=95.

Tilly, C. (2011) The impact of the economic crisis on international migration: A review. *Work, Employment & Society* 25 (4), 675–692; doi: 10.1177/0950017011421799. http://wes.sagepub.com/cgi/doi/10.1177/0950017011421799.

Tuot, D.S., Lopez, M., Miller, C. and Karliner, L.S. (2012) Impact of an easy-access telephonic interpreter program in the acute care setting: An evaluation of a quality improvement intervention. *Joint Commission Journal on Quality and Patient Safety/Joint Commission Resources* 38 (2), 81–88. http://www.ncbi.nlm.nih.gov/pubmed/22372255.

Ulmer, C., Mcfadden, B. and Nerenz, D.R. (2009) Race, Ethnicity and Language Data: Standardization for Health Care Quality Improvement. Institute of Medicine: Washington, DC.

Viruell-Fuentes, E.A., Miranda, P.Y. and Abdulrahim, S. (2012) More than culture: Structural racism, intersectionality theory, and immigrant health. *Social Science and Medicine (1982)* 75 (12), 2099–2106; doi: 10.1016/j.socscimed.2011.12.037. http://www.ncbi.nlm.nih.gov/pubmed/22386617.

Walani, S.R. (2013) Earnings of the internationally educated nurses in the US labor market. *Nursing Research* 62 (3), 169–177; doi: 10.1097/NNR.0b013e318286b7ac. http://apps.webofknowledge.com/full_record.do?product=UA&search_mode=GeneralSearch&qid=218&SID=3Bs2rCAvgga22EPHnhW&page=1&doc=3&cacheurlFromRightClick=no.

White, K., Haas, J.S. and Williams, D.R. (2012) Elucidating the role of place in health care disparities: The example of racial/ethnic residential segregation. *Health Services Research* 47 (3 Pt 2), 1278–1299; doi: 10.1111/j.1475-6773.2012.01410.x. http://www.pubmedcentral.nih.gov/articlerender.fcgi?artid=3417310&tool=pmcentrez&rendertype=abstract.

Whitman, M.V., Davis, J.A. and Terry, A.J. (2010) Perceptions of school nurses on the challenges of service provision to ESL students. *Journal of Community Health* 35 (2), 208–213; doi: 10.1007/s10900-009-9211-3. http://www.ncbi.nlm.nih.gov/pubmed/20012473.

Whittington, J.W., Nolan, K., Lewis, N. and Torres, T. (2015) Pursuing the triple aim: The first seven years. *Milbank Quarterly* 93 (2), 263–300.

2 Three Critical Steps to Enhance Delivery of Language Services in Health Care

Leah S. Karliner

Communicating across language barriers is a challenge for clinicians all across the world. Using the US as an example, the most recent American Community Survey estimated that about 20% of the adult US population speaks a language other than English at home, and almost half of these report speaking English less than very well (Johnson et al., 2010). Spanish and Chinese are the most common preferred languages for adults with limited English proficiency (LEP), but hundreds of additional languages are in use throughout the US. The rise in the number of individuals with LEP in the US in recent decades and their diffusion to geographic areas where few persons with LEP have traditionally resided present a significant challenge for healthcare systems to overcome (US Department of Health and Human Services, 2006). In addition, as the LEP population ages, they develop more chronic diseases, heightening the need for attention to language barriers to improve healthcare delivery quality and health outcomes (Center on an Aging Society, 2004).

Patients who have LEP also have poorer healthcare quality and outcomes. In multiple studies, LEP populations, compared with English-speaking populations, consistently receive worse care (Jacobs et al., 2003). Individuals with LEP are less likely to have a usual source of care (Kirkman-Liff & Mondragon, 1991; Weinick & Krauss, 2000), have less access to preventive services (Cheng et al., 2007; Jacobs et al., 2005; Pearson et al., 2008; Woloshin et al., 1997) and have worse control of diabetes (Fernandez et al., 2011). Additionally, language barriers make patients more vulnerable to serious adverse outcomes from medical errors (Divi et al., 2007), misunderstandings about medications and instructions (Andrulis et al., 2002; Flores et al., 2003; Wilson et al., 2005) and medication complications (Gandhi et al., 2000).

Poor-quality communication between patients with LEP and clinicians leads to less adherence to medication (Wilson et al., 2005; David & Rhee, 1998; Derose & Baker 2000; Orrell et al., 2003; Rivadeneyra et al., 2000), decreased patient satisfaction with care (Carrasquillo *et al.*, 1999; Lauderdale *et al.*, 2006; Morales *et al.*, 1999; Weech-Maldonado *et al.*, 2003), less patient-centered care (Karliner *et al.*, 2011) and more reports of negative clinical experiences (Hampers & McNulty, 2002). Poor communication also interferes with the quality of the patient–clinician relationship, including the development of trust and follow-up (Rivadeneyra *et al.*, 2000). This impedes patients' ability to engage in joint decision making and self-management (Wilson *et al.*, 2005; Atchison *et al.*, 2005; Wisnivesky *et al.*, 2009). These challenges in communication and care delivery contribute to health disparities for this vulnerable population.

Thankfully, professional interpreters improve quality and outcomes of clinical care for patients with LEP. Access to professional interpreters is critical for effective communication and the delivery of high-quality care (Smedley *et al.*, 2002; Betencourt, 2006; Goode *et al.*, 2006). In a comprehensive review of the literature, we found that professional interpreters improve communication, promote appropriate use of resources and significantly increase patient and clinician satisfaction (Karliner *et al.*, 2007). The use of professional interpreters also results in fewer errors in communication (Flores *et al.*, 2003), reduces disparities in utilization of services (Jacobs *et al.*, 2001) and improves clinical outcomes (Karliner *et al.*, 2007). For example, patients with LEP who had professional interpreters present for their visits had equal quality of diabetes care compared with English-speaking patients (Tocher & Larson, 1998). In one study, the perceptions of healthcare experiences of uninsured patients who had access to interpreters were comparable to or better than those of insured patients who did not need interpreters (Andrulis *et al.*, 2002). In addition, professional interpreters help bridge not only linguistic but also cultural gaps that can challenge communication between patients and providers (Tocher & Larson, 1998; Dohan & Levintova, 2007).

In the US, Federal law requires linguistic services for LEP patients. Title VI of the US Civil Rights Act states that people cannot be discriminated against as a result of their national origin, race or color, which has been extrapolated to include primary language by the US Office of Civil Rights and Department of Health and Human Services. In addition, healthcare organizations receiving US Federal funds – which most do in the form of public insurance payments (Medicaid or Medicare) for individuals with disabilities or low income, and those over age 65 – must provide services in a language that a patient with LEP can understand (Tice *et al.*, 2008). In 2000, Title VI was reinforced by US Executive Order 13166, which required that all recipients of Federal funds provide 'meaningful access' to services needed by people with LEP. The Culturally and Linguistically Appropriate Services standards (CLAS standards) in Health Care, issued by the US Department of Health and Human Services Office of Minority Health, includes the statement 'health care organizations must assure the competence of language assistance provided to limited English proficient patients/consumers by interpreters and bilingual staff' as part of its interpretation of Title VI (Karliner et al., 2008). Thus, under US Federal guidance, language access in health care can take two main forms: professional interpreter services or language concordant care by qualified professionals. Language concordant care is addressed in Chapter 7. This chapter addresses the necessary components to provision of professional interpreter services.

In the US, access to adequate language services has been stymied by multiple challenges, including the complexities of needing to meet the needs of patients speaking many different languages, hiring and maintaining a highly qualified staff in the setting of widespread lack of reimbursement for interpreter services, and deploying that staff to often physically distant clinical settings with varied clinical needs (Chen et al., 2007; Hasnain-Wynia et al., 2006; Regenstein et al., 2008; Wilson-Stronks et al., 2007). Regulations and laws mandating language assistance are important, but not sufficient to ensure that language minority patients get access to language services. For example, despite regulations in California requiring Health Maintenance Organizations (HMO) to provide language interpretation and translation services to HMO enrollees, an analysis of the California Health Interview Survey data found that HMO enrollees with LEP still encountered substantial communication barriers when seeking health care (Hadler et al., 2013).

The challenge of communicating across language barriers in health care is, of course, not limited to the US. Similar complexities have been described in multiple countries and regions ranging from the European Union to Australia to India (Jaeger et al., 2003; MacFarlane et al., 2008; Murray & Skull, 2005; Narayan, 2013). Each geographic location has specific immigrant and language groups that are traditional to that area, as well as emerging language groups related to evolving world migration patterns (Pew Research Center, 2013). However, all share similar challenges in language services delivery. In this chapter, we discuss three critical steps to enhance delivery of language access services. Those steps are: (a) identify patients with language access needs; (b) recognize the importance of trained professional interpreters; and (c) choose, and incorporate that into human resource and infrastructure planning, the modality for accessing professional interpreters.

Step 1: Identification of Patients who would Benefit from Language Access Services

Every health system requires a systematic method for identifying those patients with a language barrier, in order to understand the language access needs of its patient population. In the US, traditionally this information has been identified at the time of registration for health care, whether in the hospital or in an ambulatory setting, and entered into the demographic section of the medical record (Hasnain-Wynia & Baker, 2006). Prior to widespread use of electronic health records, language information might have been kept on a registration card used to stamp health records at each medical encounter. Historically not all health systems have collected patient language data, and those that have collected it have used a range of different fields, including 'primary language' and 'needs interpreter'. It has too frequently been left up to registration clerks to complete these fields in non-systematic ways, sometimes making assumptions about which language a patient spoke, the patient's English-language ability or their need for an interpreter, and often resulting in misinformation (Balakrishnan et al., 2005; Boscolo-Hightower et al., 2014). Even when asked, patients who know they might have to wait a long while for a professional interpreter in a given system find the question of whether they 'need' an interpreter a fraught one. If saying 'yes' means hours of sitting in a clinic waiting room or waiting in an emergency department without being attended to, then patients might answer 'no' even though their English skills are poor.

Because of its importance for provision of services and examination and elimination of disparities, the US Institute of Medicine emphasized the importance of standardizing race, ethnicity and language (REAL) data collection in its 2009 report *Race, Ethnicity, and Language Data: Standardization for Health Care Quality Improvement* (Institute of Medicine, 2009). In a benchmarking study in 2011, the Institute for Diversity in Health Management, an affiliate of the American Hospital Association (AHA), found that, although 90% of hospitals reported collecting primary language data, only 60% had analyzed the supply and demand for language services, and only 28% reported using language data to assess gaps in care (AHA, 2011). The report distinguishes between collecting demographic data and collecting REAL data that is actionable, indicating a continued need for data collection standardization in order to make it useful to hospital systems. An updated benchmarking study in 2015 showed an increase from 90% to 94% of hospitals collecting primary language data, and an increase to 38% using that data to assess gaps in care (AHA, 2015). To operationalize standardized data collection, the AHA recommends a four-step process to ensure successful REAL data collection. The four steps are: (1) determine the appropriate data categories; (2) develop a methodology for data collection; (3) train staff members on methodology for data collection; and (4) assign accountability and monitor progress of data collection efforts (HRET, 2013). Each step requires the organization to ask and answer a series of questions. For example, to achieve step 2, 'develop a methodology for data collection', the healthcare organization must decide who will collect the data (e.g. registration clerk, front desk staff, nursing staff), when the data will be collected (e.g. at check-in, over the phone prior to arrival) and in what format the data will be collected (e.g. electronic tablet/kiosk, paper, verbally). To support training, the AHA, through its research arm, the Health Research and Educational Trust (HRET) provides a free online training toolkit for REAL data collection (Hasnain-Wynia et al., 2007).

For language data, the issue of which data category to collect has evolved. In the past, it was very common for healthcare organizations in the US to record a patient's 'primary language'. This, however, did not necessarily capture whether the patient needed language access services. For example, a fully bilingual Spanish–English speaker may report their primary language to be Spanish but have no need for an interpreter or bilingual physician to communicate effectively in English. A shift has occurred to report 'preferred language for discussing healthcare'. This shift has taken place in large part because the Joint Commission, the main accreditation body for hospitals in the US, set a standard for all hospitals it accredited to collect this data category. This standard was part of their 'Patient Centered Communication Standards for Hospitals', which was fully implemented in July 2012 (TJC, 2010, 2014). In fact there is little data published on the best language data category. One study, published by this author and cited by the Institute of Medicine and The Joint Commission, described the best test characteristics for a combination of two questions (the US Census question 'how well do you speak English' and preferred language for healthcare communication) and an algorithm combining responses to the two questions in order to determine whether the patient needs language access services (Karliner et al., 2008; Institute of Medicine, 2009; TJC, 2014). However, it has proven challenging to train staff to use such an algorithm in a standardized manner. With increasing use of electronic health records, it may become feasible for the staff to collect the answers to the two questions and the computer to run the algorithm, thus automatically filling a language access data field (needs language access – interpreter or language concordant clinician – yes/no) in addition to the preferred language data field necessary to determine the best language for communicating with the patient.

Step 2: Recognizing the Importance of Professional Interpreters to Provision of Quality Health Care

Bridging language barriers requires a skilled workforce. Skills range from those necessary for language concordance – linguistic fluency to talk directly with patients and their families in a non-English (or non-culture-dominant) language (see Chapter 7 for more on language concordant care) – to the skills necessary for language interpretation – bilingual fluency and the ability to switch fluidly between two languages while interpreting the meaning and tone of what has been said from one language to another (NCIHC et al., 2010). The challenges inherent to this task contribute to the potential for errors in interpretation. Multiple studies have demonstrated that the error rate for professional interpreters is considerably lower than that of ad hoc – untrained family, friends, or non-interpreter staff – interpreters, and when errors are made, they are less likely to be clinically significant (Flores et al., 2003; Jackson *et al.*, 2011; Napoles *et al.*, 2015; Bauer & Alegria, 2010). Professional interpreters, in addition to their positive impact on process and clinical outcomes, also contribute to higher satisfaction with communication and the perceived quality of medical care for patients and physicians alike (Karliner *et al.*, 2007; Batchi *et al.*, 2011; Green *et al.*, 2005; Kuo & Fagan, 1999; Lee *et al.*, 2002).

In fact, there is some evidence that physicians and patients agree on the most important components of good language access services: accuracy, accessibility and respect for confidentiality (Kuo & Fagan, 1999). Similarly, the National Council on Interpreting in Healthcare highlights accuracy, respect and confidentiality among its standards for professionalism for interpreters (NCIHC, 2005). These components cannot be achieved through the use of ad hoc interpreters, or through online or computer-based applications; rather, they require trained, skilled people to do the interpreting whether in-person or remotely. In addition to the recognition that a skilled workforce is required to deliver high-quality care to language minority patients, health systems must contemplate decisions about how to access that workforce, which in turn impacts decisions about cost and infrastructure related to hiring and managing staff and/or investing in technology for remote interpretation.

There is no doubt that provision of interpreter services costs money. However, compared with overall healthcare expenditures, the costs are relatively small – for example provision of professional interpreters in the hospital is a fraction of the cost of a hospitalization (Jacobs *et al.*, 2007). When viewed from a healthcare value perspective in which value = outcomes achieved per dollar (or other monetary unit) spent (Porter, 2010), provision of professional interpreter services should be considered part of high-value care for patients with LEP. In fact, since professional interpreters enhance communication and outcomes for patients with LEP, including decreasing readmissions as we have found in our work, as well as decreasing errors in the hospital and improving ambulatory outcomes such as glucose control for patients with diabetes, the higher quality of care delivered and better patient outcomes achieved when a health system provides access to professional interpreters should outweigh the cost (Divi *et al.*, 2007; Tocher & Larson, 1998; Karliner *et al.*, 2015; Partida, 2007).

Nonetheless, creating a high-value language access system can be challenging and like all organizational change requires organizational will. In the case of language access and professional interpreter services, making explicit the linkage to quality for this specific patient population has been demonstrated to aid in health system leadership buy-in (Wilson-Stronks & Mutha, 2010). Additional work to engage stakeholders and physician champions, as well as bringing the Informational Technology specialists to the table early to help build systems for identifying patients who need services and when contemplating remote technologies for professional interpreter access, all are important for successful infrastructure and programmatic planning (Karliner & Mutha, 2010).

Step 3: Choosing the Communication Modality

Once a health system has identified the patients who need language access services and has come to an understanding of the importance of the human resources necessary to provide those high value services, it must choose how patients and physicians will access professional interpreters. Currently there are two general options – in-person and remote – with remote services available by telephone or videoconferencing.

In-person interpretation

In-person professional interpretation is generally considered to be the gold standard for medical interpretation owing to the ability to incorporate visual cues from both patient and physician to enhance communication as well as using the interpreter's own visual cues to ensure that the pace of conversation allows for accurate interpretation. Professional interpreters report greater understanding of patients' social and cultural backgrounds and greater ease facilitating rapport when interpreting in-person (Price et al., 2012). In-person is also the most studied communication modality for interpretation and has been demonstrated to improve satisfaction, processes and outcomes of care (Karliner et al., 2007). In-person interpretation is most feasible for either large health systems with a high number of particular language minorities or small practices which would like to train front- or back-office staff to be dual-role interpreters for a particular language group making up a large proportion of that practice's patient panel.

The major drawbacks of in-person interpretation are related to access and efficiency; in particular, limitations on the number of languages a health system can staff efficiently and time constraints on staff availability, particularly with fluctuations in demand and need to travel from one location to another between clinical encounters. As a result, while solely relying on in-person interpreters will provide high-quality communication for some patients who receive the services, it may actually reduce access for a large proportion of patients requiring services in the health system. This suggests that mixed use of multiple modalities may be a more ideal language access strategy, particularly for larger health systems.

Remote modalities: Telephone and videoconferencing

Remote interpretation increases efficiency in interpreter access by allowing for economy of scale, whether utilizing a health system's own staff in a call-center-type environment, or with staff from a contracted government or private service provider. Both approaches reduce down-time for professional interpreters waiting for physicians to see a patient, travel time between locations for interpreters, and wait time for patients (Karliner & Mutha, 2010).

With contracted service providers, both interpreters for high-demand languages (e.g. Spanish in the US) and those for less commonly requested languages (e.g. Mixtec in the US) can be accessed remotely by multiple different health systems. This allows for access without scheduling, any time of the day or night, both particularly important components of a language access service program for emergency and hospital settings.

Accessing professional interpreters via telephone has the advantage of using a ubiquitous technology which is easy to use. Telephonic interpretation does greatly increase professional interpreter use, particularly in environments that have not previously been accessing professional interpreters at all or only very little. The addition of dual-handset telephones with one-touch dialing in all hospital rooms at a children's hospital increased professional interpreter use 20% while simultaneously reducing the use of ad hoc interpreters, resulting in fewer interpretation-related delays in care (Lion et al., 2015). Likewise, in our study evaluating placement of a dual-handset interpreter telephone with quick access to a contracted service provider at every hospital bedside, we observed a 4-fold increased use in professional interpreter utilization without a decrease of in-person professional interpreter encounters (Karliner et al., 2016; Tuot et al., 2012). Nurses and physicians reported the use of the telephones particularly for brief, high-risk encounters such as medication administration and daily rounding (Tuot et al., 2012). Anecdotally, when possible, physicians continued to schedule in-person interpreters for complex family meetings and delivering bad news, and nurses scheduled them for complex teaching before hospital discharge. These are clinical scenarios that probably could benefit from remote videoconferencing, rather than telephonic, interpretation if an in-person interpreter is not available (Price et al., 2012).

Patients prefer telephonic interpreting over ad hoc or no professional interpretation (Cunningham et al., 2008); however, the data on satisfaction with communication are mixed comparing telephonic and in-person interpretation, and satisfaction of one over the other may be related to other factors such as wait-times and ease of access as well as the professionalism of the interpreter (Crossman et al., 2010; Gany et al., 2007; Garcia et al., 2004). Interpreters report telephonic interpretation to be equally good as other modalities for simple information exchange, but less satisfactory for interpersonal aspects of communication; in situations with extensive psychosocial or educational content, videoconferencing is considered better than telephonic interpretation (Price et al., 2012).

Videoconferencing, also known as Video Medical Interpretation (VMI) or Video Remote Interpretation (VRI), has the advantage over telephonic interpretation of preserving visual cues and visual expression of affect, and it provides the ability to conduct visually based teaching, for example for proper inhaler use in asthma care or dressing changes in wound care. Both clinicians and patients report the quality of VMI/VRI as equal to in-person interpretation, although in-person may still be superior for understanding cultural nuances (Jones et al., 2003; Napoles et al., 2010; Wofford et al., 2012). However, error rates for VMI/VRI appear to be equal to in-person interpretation, and both are significantly lower than for ad-hoc interpretation (Napoles et al., 2015).

As videoconferencing technology has evolved to encompass sharper visuals and high-quality audio on less bulky equipment, the uptake of this technology for professional interpretation has increased. The development of shared public-sector networks along with the entrance of private service providers into the VMI/VRI market in the US have begun to both expand the languages available and decrease the cost (Cyracom, 2015; Jacobs et al., 2011; Language-Line, 2015). However, health systems will need to invest in high-quality equipment and not rely on physicians using their own cell phones, for example, to attain the expected good outcomes from VMI/VRI use.

Internet-based applications for smartphones and tablets continue to emerge in this space to fill unmet needs for rapid interpretation and translation, but remain sorely understudied. For example, unidirectional mobile applications intended for rapid information gathering and simple communication have not been studied, and require caution. This type of application could prove useful in emergency situations when there are no other options or for use briefly while awaiting a professional interpreter; however, the very nature of communication is bidirectional and much may be missed or misconstrued when clinicians are the only ones able to express themselves in an encounter. These applications cannot replace the skilled interpretation provided by trained professionals whether in-person or remotely. Online translation tools, while promising, also require caution owing to potential errors that may leave clinicians and health systems open to liability if the translated message delivered to the patient does not match the intended message (Khanna et al., 2011). However, there remains a need for technological advances to deliver reliably accurate translations that interface with electronic health records in order to provide visit and discharge summaries and instructions to patients in their own language.

Delivering Language Access Services Enables Human Communication

In this chapter, I have made the argument that, for patients with a language barrier seeking health care, provision of language access services is necessary to achieve high-quality care. All health systems wishing to achieve this goal need to consider three critical steps: identify patients with language access needs, recognize the importance of trained professional interpreters, choose and incorporate into human resource and infrastructure planning, the modality for accessing professional interpreters. While in-person interpretation remains the gold standard against which we measure communication quality, it is not the only means of delivering language services. Remote interpretation can lead to more efficient access for a larger number of patients. Telephonic interpretation has limitations for the most complex clinical situations; these limitations seem largely to be ameliorated with videoconferencing interpretation. Some health systems will find one approach more feasible than another, and some will strive to deliver a mixture of service modalities. Ultimately it is not the technology itself that leads to better communication and outcomes for our patients, but rather the people leveraging those tools to ensure that we can engage with our patients in the very human act of communicating.

References

AHA (2011) *Diversity and Disparities: A Benchmark Study of US Hospitals*. Chicago, IL: American Hospital Association. Available from http://www.diversityconnection.org/diversityconnection/leadership-conferences/Benchmarking-Survey.jsp?fll=S1.

AHA (2015) *Diversity and Disparities: A Benchmark Sudy of US Hospitals*. Chigago, IL: American Hospital Association. Available from http://www.diversityconnection.org/diversityconnection/leadership-conferences/Benchmarking-Survey.jsp?fll=S1.

Andrulis, D., Goodman, N. and Pryor C. (2002) What a difference an interpreter can make: Health care experiences of uninsured with limited English proficiency. Boston, MA: The Access Project.

Atchison, K.A., Black, E.E., Leathers, R., Belin, T.R., Abrego, M., Gironda, M.W., Wong, D., Shetty, V. and DerMartirosian, C. (2005) A qualitative report of patient problems and postoperative instructions. *Journal of Oral and Maxillofacial Surgery: Official Journal of the American Association of Oral and Maxillofacial Surgeons* 63 (4), 449–456; Epub 2005/03/25; doi: 10.1016/j.joms.2004.07.019. PubMed PMID: 15789315.

Bagchi, A.D., Dale, S., Verbitsky-Savitz, N., Andrecheck, S., Zavotsky, K. and Eisenstein, R. (2011) Examining effectiveness of medical interpreters in emergency departments for Spanish-speaking patients with limited English proficiency: Results of a randomized controlled trial. *Annals of Emergency Medicine* 57 (3), 248–256, e1–4; Epub 2010/08/04; doi: 10.1016/j.annemergmed.2010.05.032. PubMed PMID: 20678825.

Balakrishnan, V., Roper, J., Cossey, K., Roman, C. and Jeanmonod, R. Misidentification of English Language Proficiency in Triage: Impact on (2015) Satisfaction and door-to-room time. *Journal of Immigrant and Minority Health/Center for Minority Public Health*; Epub 2015/03/10; doi: 10.1007/s10903-015-0174-4. PubMed PMID: 25750135.

Bauer, A.M. and Alegria, M. (2010) Impact of patient language proficiency and interpreter service use on the quality of psychiatric care: A systematic review. *Psychiatric Services* 61 (8), 765–773; Epub 2010/08/03; doi: 10.1176/appi.ps.61.8.765. PubMed PMID: 20675834; PMCID: PMC2946248.

Betencourt, J. (2006) Improving quality and achieving equity: The role of cultural competence in reducing racial and ethnic disparities in health care. The Commonwealth Fund, October.

Boscolo-Hightower, A., Rafton, S.A., Tolman, M., Zhou, C. and Ebel, B.E. (2014) Identifying families with limited English proficiency using a capture-recapture approach. *Hospital Pediatrics* 4 (1), 16–22; Epub 2014/01/18; doi: 10.1542/hpeds.2013-0040. PubMed PMID: 24435596.

Carrasquillo, O., Orav, E.J., Brennan, T.A. and Burstin, H.R. (1999) Impact of language barriers on patient satisfaction in an emergency department. *Journal of General Internal Medicine* 14 (2), 82–87; Epub 1999/03/03. PubMed PMID: 10051778.

Center on an Aging Society (2004) *Cultural Competence In Health Care: Is It Important for People with Chronic Conditions*. Washington, DC: Center on an Aging Society, Georgetown University.

Chen, A.H., Youdelman, M.K. and Brooks, J. (2007) The legal framework for language access in healthcare settings: Title VI and beyond. *Journal of General Internal Medicine* 22 (Suppl 2), 362–367; PubMed PMID: 17957427.

Cheng, E.M., Chen, A. and Cunningham, W. (2007) Primary language and receipt of recommended health care among Hispanics in the United States. *Journal of General Internal Medicine* 22 (Suppl 2), 283–288; Epub 2007/11/28; doi: 10.1007/s11606-007-0346-6. PubMed PMID: 17957412; PMCID: Pmc2078546.

Crossman, K.L., Wiener, E., Roosevelt, G., Bajaj, L. and Hampers, L.C. (2010) Interpreters: telephonic, in-person interpretation and bilingual providers. *Pediatrics* 125 (3), e631–638; Epub 2010/02/24; doi: 10.1542/peds.2009-0769. PubMed PMID: 20176670.

Cunningham, H., Cushman, L.F., Akuete-Penn, C. and Meyer, D.D. (2008) Satisfaction with telephonic interpreters in pediatric care. *Journal of Natural Medicine Association* 100 (4), 429–434; Epub 2008/05/17. PubMed PMID: 18481483.

Cyracom (2015) See http://www.cyracom.com/vri/ (accessed 13 June 2015).

David, R.A. and Rhee, M. (1998) The impact of language as a barrier to effective health care in an underserved urban Hispanic community. *The Mount Sinai Journal of Medicine, New York* 65 (5–6), 393–397; Epub 1998/12/09. PubMed PMID: 9844369.

Derose, K.P. and Baker, D.W. (2000) Limited English proficiency and Latinos' use of physician services. *Medical Care Research and Review* 57 (1), 76–91; Epub 2000/03/08. PubMed PMID: 10705703.

Divi, C., Koss, R.G., Schmaltz, S.P. and Loeb, J.M. (2007) Language proficiency and adverse events in US hospitals: A pilot study. *International Journal of Qualitative Health Care* 19 (2), 60–67; Epub 2007/02/06; doi: 10.1093/intqhc/mzl069. PubMed PMID: 17277013.

Dohan, D. and Levintova, M. (2007) Barriers beyond words: cancer, culture, and translation in a community of Russian speakers. *Journal of General Internal Medicine* 22 (Suppl 2), 300–305; Epub 2007/11/28; doi: 10.1007/s11606-007-0325-y. PubMed PMID: 17957415; PMCID: Pmc2078549.

Fernandez, A., Schillinger, D., Warton, E.M., Adler, N., Moffet, H.H., Schenker, Y., Salgado, M.V., Ahmed, A. and Karter, A.J. (2011) Language barriers, physician–patient language concordance, and glycemic control among insured Latinos with diabetes: The Diabetes Study of Northern California (DISTANCE). *Journal of General Internal Medicine* 26 (2), 170–176; doi: 10.1007/s11606-010-1507-6. PubMed PMID: 20878497; PMCID: 3019330.

Flores, G., Laws, M.B., Mayo, S.J., Zuckerman, B., Abreu, M., Medina, L. and Hardt, E.J. (2003) Errors in medical interpretation and their potential clinical consequences in pediatric encounters. *Pediatrics* 111 (1), 6–14; Epub 2003/01/02. PubMed PMID: 12509547.

Gandhi, T.K., Burstin, H.R., Cook, E.F., Puopolo, A.L., Haas, J.S., Brennan, T.A. *et al.* (2000) Drug complications in outpatients. *Journal of General Internal Medicine* 15 (3), 149–154.

Gany, F., Leng, J., Shapiro, E., Abramson, D., Motola, I., Shield, D.C. and Changrani, J. (2007) Patient satisfaction with different interpreting methods: a randomized controlled trial. *Journal of General Internal Medicine* 22 (Suppl 2), 312–318; Epub 2007/11/28; doi: 10.1007/s11606-007-0360-8. PubMed PMID: 17957417; PMCID: PMC2078551.

Garcia, E.A., Roy, L.C., Okada, P.J., Perkins, S.D. and Wiebe, R.A. (2004) A comparison of the influence of hospital-trained, ad hoc, and telephone interpreters on perceived satisfaction of limited English-proficient parents presenting to a pediatric emergency department. *Pediatric Emergency Care* 20 (6), 373–378; Epub 2004/06/05. PubMed PMID: 15179145.

Goode, R., Dunne, M. and Bronheim, S. (2006) The evidence base for cultural and linguistic competency in health care. The Commonwealth Fund, October.

Green, A.R., Ngo-Metzger, Q., Legedza, A.T., Massagli, M.P., Phillips, R.S. and Iezzoni, L.I. (2005) Interpreter services, language concordance, and health care quality. Experiences of Asian Americans with limited English proficiency. *Journal of General Internal Medicine* 20 (11), 1050–1056; Epub 2005/11/26; doi: 10.1111/j.1525-1497.2005.0223.x. PubMed PMID: 16307633; PMCID: Pmc1490255.

Hadler, M.W., Chen, X., Gonzalez, E. and Roby, D.H. (2013) Limited English proficient HMO enrollees remain vulnerable to communication barriers despite language assistance regulations. Policy Brief UCLA Cent Health Policy Research (PB2013-1), 1–8; Epub 2013/04/05. PubMed PMID: 23550321.

Hampers, L.C. and McNulty, J.E. (2002) Professional interpreters and bilingual physicians in a pediatric emergency department: Effect on resource utilization. *Archives of Pediatric Adolescence Medicine* 156 (11), 1108–1113; Epub 2002/11/07. PubMed PMID: 12413338.

Hasnain-Wynia, R. and Baker, D.W. (2006) Obtaining data on patient race, ethnicity, and primary language in health care organizations: Current challenges and proposed solutions. *Health Services Research* 41, 1501–1518.

Hasnain-Wynia, R., Yonek, J., Pierce, D., Kang, R. and Greising, C. (2006) Hospital langague services for patients with limited English proficiency: Results from a national survey. Health Research and Educational Trust and National Health Law Program, October.

Hasnain-Wynia, R., Pierce, D., Haque, A., Hedges Greising, C., Prince, V. and Reiter, J. (2007) Health Research and Educational Trust Disparities Toolkit.

HRET (2013) *Reducing Health Care Disparities: Collection and Use of Race, Ethnicity and Language Data*. Chicago, IL: Health Research and Educational Trust.

Institute of Medicine (2009) *Subcommittee on Standardized Collection of Race/Ethnicity Data for Healthcare Quality Improvement. Race, Ethnicity, and Language Data: Standardization for Health Care Quality Improvement*. Washington, DC: The National Academies Press.

Jacobs, E.A., Lauderdale, D.S., Meltzer, D., Shorey, J.M., Levinson, W. and Thisted, R.A. (2001) Impact of interpreter services on delivery of health care to limited-English-proficient patients. *Journal of General Internal Medicine* 16 (7), 468–474; Epub 2001/08/25. PubMed PMID: 11520385; PMCID: Pmc1495243.

Jacobs, E., Agger-Gupta, N., Chen, A.H., Piotrowski, A. and Hardt, E.J. (2003) *Langue Barrieres in Health Care Settings: An Annotated Bibliography of the Research*. The California Endowment.

Jacobs, E.A., Karavolos, K., Rathouz, P.J., Ferris, T.G. and Powell, L.H. (2005) Limited English proficiency and breast and cervical cancer screening in a multiethnic population. *American Journal of Public Health* 95 (8), 1410–1416; Epub 2005/07/27; doi: 10.2105/ajph.2004.041418. PubMed PMID: 16043670; PMCID: Pmc1449374.

Jacobs, E.A., Sadowski, L.S. and Rathouz, P.J. (2007) The impact of an enhanced interpreter service intervention on hospital costs and patient satisfaction. *Journal of General Internal Medicine* 22 (Suppl 2), 306–311; Epub 2007/11/28; doi: 10.1007/s11606-007-0357-3. PubMed PMID: 17957416; PMCID: PMC2078550.

Jacobs, E.A., Leos, G.S., Rathouz, P.J. and Fu, P., Jr. (2011) Shared networks of interpreter services, at relatively low cost, can help providers serve patients with limited english skills. *Health Affairs (Millwood)* 30 (10), 1930–1938; Epub 2011/10/07; doi: 10.1377/hlthaff.2011.0667. PubMed PMID: 21976337.

Jackson, J.C., Nguyen, D., Hu, N., Harris, R. and Terasaki, G.S. (2011) Alterations in medical interpretation during routine primary care. *Journal of General Internal Medicine* 26 (3), 259–264; Epub 2010/10/06; doi: 10.1007/s11606-010-1519-2. PubMed PMID: 20922496; PMCID: PMC3043197.

Jaeger, F.N., Kiss, L., Hossain, M. and Zimmerman, C. (2013) Migrant-friendly hospitals: A paediatric perspective – improving hospital care for migrant children. *BMC Health Services Research* 13, 389; Epub 2013/10/08; doi: 10.1186/1472-6963-13-389. PubMed PMID: 24093461; PMCID: PMC3852418.

Johnson, T.D.R.M., Drewery, M.P., Ennis, S.R. and Kim, M.O. (2010) *People Who Spoke a Language Other Than English at Home by Hispanic Origin and Race: 2009* (pp. 9–19). Washington DC: US Census Bureau.

Jones, D., Gill, P., Harrison, R., Meakin, R. and Wallace, P. (2003) An exploratory study of language interpretation services provided by videoconferencing. *Journal of Telemedicine and Telecare* 9 (1), 51–56; Epub 2003/03/19. PubMed PMID: 12641894.

Karliner, L.S. and Mutha, S. (2010) Achieving quality in health care through language access services: Lessons from a California public hospital. *American Journal of Medical Quality* 25 (1), 51–59; Epub 2009/12/04; doi: 10.1177/1062860609351237. PubMed PMID: 19955512.

Karliner, L.S., Jacobs, E.A., Chen, A.H. and Mutha, S. (2007) Do professional interpreters improve clinical care for patients with limited English proficiency? A systematic review of the literature. *Health Services Research* 42 (2), 727–754; doi: 10.1111/j.1475-6773.2006.00629.x. PubMed PMID: 17362215; PMCID: 1955368.

Karliner, L.S., Napoles-Springer, A.M., Schillinger, D., Bibbins-Domingo, K. and Perez-Stable, E.J. (2008) Identification of limited English proficient patients in clinical care. *Journal of General Internal Medicine* 23 (10), 1555–1560; Epub 2008/07/12; doi: 10.1007/s11606-008-0693-y. PubMed PMID: 18618200; PMCID: 2533382.

Karliner, L.S., Hwang, E.S., Nickleach, D. and Kaplan, C.P. (2011) Language barriers and patient-centered breast cancer care. *Patient Education Counseling* 84 (2), 223–228; Epub 2010/08/06; doi: 10.1016/j.pec.2010.07.009. PubMed PMID: 20685068.

Karliner, L., Perez-Stable, E.J. and Gregorich, S.E. (2016) Easy access to professional interpreters in the hospital decreases readmission rates and estimated hospital expenditures for patients with limited English proficient. Med Care; Epub Aug 30, 2016.

Khanna, R.R., Karliner, L.S., Eck, M., Vittinghoff, E., Koenig, C.J. and Fang, MC. (2011) Performance of an online translation tool when applied to patient educational material. *Journal of Hospital Medicine* 6 (9), 519–525; Epub 2011/10/29; doi: 10.1002/jhm.898. PubMed PMID: 22034196.

Kirkman-Liff, B. and Mondragon, D. (1991) Language of interview: relevance for research of southwest Hispanics. *American Journal of Public Health* 81 (11), 1399–1404; Epub 1991/11/01. PubMed PMID: 1951794; PMCID: Pmc1405679.

Kuo, D. and Fagan, M.J. (1999) Satisfaction with methods of Spanish interpretation in an ambulatory care clinic. *Journal of General Internal Medicine* 14 (9), 547–550; Epub 1999/09/22. PubMed PMID: 10491243; PMCID: PMC1496734.

Language-Line (2015) See http://www.languageline.com/solutions/video-interpretation/ (accessed 13 June 2015).

Lauderdale, D.S., Wen, M., Jacobs, E.A. and Kandula, N.R. (2003) Immigrant perceptions of discrimination in health care: The California Health Interview Survey 2003. *Medical Care* 44 (10), 914–920; Epub 2006/09/27; doi: 10.1097/01.mlr.0000220829.87073.f7. PubMed PMID: 17001262.

Lee, L.J., Batal, H.A., Maselli, J.H. and Kutner, J.S. (2002) Effect of Spanish interpretation method on patient satisfaction in an urban walk-in clinic. *Journal of General Internal Medicine* 17 (8), 641–645; Epub 2002/09/06. PubMed PMID: 12213146; PMCID: PMC1495083.

Lion, K.C., Ebel, B.E., Rafton, S., Zhou, C., Hencz, P. and Mangione-Smith, R. (2015) Evaluation of a quality improvement intervention to increase use of telephonic interpretation. *Pediatrics* 135 (3), e709–716; Epub 2015/02/26; doi: 10.1542/peds.2014-2024. PubMed PMID: 25713276.

MacFarlane, A., Glynn, L.G., Mosinkie, P.I. and Murphy, A.W. (2008) Responses to language barriers in consultations with refugees and asylum seekers: A telephone survey of Irish general practitioners. *BMC Family Practice* 9, 68; Epub 2008/12/24; doi: 10.1186/1471-2296-9-68. PubMed PMID: 19102735; PMCID: PMC2637872.

Morales, L.S., Cunningham, W.E., Brown, J.A., Liu, H. and Hays, R.D. (1999) Are Latinos less satisfied with communication by health care providers? *Journal of General Internal Medicine* 14 (7), 409–417; Epub 1999/07/27. PubMed PMID: 10417598; PMCID: Pmc1496614.

Murray, S.B. and Skull, S.A. (2005) Hurdles to health: Immigrant and refugee health care in Australia. *Australian Health Review* 29 (1), 25–29; Epub 2005/02/03. PubMed PMID: 15683352.

Napoles, A.M., Santoyo-Olsson, J., Karliner, L.S., O'Brien, H., Gregorich, S.E. and Perez-Stable, E.J. (2010) Clinician ratings of interpreter mediated visits in underserved primary care settings with ad hoc, in-person professional, and video conferencing modes. *Journal of Health Care: Poor Underserved* 21 (1), 301–317; Epub 2010/02/23; doi: 10.1353/hpu.0.0269. PubMed PMID: 20173271; PMCID: 3576468.

Napoles, A.M., Santoyo-Olsson, J., Karliner, L.S., Gregorich, S.E. and Perez-Stable, E.J. (2015) Inaccurate language interpretation in medical encounters and its clinical significance in the medical encounters of Spanish-speaking Latinos. *Medical Care* 53 (11), 940–947.

Narayan, L. (2013) Addressing language barriers to healthcare in India. *National Medical Journal of India* 26 (4), 236–238; Epub 2014/04/25. PubMed PMID: 24758452.

NCIHC (2005) National Standards of Practice for Interpreters in Health Care.

NCIHC, NHELP and ATA (2010) What's In A Word? A Guide to Understanding Interpreting and Translation in Healthcare.

Orrell, C., Bangsberg, D.R., Badri, M. and Wood, R. (2003) Adherence is not a barrier to successful antiretroviral therapy in South Africa. *Aids* 17 (9), 1369–1375; Epub 2003/06/12; doi: 10.1097/01.aids.0000060398.18106.f6. PubMed PMID: 12799558.

Partida, Y. (2007) Addressing language barriers: Building response capacity for a changing nation. *Journal of General Internal Medicine* 22 (Suppl 2), 347–349; Epub 2007/11/28; doi: 10.1007/s11606-007-0367-1. PubMed PMID: 17957423; PMCID: PMC2078541.

Pearson, W.S., Ahluwalia, I.B., Ford, E.S. and Mokdad, A.H. (2008) Language preference as a predictor of access to and use of healthcare services among Hispanics in the United States. *Ethnicity and Disease* 18 (1), 93–97; Epub 2008/05/02. PubMed PMID: 18447107.

Pew Research Center (2013) 7 Facts About World Migration 2013. See http://www.pewresearch.org/fact-tank/2014/09/02/7-facts-about-world-migration/.

Porter, M.E. (2010) What is value in health care. *New England Journal of Medicine* 363, 2477–2481.

Price, E.L., Perez-Stable, E.J., Nickleach, D., Lopez, M. and Karliner, L.S. (2012) Interpreter perspectives of in-person, telephonic, and videoconferencing medical interpretation in clinical encounters. *Patient Education Counseling* 87 (2), 226–232; Epub 2011/09/21; doi: 10.1016/j.pec.2011.08.006. PubMed PMID: 21930360; PMCID: 4059012.

Regenstein, M., Trott, J., West, C. and Huang, J. (2008) *In Any Language: Improving the Quality and Availability of Language Services in Hospitals*. Washington, DC: Robert Wood Johnson Foundation, May.

Rivadeneyra, R., Elderkin-Thompson, V., Silver, R.C. and Waitzkin, H. (2000) Patient centeredness in medical encounters requiring an interpreter. *American Journal of Medicine* 108 (6), 470–474; Epub 2000/04/27. PubMed PMID: 10781779.

Smedley, B., Stith, A. and Nelson, A. (eds) (2002) *Unequal Treatment: Confronting Racial And Ethnic Disparities In Health Care*. Institute of Medicine of the National Academies.

Tice, J.A., Karliner, L., Walsh, J., Petersen, A.J. and Feldman, M.D. (2008) Gastric banding or bypass? A systematic review comparing the two most popular bariatric procedures. *American Journal of Medicine* 121 (10), 885–893; Epub 2008/10/01; doi: 10.1016/j.amjmed.2008.05.036. PubMed PMID: 18823860.

TJC (2010) *Advancing Effective Communication, Cultural Competence and Patient- and Family-Centered Care: A Roadmap for Hospitals*. Oakbrook Terrace, IL: The Joint Commission.

TJC (2014) *The Joint Commission: Advancing Effective Communication, Cultural Competence, and Patient- and-Family-Centered Care 2014*. (Updated 24 November 2014 and 3 April 2015.) See http://www.jointcommission.org/Advancing_Effective_Communication/.

Tocher, T.M. and Larson, E. (1998) Quality of diabetes care for non-English-speaking patients. A comparative study. *Western Journal of Medicine* 168 (6), 504–511; Epub 1998/07/10. PubMed PMID: 9655991; PMCID: Pmc1305066.

Tuot, D.S., Lopez, M., Miller, C. and Karliner, L.S. (2012) Impact of an easy-access telephonic interpreter program in the acute care setting: An evaluation of a quality improvement intervention. *Joint Commission: Journal of Qualitative Patient Safety* 38 (2), 81–88; Epub 2012/03/01. PubMed PMID: 22372255.

US Department of Health and Human Services (2006) National Healthcare Disparities Report. AHRQ Publication No. 070012.

Weech-Maldonado, R., Morales, L.S., Elliott, M., Spritzer, K., Marshall, G. and Hays, R.D. (2003) Race/ethnicity, language, and patients' assessments of care in Medicaid managed care. *Health Services Research* 38 (3), 789–808; Epub 2003/06/26. PubMed PMID: 12822913; PMCID: Pmc1360917.

Weinick, R.M. and Krauss, N.A. (2000) Racial/ethnic differences in children's access to care. *American Journal of Public Health* 90 (11), 1771–1774; Epub 2000/11/15. PubMed PMID: 11076248; PMCID: Pmc1446405.

Wilson, E., Chen, A.H., Grumbach, K., Wang, F. and Fernandez, A. (2005) Effects of limited English proficiency and physician language on health care comprehension. *Journal of General Internal Medicine* 20 (9), 800–806; Epub 2005/08/25; doi: 10.1111/j.1525-1497.2005.0174.x. PubMed PMID: 16117746; PMCID: Pmc1490205.

Wilson-Stronks, A. and Galvez, E. (2007) *Hospitals, Language, and Culture: A Snapshot of the Nation*. Oakbrook Terrace, IL: The Joint Commission and The California Endowment, 2007.

Wilson-Stronks, A. and Mutha, S. (2010) From the perspective of CEOs: What motivates hospitals to embrace cultural competence? *Journal of Healthcare Management* 55 (5), 339–351; discussion 51-2. PubMed PMID: 21077583.

Wisnivesky, J.P., Kattan, M., Evans, D., Leventhal, H., Musumeci-Szabo, T.J., McGinn, T. and Halm, E.A. (2009) Assessing the relationship between language proficiency and asthma morbidity among inner-city asthmatics. *Medical Care* 47 (2), 243–249; Epub 2009/01/27; doi: 10.1097/MLR.0b013e3181847606. PubMed PMID: 19169126.

Wofford, J.L., Campos, C.L., Johnson, D.A. and Brown, M.T. (2012) Providing a Spanish interpreter using low-cost videoconferencing in a community health centre: A pilot study using tablet computers. *Informal Primary Care* 20 (2), 141–146; Epub 2012/01/01. PubMed PMID: 23710778.

Woloshin, S., Schwartz, L.M., Katz, S.J. and Welch, H.G. (1997) Is language a barrier to the use of preventive services? *Journal of General Internal Medicine* 12 (8), 472–477; Epub 1997/08/01. PubMed PMID: 9276652; PMCID: Pmc1497155.

3 Conceptualizing Bilingual Health Communication: A Theory-based Approach to Interpreter-mediated Medical Encounters

Elaine Hsieh

The field of interpreter-mediated interactions appears to have plateaued in terms of its theoretical development. Since the important breakthrough in recognizing interpreters as active participants in discursive events (Metzger, 1999; Pöchhacker & Shlesinger, 2005; Roy, 2000; Wadensjö, 1998), researchers have examined interpreters' visibility (Angelelli, 2004), strategic management of medical encounters (Greenhalgh *et al.*, 2006; Leanza *et al.*, 2010), and impacts on patients' health outcomes (Butow *et al.*, 2011; Flores *et al.*, 2012). What is implied in these lines of research is the recognition that interpreters influence the process, content, and outcome of provider–patient interactions. However, they do not provide theoretical explanations about how or why interpreters consciously and unconsciously influence medical encounters in one way or the other. Similarly, both researchers and practitioners increasingly emphasize the role of other speakers (e.g. physicians and patients) in interpreter-mediated medical encounters in ensuring quality of care, but little has been done to incorporate these conversational others into the theoretical conceptualization of interpreter-mediated medical encounters.

These two issues prompted me to consider interpreter-mediated medical encounters from a different angle. Rather than focusing on interpreter behaviors, I am interested in examining how these interpersonal dynamics may shape the process and content of interpreter-mediated interactions. If interpreters act as active participants in medical encounters along with at least two other speakers (i.e. the provider and the patient), researchers should conceptualize interpreter-mediated medical encounters as triadic interactions (Laidsaar-Powell *et al.*, 2013; Valero-Garcés, 2005). More importantly, the examination of the interpreter-mediated medical encounter should explore how the participants coordinate with one another throughout the emergent and dynamic processes of cross-cultural care, responding to challenges and tensions in provider–patient interactions. In other words, the focus of our analysis should be how each participant coordinates and collaborates with one other as a communicative accomplishment during medical encounters.

It is from this perspective that I adopt a normative approach to interpreter-mediated medical encounters (Baumslag, 1998). By normative, I mean a theoretical account designed to predict and explain the meanings and evaluations of communicative responses during interpreter-mediated medical encounters. Goldsmith (2001: 515) explained, 'One important goal of a normative theory is to provide a basis for recommendations about how communicators can achieve desirable outcomes'. Rather than focusing on the accuracy and fidelity of interpreted texts, I ask, 'How do different participants coordinate with each other during the communicative event of provider–patient interactions?' This approach also takes into account the variations of communicative practices and their corresponding impacts. By assuming that individuals coordinate their competing goals through communicative practices, I propose that certain practices can be more effective and appropriate than others owing to the unique values and preferences within specific contexts, including clinical contexts (e.g. end-of-life care) and sociocultural contexts (e.g. organizational hierarchy and cultural preferences). Goldsmith (2001: 518) explained:

> Both speech community and speech event are defined by expectations about how communication is structured (e.g., who speaks to whom, how, in what setting, for what purposes?) and about how communication is evaluated (e.g., what is the purpose of the episode, what are the appropriate identities and relational definitions for carrying out such an episode, what values are enacted in these episodes?). Any particular individual may be more or less attuned to these expectations and the degree to which particular episodes embody these expectations may vary; nonetheless, it is possible to abstract from observed practice and from participants' articulation of their expectations a description of the social norms that define speech communities and speech events.

Taking inspiration from Goldsmith's normative approach (Goldsmith, 2001; Goldsmith & Fitch, 1997), I propose to ask: (a) how people should behave if they wish to achieve desired outcomes and why; and (b) how people will be evaluated when they behave in a particular way.

The meanings, significance, and processes of interpreter-mediated medical discourse in a particular context may evoke multiple and potentially conflicting goals. Following the traditions of dialectic theorists (Bakhtin, 1981;

Baxter & Montgomery, 1996; Houtlosser & van Rees, 2006), I conceptualize interpreter-mediated medical encounters within the contexts of potentially conflicting goals and the dilemmas these can create. By recognizing that each participant in interpreter-mediated encounters may have distinctive goals regarding tasks, identity, and relationships and that these goals often are: (a) implicitly coordinated between participants; and (b) mediated by an interpreter (Tracy, 2013), I explore situations in which the tensions between individuals' management of these goals are high, in order to understand how communication serves as a way to manage these competing goals.

This new approach allows researchers to ask interesting research questions regarding: (a) the meanings and functions of interpreter-mediated medical encounters within specific contexts and the potentially conflicting goals speakers may have as they seek to honor competing values such as control over the discursive processes, patient autonomy and shared decision-making, among others (e.g. providers may believe that end-of-life disclosure empowers a patient to make informed decision; in contrast, a patient's family member may argue that the act of disclosure contradicts the value of beneficence, i.e. do no harm); (b) the interrelationships among communicative behaviors that are related to individuals' management of these goals and the ways in which these form meaningful practices (e.g. the different strategies an interpreter adopts to coordinate with others to empower patient without causing additional harm during an end-of-life disclosure); and (c) the ways in which the meanings and functions of interpreter-mediated medical encounters provide an account for why certain behaviors are judged to be more appropriate and effective than others (e.g. what are the guiding values that influence a provider's or a patient's evaluation about the appropriateness and effectiveness of an interpreters' strategy?).

Goldsmith (2001: 530) explained:

> A normative theory poses questions such as the following: When a social actor wishes to accomplish some purpose in a particular kind of social contexts, what are the constraints to accomplishing that purpose, what are the discursive resources that are available for addressing those constraints, and what are the evaluative criteria by which the effectiveness and appropriateness of the actor's efforts may be judged.

This line of questions presents two major shifts in research focus, moving away from the text-centered, interpreter-oriented approach to one focusing on interpreter-mediated medical encounters. The first shift is to focus attention not simply on the frequency of individual communicative behaviors (e.g. interpreter alterations or mistakes), but on the *meanings* of such practices. The end goal of a normative approach is to account for judgments that some communicative practices in interpreter-mediated medical encounters are 'better' than others. These judgments are embedded in cultural systems of meaning and belief, including individual assumptions about the competing goals and values as well as the expected norms in managing them. By identifying the cultural systems that facilitate the interpretation and evaluation of these practices, researchers can predict why certain practices would be preferred over others. For example, by identifying providers' preferences for in-person intimacy when disclosing a poor prognosis (Hsieh, 2015), we can speculate that providers may opt for less-qualified non-professional interpreters even when professional telephone interpreters are readily available. In other words, by identifying the values that shape individuals' interpretation and drive their communicative behaviors, researchers can prescribe communicative interventions and practices that are likely to be adopted as they are consistent with the values or goals of the participants.

The second shift is to move from a linear, positivistic view in prescribing appropriate behaviors in interpreter-mediated medical encounters to an interpretive, heuristic approach to predict and explain the evaluations of behaviors as more or less appropriate and effective. My goal is not to define, identify, or regulate the particular behavior that is deemed appropriate or effective in a given provider–patient interaction in a top-down manner. Rather, I aim to explore why certain behaviors are evaluated more favorably than others by examining how well these practices adapt to the potentially conflicting values which emerge in provider–patient interactions. To understand the conflicting values to which participants in interpreter-mediated medical encounters orient, we need to identify the meanings and functions of interpreter-mediated medical encounters. To understand the wide range of communicative strategies that can be employed to respond to interactional dilemmas, we need to first identify the communicative practices within the specific contexts.

By examining the underlying values and principles that shape participants' evaluation and interpretation of communicative behaviors, we can identify some basic features of discourse that can serve as resources to address conflicting goals. Because discursive resources are often language-specific and contextually situated, this approach allows researchers to explore the socially defined contexts (e.g. linguistic, cultural, political and clinical contexts, among others) that shape individuals' evaluation and interpretation. This approach also provides opportunities for researchers to hypothesize how and why certain discursive practices are associated with situated evaluations, investigating both the correlation and the specific processes that connect these two. For example, should interpreters relay other speakers' emotions and affective attitudes in their interpretation? Why do we think it would be necessary and valuable for an interpreter to relay a providers' positive emotions and supportive attitudes when interacting with a patient? How about a providers' prejudicial comments? What are the values or underlying principles that motivate an interpreter to screen out a provider's stigmatizing attitudes (Seale et al., 2013)?

A Model of Bilingual Health Communication

The normative approach to interpreter-mediated medical encounters forms the basis of my Model of Bilingual Health Communication (the BHC Model). I have reported and synthesized evidence-based findings related to the Model elsewhere (Hsieh, 2016). In this section, I will focus on delineating the theoretical aspects of the Model: (a) the individual-level constructs; (b) interpersonal-level constructs; and (c) propositions of this Model.

The individual-level constructs are factors that shape individual behaviors and evaluations of the interpreter-mediated medical encounter (see Figure 3.1). The four constructs are: Communicative Goals, Individual Agency, System Norms, and Quality and Equality of Care. It is important to note that all these constructs are applicable to all participants in the medical encounter. However, individuals' understanding, assessment and skill level for these constructs may differ. In addition, individuals may hold competing (and potentially conflicting) understanding of these constructs, resulting in tensions and challenges in interpreter-mediated medical encounters.

Communicative goals

Fundamental to the BHC Model is my assumption that interpreter-mediated medical encounters are goal-oriented communicative activities. In everyday talk, individuals hold multiple goals (e.g. task, identity and relationship goals) that are often negotiated and coordinated rather than explicitly discussed (Tracy, 2013). All participants in interpreter-mediated interactions, including the interpreter, have communicative goals. For example, an

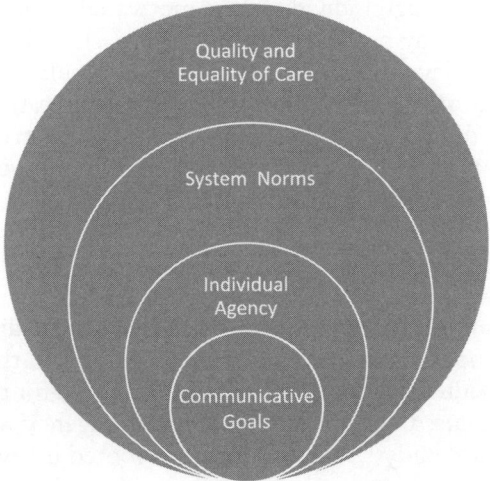

Figure 3.1 Individual-level constructs within the Model of Bilingual Health Communication

interpreter may wish to appear neutral, maintain job security or ensure the quality of care. The communicative goals can be inherent in the communicative activity but can also emerge during the dynamic discursive process. For example, although an interpreter may wish to maintain neutrality in medical encounters, the patient's lack of communicative competence may prompt the interpreter to address the imbalance of provider–patient communication by adopting a more active role in mediating provider–patient interactions.

Although individuals in interpreter-mediated interactions may share some goals (e.g. improving a patient's health), they also have unique individual goals. For example, providers may hold specific interpersonal goals (e.g. developing trust and rapport), in addition to their therapeutic goals. Individuals' multiple goals may not be compatible with one another or with others' goals. For example, patients may wish to receive Western biomedical care without giving up their cultural health practices (e.g. taking herbal medicine). On the other hand, a provider may refuse to offer treatment to a patient who insists on continuing to take herbal medicine for fear of potential interactions with the prescribed medication.

Individuals' interpretation and evaluation about the meaning and quality of interpreter-mediated medical encounters are fundamental to their understanding of their goals. A provider who wishes to show empathy with a patient may feel frustrated by an interpreter who focuses on medical information while neglecting rapport talk (Aranguri *et al.*, 2006). Finally, the ability of individuals to fulfill their communicative goals may be dependent on their and others' communicative competence as well as other contextual factors during the communicative event. For example, an interpreter may find it difficult to maintain a passive presence when a provider engages the interpreter in a conversation by asking a question directed to the interpreter (Hsieh, 2006).

In summary, although individuals are motivated to fulfill their communicative goals, they may need to reconcile their own and others' competing goals. Failure to achieve their intended goals may result in problematic outcomes (e.g. frustration, dissatisfaction and miscommunication). Nevertheless, because goals are dynamic and can be interactively constructed/negotiated, all individuals can actively collaborate and coordinate with each other to identify and fulfill each other's communicative goals.

Individual agency

Whereas communicative goals emphasize individuals' differences in their agendas, they do not address individuals' ability to fulfill those goals. In the BHC, I view individual agency as the condition needed for the fulfillment of communicative goals. I conceptualize individual agency as a socially constructed and contextually situated self that is rooted in 'everyday practices and sites that call forth and supply its meanings' (Gubrium & Holstein, 1995: 566). The meanings and functions of individual agency cannot be separated from actors or the participants in the communicative event. From this perspective, individual agency is not just an inherent or fixed ability the human agent holds, but a quality that can be interactively negotiated and socially enacted (De Jaegher & Froese, 2009).

Why is this social constructionist approach to individual agency important to BHC? In health care settings, not all individuals have the same kinds or degree of agency. From an institutional perspective, individual agency can be shaped by power structure, institutional hierarchy, access to resources and professionalism. For example, physicians are likely to have more agency than nurses as they are at the head of a healthcare team, entitled with higher institutional power. In contrast, compared with nurses, interpreters can have even less individual agency as they do not always have an institutionalized office (e.g. interpreter services), can be outsourced to external agencies or are considered to be low-ranked or low-priority workers. As a result, a physician is likely to exert their own communicative goals over those of the interpreter when their goals conflict with one another. On the other hand, because interpreters are often trained to assume a neutral, passive presence in provider–patient interactions, they may actively refrain from intervening in the medical discourse even when they have observed problematic interactions.

At an individual level, agency is shaped by individuals' educational background, self-efficacy skills, communicative competence, emotional status and motivational relevance (Bandura, 2001). A patient with high health literacy is more likely to actively participate in the medical discourse than a patient who has minimal education and is terrified about seeking care in a cultural system that is completely foreign to him or her (Shaw et al., 2009; Sudore et al., 2009). Compared to a telephone interpreter who provide services at a remote location, a patient's family member is more likely to intervene in the provider–patient communication and exert their communicative goals when acting as an interpreter because s/he is are more motivated to ensure high-quality care (Greenhalgh et al., 2006). Physicians with low self-efficacy admitted that they actively avoided communicating with language-discordant patients (O'Leary et al., 2003); fortunately, physician self-efficacy can be enhanced through training and experiences of working with language-discordant patients (Hernandez et al., 2014; Thompson et al., 2013).

At an interpersonal level, individual agency can be shaped by interpersonal relationships, social obligations and interactional dynamics. For example, an interpreter who is familiar with and trusted by the provider is likely to have higher individual agency to pursue his or her communicative goals than an interpreter who does not know anyone in the clinic. A family member acting as an interpreter may feel obligated to insist on specific ways of communication (e.g. do not disclose a poor prognosis to the patient) than a professional interpreter. An interpreter may become more aggressive in seeking information upon a patient's request (e.g. 'I don't know what questions to ask. Can you help me? Ask whatever is important').

Finally, it is important to note that individual agency also can be challenged. For example, a provider may ask an interpreter to interpret only what the patient has said and not to add additional personal opinions when conducting interpreting, which is consistent with the default interpreting model in interpreter training (i.e. interpreter-as-conduit). An interpreter may inform a provider that a particular line of questioning is culturally inappropriate and unlikely to get a truthful answer from the patient. Although individual agency is about individuals' ability and willingness to assert their communicative goals, the appropriateness and effectiveness of individuals' enactment or embodiment of individual agency is still subject to others' evaluation.

In summary, I view individual agency as a necessary condition for individuals involved in a medical encounter to pursue their communicative goals. Individual agency can be inherent in institutional structures (e.g. as a part of institutional hierarchy) as well as individuals' skills and competence. However, it also can be socially constructed (e.g. compromised, enhanced, negotiated, and resisted) through interpersonal interactions. A successful communicator can leverage others' support and contextual factors to gain more individual agency; in contrast, a less successful communicator may fail to utilize the resources available to maintain their individual agency.

System norms

System norms move the understanding of interpreter-mediated interactions beyond the examination of individual performances and behaviors to a larger context. Each individual in interpreter-mediated medical encounters assumes certain roles, functions, and behaviors under the influences and frames of the system(s). I view the system as social systems and cultures, in which there are specific norms, values, and worldviews that are imposed upon individuals within the system. In other words, individuals interpret meaning through the system to which they subscribe. From this perspective, we can argue that providers are within the culture of (Western) medicine, in which there are specific views about conceptualizing health and illness (e.g. principle of verification, germ theory and Cartesian dualism) that make a patient's cultural illness ideology (e.g. an illness caused by spirits stealing one's souls) incompatible if not incomprehensible.

System norms guide the behaviors of individuals within the system. For example, because professional interpreters are trained to value neutrality and to view the provider–patient relationship as the primary relationship in medical encounters, they adopt specific behaviors (e.g. interpreting in first-person style and avoiding eye contact with others) in an effort to minimize their presence during the interpreter-mediated medical encounters. A provider expects to assume the leading and controlling role in provider–patient interactions as they are trained to take charge of the flow of medical discourse. From this perspective, individuals' behaviors almost always are coherent and consistent within the meaning structure of the system. In fact, when individuals fail to observe system norms, they are often made aware of their violations through social sanctions.

However, because not all individuals share the same system, participants in bilingual/cross-cultural medical encounters may experience problematic interactions. For example, a provider may have a hard time understanding why an interpreter insists on avoiding eye contact when providing interpreting services or why a patient continues to complain about haunting spirits when seeking biomedical care (Hsieh, 2006, 2010). Miscommunication can arise as a result of competing systems.

Because individuals in interpreter-mediated medical encounters are not necessarily regulated by the same systems and the systems involved may not be compatible with each other, individuals may struggle to: (a) identify the systems at play during the medical encounter; and (b) prioritize and negotiate the system that gives meaning to the current interaction. For example, a patient may choose to ignore a provider's treatment recommendation if s/he believes the provider has failed to provide an accurate diagnosis. However, a provider can contact child protective services and take away a pediatric patient from a parent if s/he suspects that the parent has endangered the child by providing substandard care (Fadiman, 1997). In other words, not all systems are of equal footing (e.g. some systems may have higher institutional, legal or moral hierarchies than others). Although the parents are considered dutiful parents in their own ethnic culture, a physician using the biomedical system to identify parents' failure in providing proper dosing for treatment can access the legal system to exert his/her control not just over the minor patient's illness experiences but also the parents' control over the child. Miscommunication owing to incompatibilities between systems can result in problematic outcomes, including intense conflicts.

The identification and prioritization of systems may prompt individuals to ignore or overrule other participants' needs and preferences. For example, although attending to patient preference is an important component in patient-centered care, a provider may decide that the legal obligation for informed consent supersedes a patient's family members' preferences about end-of-life disclosure. In other words, by aligning oneself with a system of higher power/value (e.g. the legal system supersedes the healthcare system), a person may feel legitimized to adopt behaviors that override the values of other systems (e.g. imposing informed consent against patient or family member preference). Similarly, when an interpreter prioritizes institutional goals (e.g. conserving limited resources and maintaining organizational ethics) over interpreter neutrality, an interpreter may choose to editorialize other participants' narratives and thus act as an institutional gatekeeper (e.g. keeping a patient's interview narrative on-track to avoid 'wasting' a physician's time; Davidson, 2000) or as a moral mediator to ensure the quality of care (e.g. omitting a nurse's stigmatizing comment to protect a patient; Seale *et al.*, 2013).

Finally, although all systems have their internal values and structures, systems can also be adaptive to changes as well as influences and impositions from other systems. Granted, not all systems are equally adaptive. For example, the legal system is much more rigid because any changes require legislative efforts to modify laws and regulations. However, a provider who originally subscribed to the values and norms of a biomedical system may become increasingly aware and even appreciative of the patients' cultural understanding of their illness. In fact, the ability of providers to incorporate patients' cultural worldviews in the treatment process is essential in gaining patient compliance and improving health outcomes (Dutta, 2007; Dutta & Basu, 2007). This does not mean that the provider abandons his/her original system norms. Rather, the provider learns to integrate two different systems by developing skills to communicate with the patient, using the system norms that construct meanings and guide behaviors for the patient. In cross-cultural care, an interpreter is presumed to be aware of such diverging system norms that guide both the provider and the patient's understanding and behaviors of the medical encounter. As a result, interpreters are encouraged to serve as cultural brokers in cross-cultural care (Butow *et al.*, 2012; Dohan & Levintova, 2007).

What happens when individuals' system norms conflict with one another in interpreter-mediated medical encounters? Which system gets to be prioritized over other systems? Within the context of the BHC model, answers to these questions come from a higher guiding value for provider–patient communication and cross-cultural care: quality and equality of care.

Quality and equality of care

I list Quality and Equality of Care as the overarching value for the BHC Model. While in the literature, quality of care and equality of care have been identified as two separate values, I view it as an integrated value under the BHC Model. Quality of care cannot exist without equality of care for marginalized and underserved populations. Although Quality and Equality of Care can be a communicative goal when applied in context, it also serves as an all-encompassing value that integrates differences between systems, providing the ultimate value that guides the adjudication of competing systems. In other words, when participants in an interpreter-mediated medical encounters experience conflicts owing to competing or conflicting system norms, they rely on the guiding value of Quality and Equality of Care to resolve their differences.

Traditionally, quality of care has been conceptualized using three components: structure (i.e. the organizational factors that define the healthcare system under which care is provided), process (i.e. the clinical and interpersonal care given to the patient) and outcomes (i.e. consequences of care) (Donabedian, 1980). Individuals' quality of care can be evaluated through their access (i.e. whether individuals can access healthcare structures and process of care which they need) and effectiveness (i.e. the extent to which care delivers its intended outcome or results in a desired process, in response to needs) of structure, process and outcomes (Campbell *et al.*, 2000). Within the BHC model, I am particularly interested in process as an indicator of quality care. Interpreters are essential to ensuring access (e.g. making information and resources available to patients) and effectiveness (e.g. allowing providers to provide culturally sensitive care to achieve optimal outcomes) of clinical and interpersonal care, in which patients and clinicians rely on interpreters to communicate needs, coordinate tasks, and perform identities (e.g. an interpreter may adopt a supportive tone when interpreting to highlight the provider's friendliness).

I recognize that quality of care can be a cultural (and system) construct (Harmsen *et al.*, 2008). Individuals from different systems are likely to define and perceive quality of care differently (Campbell *et al.*, 2000). For example, for Jehovah's witnesses, not accepting blood transfusions even in life-or-death situations is essential to their faith and, thus, does not constitute a threat to quality of care for them. A Chinese patient may consider Chinese food therapy (i.e. consuming food that has specific medical effects) to be a dietary health practice that defines his/her cultural identity and cannot be separated from his/her everyday life (Kong & Hsieh, 2012). Quality of care cannot be separated from one's understanding of their well-being, which is always culturally and socially situated (Ryan & Deci, 2011; Williams *et al.*, 2011). There is a possibility that a patient, a provider, and/or an interpreter do not share the same understanding of quality of care.

In fact, some bioethicists have argued that imposing Western biomedical values on patients who do not share the same values can be problematic, if not unethical (Ho, 2008). For example, European American and African American patients were more likely to view truth-telling as empowering, enabling the patient to make choices; in contrast, Korean American and Mexican American patients were more likely to see the truth-telling as cruel, and even harmful, to the patients (Blackhall *et al.*, 2001). The differences in the functions and meanings of 'truths' in various communities can result in diverging practices. For example, Korean American and Mexican American populations are more likely to shelter patients from information about a poor prognosis and adopt a family-centered model of medical decision making; in contrast, European American and African American populations are more likely to emphasize individual autonomy and informed decision-making of the patient (Blackhall *et al.*, 1995). If a physician insists on disclosing a poor prognosis to a Korean American or Mexican American patient despite his/her family's objection, the physician is likely to increase the patient's suffering and distress, potentially causing disruption in the patient's social network. Such practices ignore the cultural meanings, functions, and practices of truth-telling.

In cross-cultural care, interpreters are faced with challenges regarding cultural differences with regard to disclosure practices and information management, which are fused with meanings about identity and relationships. For example, in Chinese culture, if a son fails to assume the responsibilities of information management for the parent as patient (e.g. seeking information about treatment options or concealing information from the patient), he may face public criticism that he is inadequate as a son (Muller & Desmond, 1992). On the other hand, if a Chinese father gives permission for his son to take over the responsibilities of information management and to be a proxy decision maker (e.g. making decisions about treatments), the father is demonstrating his commitment to his family and community (Ellerby et al., 2000). Rees and Bath (2000) found that, when mothers with breast cancer withheld information from their daughters, it often was motivated by their identity as a mother because they wanted to protect their daughters. Miller and Zook (1997) noted that AIDS patients' care partners negotiated and legitimized their roles through actively seeking information from physicians. Therefore, information management in a family is not just about patient autonomy but also about family members' identities as part of the family (Blackhall et al., 2001). Failing to respect these cultural meanings of health practices can result in major disruptions in patients' well-being. From this perspective, quality of care cannot be achieved without considering the cultural construction and meanings of patients' sense of well-being.

For marginalized and underserved populations, including language-discordant populations, quality of care cannot be separated from equality of care (Aligning Forces for Quality, 2010). For the BHC model, I define equality of care as the extent to which the language-discordant populations share comparable access to and effectiveness of care as language-concordant populations. More importantly, equality of health is 'conditional upon a respect for personal preferences [or in medical ethics, the principle of 'autonomy'] and upon a prohibition on reductions in current health' (Culyer & Wagstaff, 1993: 455). From this perspective, like quality of care, equality of care is not beyond the influence of system as individual preferences are often shaped by their cultural norms.

In reality, all participants in interpreter-mediated medical encounters often need to manage a potentially delicate and complicated balance between personal preference and health outcomes. Despite the fact that Quality and Equality of Care cannot escape the influences of (cultural) systems, individuals within different systems can learn to recognize and acknowledge the transcending values of Quality and Equality of Care. For example, a provider can recognize and respect a parent's desire to provide the best care for his/her child, despite their disagreement on the treatment procedures. Similarly, interpreters can educate providers, patients, and their family members about the cultural differences in the meanings and functions of truth-telling in end-of-life care, allowing all participants to become aware of other participants' legal obligations and social needs. Rather than advocating universalistic values of quality of care (Beauchamp, 2004), I propose that individuals from different (cultural) systems can generate an integrated value of Quality and Equality of Care. Because the participants are from different cultural systems, the values they bring to the integrated value meta-system may not always be compatible or consistent with each other. Different groups of participants may agree on different definitions of Quality and Equality of Care depending on the situational/interactional contexts. As a result, what really constitutes the integrated value of Quality and Equality of Care is not a fixed value. Rather, it is constantly co-constructed and negotiated among multiple parties and is meaningful and appropriate at the particular point in time and place. All participants should collaborate to develop a prioritized list of diverse values, accessing resources to strengthen their claim and control over the definition of Quality and Equality of Care.

In summary, I view Quality and Equality of Care as a value system that guides the practices of all involved in interpreter-mediated medical encounters. The value is not a fixed, preexisting, or universal value. Rather, it is contextually situated, interactionally managed, and locally defined in the communicative process (i.e. the meanings of Quality and Equality of Care are shaped by the contexts in which participants negotiated its meanings during their social interaction that is situated in a specific time and place). Nevertheless, it allows individuals with competing systems to acknowledge others' perspectives and forces all participants to subject themselves to the meta-value of Quality and Equality of Care that is co-constructed by all involved in the medical encounter.

Interpersonal-level constructs within the model of bilingual health communication

Whereas individual-level constructs shape individual behaviors and evaluations of the interpreter-mediated medical encounter, interpersonal-level constructs delineate the dimensions through which these individual-level constructs operate. Based on the literature and my own research, I have included two interpersonal-level constructs: (a) Trust–Control–Power; and (b) the Temporal Dimension.

Trust–Control–Power

Trust–Control–Power has been identified as a major theme in bilingual health care. This dynamic can exist at the micro, interpersonal level of provider–patient–interpreter interactions and at the macro, system/cultural level of healthcare institutions and the society at large (Brisset et al., 2013). By recognizing interpreters' active role in bilingual health care, recent studies have highlighted the importance of *relational contexts* (e.g. interpersonal trust and therapeutic alliances) in shaping providers' and interpreters' collaboration with each other (Gray et al., 2011; Hsieh et al., 2010; Robb & Greenhalgh, 2006). In addition, providers and interpreters often compete for control over the communicative process by monitoring others' performance, setting boundaries of time, space and content of provider–patient interactions, and adopting specific verbal and nonverbal strategies to control others' behaviors (Hsieh, 2010; Mason & Ren, 2012; Zimányi, 2013).

Trust–Control–Power as a dimension shapes how participants negotiate the various individual-level constructs with respect to one another. For example, when individuals have diverging communicative goals, individual agency or system norms, who gets to control the provider–patient interaction? Does the person with the most power get to control the interaction? What kinds of power? The provider has legitimate power (i.e. institutional hierarchy) and expert power (i.e. medical expertise); in contrast, the interpreter has expert power with regard to language and culture and the informational power, as they control the content and process of communication through their interpretation (Mason & Ren, 2012; Nugus et al., 2010; Raven, 1993). On the other hand, the patient has reward power (e.g. offer more business through repeated visits) and coercive power (e.g. threats of terminating provider–patient relationships) as they can always choose to find a different provider if the provider fails to respect the patients' request to use a family interpreter, who maintains social power with the patient through long-term relational trust. In other words, Trust–Control–Power is not fixed; rather, it is constantly enacted and resisted in the communicative process.

From this perspective, Trust–Control–Poweras a dimension reflects individuals' efforts and competition in defining their interactional (and professional) boundaries. This can be particularly tricky in cross-cultural care because the boundaries of medicine, language, and culture are often overlapping and blurred because patients' illness experiences cannot be separated from their culture or language. For example, a Chinese male patient may use the term '腎虛' (pronounced shenshu) to describe his illness, which literally means 'weak kidney' in English. However, for male patients, this term can be used to describe various symptoms, including bodily coldness, poor memory, defective cognition, palpitations, dizziness, premature ejaculation, poor erectile function, back pain, and urinary frequency and weakness (Hinton et al., 2005). Patients' understanding of their illness and illness symptoms are situated in their lifeworld (Lo & Bahar, 2013; Todres et al., 2007), which is infused with their cultural beliefs, social experiences, and folk ideologies. As interpreters assist in cross-cultural care, they inevitably need to tread on the boundaries of medicine as they bridge the blurry boundaries of medicine, language, and culture. Despite the providers' claim and power over medical expertise, they face challenges in sharing their control over the process of care and meanings of medicine with interpreters in cross-cultural care.

In addition, trust, control, and power are interdependent and intertwined. For example, as an interpreter develops more trust with the provider, the interpreter is able to have more power to control the process and content of provider–patient interactions (Hsieh, 2010). On the other hand, when a provider adopts a utilitarian view of interpreters' roles and function (i.e. treating an interpreter as a utility to be wielded at the will of a provider), interpreters' relationships with patients can be viewed as resources to be exploited for therapeutic objectives (Hsieh & Kramer, 2012). In other words, even interpreters' goals and relationships are subject to providers' control.

Temporal Dimension

Time is a theoretical dimension (e.g. how time affects the ongoing relationships and the quality of care in interpreter-mediated medical encounters) that has rarely been discussed in the literature of bilingual health care. This can be partially attributed to the conduit model of interpreting, in which interpreters are often viewed as translation machines. If interpreters are no more than conduits, providing mechanical and faithful relay of information from one language to another, time would not make any difference in the quality of interpreting or the quality of care. After all, a good hammer remains the same tool, regardless of the time elapsed. A user is unlikely to develop a closer bond or relationship with a certain tool, resulting in different usage patterns when using an old machine versus a new one. In short, in the traditional literature of healthcare interpreting, the Temporal Dimension in interpreter-mediated health care is irrelevant and thus undertheorized. Nevertheless, we know that even the analogy of a hammer is problematic. Even with a tool as rigid as a hammer, we do become more comfortable with the one we have grown accustomed to using. We learn its unique characteristics and develop tricks that make the specific hammer work better in different situations.

However, when researchers and practitioners do consider the temporal dimension in interpreter-mediated interactions, time is often perceived to be an enemy, a point of human weaknesses, of interpreter-mediated medical encounters. For example, the Temporal Dimension of interpreter-mediated health care makes it possible for interpreters to develop relationships with their clients, making them susceptible to the corruption and pressure of interpersonal relationships. Traditionally, the industry has developed specific strategies to prevent potential problems as a result of the Temporal Dimension of interpreter-mediated health care. For example, to avoid interpreter–patient bonding, some interpreting agencies establish internal rules to minimize repeatedly pairing the same interpreter with the same patient. In contrast, there seems to be less anxiety about and no internal rules against pairing the same interpreter with the same provider. In fact, recent studies have suggested important benefits when the provider–interpreter pair can develop effective patterns of collaboration over time (Hsieh *et al.*, 2010). I am intrigued by the tensions within the normative assumptions: time as a point of corruption to the patient–interpreter relationship versus a point of enhancement to the provider–interpreter relationship. It is possible that such tensions in thinking about the impacts and functions of time reflect an emphasis on institutional control (e.g. prioritizing providers' control and needs over that of patients) in healthcare settings.

Time is an important dimension in any system. Most systems are open systems that develop adaptive changes in response to outside influences as well as internal tensions. Because interpreter-mediated provider–patient interactions simultaneously involve several different systems, each of which entails its own unique values and norms, the participants are likely to face tensions, challenges, and conflicts owing to the diverse systems, including practices and values, in play. However, time as a dimension makes integrations of diverging systems possible, at the individual, organizational, and even cultural levels. For example, interpreters intentionally develop a particular way of speaking (e.g. first-person interpreting styles and avoiding eye contact when interpreting) to systematically reinforce the provider–patient relationship and to claim an invisible role (Hsieh, 2009). For a person who is not aware of the meanings of such practices, interpreters' performance may appear strange, rude or even disruptive. Because of the institutional pressure to conserve providers' time, interpreters often feel that they do not have sufficient time to educate providers about their specialized practices (Hsieh, 2008). However, when a provider learns the meanings and functions of such practices in an interpreter's speech community, a provider may come to appreciate the interpreter's performance (Hsieh, 2010).

Similarly, time makes it possible for people who are initially unfamiliar with each other's behaviors and intentions to develop rapport and trust, allowing them to be more flexible and adaptive to each other's needs and expectations. For example, as physicians become more familiar with patients' cultural values, they may be more willing to modify their communicative practices to accommodate patients' needs. This is the basis of interpreters' role as a cultural broker. We assume that, as participants in interpreter-mediated medical encounters become more knowledgeable about different cultural norms and values, all will become better at understanding and interacting with one another.

It is important to note that recent literature on acculturation has demonstrated that individuals are unlikely to abandon their own cultural values once they become familiar with or even adaptive to the new cultural practices (Kramer, 2013; Wade et al., 2007). Rather, individuals tend to develop layers of consciousness and pluralistic approaches to managing different areas of life. Time does not make a person forget or abandon his or her original cultural norms. Several studies have demonstrated that acculturation level does not predict individuals' health practices in abandoning prior health beliefs and health practices (Ma, 1999; Wade et al., 2007); rather, interactions between systems allow individuals to develop multiple repertoires. For example, a Chinese patient may prefer to adopt a biomedical model for acute conditions but rely on traditional Chinese medicine for chronic illnesses (Chung et al., 2012). An American physician may welcome shamanistic practices for patients' spiritual well-being but feel strongly about ensuring accurate medication and dosing practices (Brown, 2009).

Finally, rather than painting a rosy picture of time as a theoretical dimension, researchers also need to recognize that, without meaningful interactions, time may perpetuate miscommunication. For example, patients may become increasingly agitated when a provider fails to acknowledge or accommodate their cultural practices and values after repeated interactions. Such feelings may prompt a patient to avoid care and minimize interactions with clinicians. When a problematic performance by an interpreter becomes an institutional cautionary tale shared among healthcare providers over time, there can be increasing distrust of all interpreters that may result in widespread distrust for inter-professional collaboration within the organization (Hsieh et al., 2010). In short, the Temporal Dimension within interpreter-mediated health care does not guarantee improved interactions over time.

Propositions of the Bilingual Health Communication Model

By adopting a heuristic approach, I have sought to generate a theoretical framework for conceptualizing interpreter-mediated medical encounters as interactive, goal-oriented communicative activities that are situated in the larger communicative event of provider–patient interactions. In addition, the BHC model presumes that Quality and Equality of Care is a shared value that guides all participants' interpretation of and practices in interpreter-mediated medical encounters.

Given the individual-level and interpersonal-level constructs proposed in the BHC Model, I propose the following general propositions that guide the understanding and assessment of interpreter-mediated medical encounters:

(1) Successful BHC is dependent on the ability and agency of individuals to negotiate and adapt to competing and/or emerging goals. Moving away from the focus on interpreter performance, this proposition views interpreter-mediated medical encounters as a collaborative achievement among all participants.
(2) Evaluation of the appropriateness and effectiveness of the strategies used by interpreters requires considerations for their corresponding short-term and long-term impacts. One strategy may have desirable short-term impacts in clinical care but entail problematic consequences for long-term provider–patient trust.
(3) The desired interpreting style is dependent on contexts. Rather than adopting a positivist stance in pursuing the ideal interpretation through equivalences between two languages, the BHC Model acknowledges that several contexts are essential in participants' understanding of and preference interpreter-mediated interactions and interpreters' performances. These contexts can include but are not limited to the clinical, interpersonal, and sociocultural contexts.

Conclusion

A successful interpreter-mediated medical encounter is a coordinated achievement among all participants involved. By recognizing that the communicative process, meanings of an illness event, and even the quality of care are socially constructed, the Bilingual Health Communication Model provides multiple opportunities and entry points for theory development and practice implications.

The best practice for interpreter-mediated medical encounters is not a fixed formula that can predict standardized results. Rather, optimal interpreter-mediated encounters take place when all participant are able to appropriately and effectively identify and negotiate their communicative goals, exercise individual agency, acknowledge differences in their normative expectations *and* find ways to generate compatible, if not shared, understanding of Quality and Equality of Care. The best bilingual health communication does not rely on the interpreter to do a perfect job; rather, it counts on all individuals to be problem-solvers, adopting flexible and adaptive strategies to meet the challenges emerged during the communicative process of cross-cultural care.

References

Aligning Forces for Quality (2010) Quality and equality in US health care: A message handbook. See http://www.rwjf.org/content/dam/farm/reports/reports/2010/rwjf69340 (accessed 14 March 2015).

Angelelli, C.V. (2004) *Medical Interpreting and Cross-cultural Communication*. Cambridge: Cambridge University Press.

Aranguri, C., Davidson, B. and Ramirez, R. (2006) Patterns of communication through interpreters: A detailed sociolinguistic analysis. *Journal of General Internal Medicine* 21 (6), 623–629.

Bakhtin, M.M. (1981) *The Dialogic Imagination: Four Essays by M. M. Bakhtin* (M. Holquist and C. Emerson, Trans.). Austin, TX: University of Texas Press.

Bandura, A. (2001) Social cognitive theory: An agentic perspective. *Annual Review of Psychology* 52, 1–26.

Baumslag, D. (1998) Choosing scientific goals: The need for a normative approach. *Studies in History and Philosophy of Science* 29 (1), 81–96.

Baxter, L.A. and Montgomery, B.M. (1996) *Relating: Dialogues and Dialectics*. New York: Guilford Press.

Beauchamp, T.L. (2004) Does ethical theory have a future in bioethics? *Journal of Law, Medicine and Ethics* 32 (2), 209–217.

Blackhall, L.J., Murphy, S.T., Frank, G., Michel, V. and Azen, S. (1995) Ethnicity and attitudes toward patient autonomy. *Journal of the American Medical Association* 274 (10), 820–825.

Blackhall, L.J., Frank, G., Murphy, S. and Michel, V. (2001) Bioethics in a different tongue: The case of truth-telling. *Journal of Urban Health* 78 (1), 59–71.

Brisset, C., Leanza, Y. and Laforest, K. (2013) Working with interpreters in health care: A systematic review and meta-ethnography of qualitative studies. *Patient Education and Counseling* 91 (2), 131–140.

Brown, P.L. (2009) A doctor for disease, a shaman for the soul. *The New York Times*, 20 September, p. A20. See http://www.nytimes.com/2009/09/20/us/20shaman.html

Butow, P.N., Goldstein, D., Bell, M.L., Sze, M., Aldridge, L.J., Abdo, S., Tanious, M., Dong, S., Iedema, R., Vardy, J., Ashgari, R., Hui, R. and Eisenbruch, M. (2011) Interpretation in consultations with immigrant patients with cancer: How accurate is it? *Journal of Clinical Oncology* 29 (20), 2801–2807.

Butow, P.N., Lobb, E., Jefford, M., Goldstein, D., Eisenbruch, M., Girgis, A., King, M., Sze, M., Aldridge, L. and Schofield, P. (2012) A bridge between cultures: Interpreters' perspectives of consultations with migrant oncology patients. *Supportive Care in Cancer* 20 (2), 235–244.

Campbell, S.M., Roland, M.O. and Buetow, S.A. (2000) Defining quality of care. *Social Science and Medicine* 51 (11), 1611–1625.

Chung, V.C.H., Ma, P.H.X., Lau, C.H., Wong, S.Y.S., Yeoh, E.K. and Griffiths, S.M. (2012) Views on traditional Chinese medicine amongst Chinese population: A systematic review of qualitative and quantitative studies. *Health Expectations*.

Culyer, A.J. and Wagstaff, A. (1993) Equity and equality in health and health care. *Journal of Health Economics* 12 (4), 431–457.

Davidson, B. (2000) The interpreter as institutional gatekeeper: The social–linguistic role of interpreters in Spanish–English medical discourse. *Journal of Sociolinguistics* 4 (3), 379–405.

De Jaegher, H. and Froese, T. (2009) On the role of social interaction in individual agency. *Adaptive Behavior* 17 (5), 444–460.

Dohan, D. and Levintova, M. (2007) Barriers beyond words: Cancer, culture, and translation in a community of Russian speakers. *Journal of General Internal Medicine* 22 (Suppl 2), S300–305.

Donabedian, A. (1980) *The Definition of Quality and Approaches to its Assessment*. Chicago, IL: Health Administration Press.

Dutta, M.J. (2007) Communicating about culture and health: Theorizing culture-centered and cultural sensitivity approaches. *Communication Theory* 17 (3), 304–328.

Dutta, M.J. and Basu, A. (2007) Health among men in rural Bengal: Exploring meanings through a culture-centered approach. *Qualitative Health Research* 17 (1), 38–48.

Ellerby, J.H., McKenzie, J., McKay, S., Gariepy, G.J. and Kaufert, J.M. (2000) Bioethics for clinicians: 18. Aboriginal cultures. *Canadian Medical Association Journal* 163 (7), 845–850.

Fadiman, A. (1997) *The Spirit Catches You and You Fall Down*. New York: Farrar, Straus and Giroux.

Flores, G., Abreu, M., Barone, C.P., Bachur, R. and Lin, H. (2012) Errors of medical interpretation and their potential clinical consequences: A comparison of professional versus ad hoc versus no interpreters. *Annals of Emergency Medicine* 60 (5), 545–553.

Goldsmith, D.J. (2001) A normative approach to the study of uncertainty and communication. *Journal of Communication* 51 (3), 514–533.

Goldsmith, D.J. and Fitch, K. (1997) The normative context of advice as social support. *Human Communication Research* 23 (4), 454–476.

Gray, B., Hilder, J. and Donaldson, H. (2011) Why do we not use trained interpreters for all patients with limited English proficiency? Is there a place for using family members? *Australian Journal of Primary Health* 17 (3), 240–249.

Greenhalgh, T., Robb, N. and Scambler, G. (2006) Communicative and strategic action in interpreted consultations in primary health care: A Habermasian perspective. *Social Science and Medicine* 63 (5), 1170–1187.

Gubrium, J.F. and Holstein, J.A. (1995) Individual agency, the ordinary, and postmodern life. *Sociological Quarterly* 36 (3), 555–570.

Harmsen, J.A.M., Bernsen, R.M.D., Bruijnzeels, M.A. and Meeuwesen, L. (2008) Patients' evaluation of quality of care in general practice: What are the cultural and linguistic barriers? *Patient Education and Counseling* 72 (1), 155–162.

Hernandez, R.G., Cowden, J.D., Moon, M., Brands, C.K., Sisson, S.D. and Thompson, D.A. (2014) Predictors of resident satisfaction in caring for limited English proficient families: A multisite study. *Academic Pediatrics* 14 (2), 173–180.

Hinton, D.E., Nguyen, L., Tran, M. and Quinn, S. (2005) Weak kidney and panic attacks in a traumatized vietnamese male. *Culture, Medicine and Psychiatry* 29 (1), 125–135.

Ho, A. (2008) Using family members as interpreters in the clinical setting. *Journal of Clinical Ethics* 19 (3), 223–233.

Houtlosser, P. and van Rees, A. (eds) (2006) *Considering Pragma-dialectics*. Mahwah, NJ: Erlbaum.

Hsieh, E. (2006) Conflicts in how interpreters manage their roles in provider–patient interactions. *Social Science and Medicine* 62 (3), 721–730.

Hsieh, E. (2008) 'I am not a robot!' Interpreters' views of their roles in health care settings. *Qualitative Health Research* 18 (10), 1367–1383.

Hsieh, E. (2009) Moving beyond a conduit model: Medical interpreters as mediators. In D.E. Brashers and D.J. Goldsmith (eds) *Communicating to Manage Health and Illness* (pp. 121–146). New York: Routledge.

Hsieh, E. (2010) Provider–interpreter collaboration in bilingual health care: Competitions of control over interpreter-mediated interactions. *Patient Education and Counseling* 78 (2), 154–159.

Hsieh, E. (2015) Not just 'getting by': Factors influencing providers' choice of interpreters. *Journal of General Internal Medicine* 30 (1), 75–82.

Hsieh, E. (2016) *Bilingual Health Communication: Working with Interpreters in Cross-cultural Care*. New York: Routledge.

Hsieh, E. and Kramer, E.M. (2012) Medical interpreters as tools: Dangers and challenges in the utilitarian approach to interpreters' roles and functions. *Patient Education and Counseling* 89 (1), 158–162.

Hsieh, E., Ju, H. and Kong, H. (2010) Dimensions of trust: The tensions and challenges in provider–interpreter trust. *Qualitative Health Research* 20 (2), 170–181.

Kong, H. and Hsieh, E. (2012) The social meanings of traditional Chinese medicine: Elderly Chinese immigrants' health practice in the United States. *Journal of Immigrant and Minority Health* 14 (5), 841–849.

Kramer, E.M. (2013) Dimensional accrual and dissociation: An introduction. In J. Grace and E.M. Kramer (eds) *Communication, Comparative Cultures, and Civilizations* (Vol. 3, pp. 123–184). New York: Hampton.

Laidsaar-Powell, R.C., Butow, P.N., Bu, S., Charles, C., Gafni, A., Lam, W.W.T., Jansen, J. McCaffery, K.J., Shepherd, H.L., Tattersall, M.H. and Juraskova, I. (2013) Physician–patient–companion communication and decision-making: A systematic review of triadic medical consultations. *Patient Education and Counseling* 91 (1), 3–13.

Leanza, Y., Boivin, I. and Rosenberg, E. (2010) Interruptions and resistance: A comparison of medical consultations with family and trained interpreters. *Social Science and Medicine* 70 (12), 1888–1895.

Lo, M.C. and Bahar, R. (2013) Resisting the colonization of the lifeworld? Immigrant patients' experiences with co-ethnic healthcare workers. *Social Science and Medicine* 87, 68–76.

Ma, G.X. (1999) Between two worlds: The use of traditional and Western health services by Chinese immigrants. *Journal of Community Health* 24 (6), 421–437.

Mason, I. and Ren, W. (2012) Power in face-to-face interpreting events. *Translation and Interpreting Studies* 7 (2), 234–253.

Metzger, M. (1999) *Sign Language Interpreting: Deconstructing the Myth of Neutrality*. Washington, DC: Gallaudet University Press.

Miller, K. and Zook, E.G. (1997) Care partners for persons with AIDS: Implications for health communication. *Journal of Applied Communication Research* 25 (1), 57–74.
Muller, J.H. and Desmond, B. (1992) Ethical dilemmas in a cross-cultural context: A Chinese example. *Western Journal of Medicine* 157 (3), 323–327.
Nugus, P., Greenfield, D., Travaglia, J., Westbrook, J. and Braithwaite, J. (2010) How and where clinicians exercise power: Interprofessional relations in health care. *Social Science and Medicine* 71 (5), 898–909.
O'Leary, S.C.B., Federico, S. and Hampers, L.C. (2003) The truth about language barriers: One residency program's experience. *Pediatrics* 111 (5 Pt 1), e569–573.
Pöchhacker, F. and Shlesinger, M. (2005) Introduction: Discourse-based research on healthcare interpreting. *Interpreting* 7 (2), 157–165.
Raven, B.H. (1993) The bases of power: Origins and recent developments. *Journal of Social Issues* 49 (4), 227–251.
Rees, C.E. and Bath, P.A. (2000) Meeting the information needs of adult daughters of women with early breast cancer: Patients and health care professionals as information providers. *Cancer Nursing* 23 (1), 71–79.
Robb, N. and Greenhalgh, T. (2006) 'You have to cover up the words of the doctor': The mediation of trust in interpreted consultations in primary care. *Journal of Health Organization and Management* 20 (5), 434–455.
Roy, C.B. (2000) *Interpreting as a Discourse Process*. New York: Oxford University Press.
Ryan, R.M. and Deci, E.L. (2011) A self-determination theory perspective on social, institutional, cultural, and economic supports for autonomy and their importance for well-being. In V.I. Chirkov, R.M. Ryan and K.M. Sheldon (eds) *Human Autonomy in Cross-cultural Context* (Vol. 1, pp. 45–64). New York: Springer.
Seale, C., Rivas, C., Al-Sarraj, H., Webb, S. and Kelly, M. (2013) Moral mediation in interpreted health care consultations. *Social Science and Medicine* 98, 141–148.
Shaw, S.J., Huebner, C., Armin, J., Orzech, K. and Vivian, J. (2009) The role of culture in health literacy and chronic disease screening and management. *Journal of Immigrant and Minority Health* 11 (6), 460–467.
Sudore, R.L., Landefeld, C.S., Pérez-Stable, E.J., Bibbins-Domingo, K., Williams, B.A. and Schillinger, D. (2009) Unraveling the relationship between literacy, language proficiency, and patient–physician communication. *Patient Education and Counseling* 75 (3), 398–402.
Thompson, D.A., Hernandez, R.G., Cowden, J.D., Sisson, S.D. and Moon, M. (2013) Caring for patients with limited English proficiency: Are residents prepared to use medical interpreters? *Academic Medicine* 88 (10), 1485–1492.
Todres, L., Galvin, K. and Dahlberg, K. (2007) Lifeworld-led healthcare: Revisiting a humanising philosophy that integrates emerging trends. *Medicine, Health Care and Philosophy* 10 (1), 53–63.
Tracy, K. (2013) *Everyday Talk: Building and Reflecting Identities* (2nd ed.). New York: Guilford.
Valero-Garcés, C. (2005) Doctor–patient consultations in dyadic and triadic exchanges. *Interpreting* 7 (2), 193–210.
Wade, C., Chao, M.T. and Kronenberg, F. (2007) Medical pluralism of Chinese women living in the United States. *Journal of Immigrant and Minority Health* 9 (4), 255–267.
Wadensjö, C. (1998) *Interpreting as Interaction*. London: Longman.
Williams, G., Teixeira, P., Carraça, E. and Resnicow, K. (2011) Physical wellness, health care, and personal autonomy. In V.I. Chirkov, R.M. Ryan and K.M. Sheldon (eds) *Human Autonomy in Cross-cultural Context* (Vol. 1, pp. 133–162). New York: Springer.
Zimányi, K. (2013) Somebody has to be in charge of a session: On the control of communication in interpreter-mediated mental health encounters. *Translation and Interpreting Studies* 8 (1), 94–111.

4 Challenges to and Recommendations for Working with a Community Interpreter in Mental Health: A Canadian Perspective

Yvan Leanza, Camille Brisset, Rhéa Rocque and Alexandra Boilard

Introduction

World migration is perpetually increasing and will reach the spectacular number of 1 billion people by 2050,[1] according to the United Nations Development Programme (2009); one-third of this population will be international migrants. These migration trends have major impacts on host societies requiring them to re-evaluate their migration and integration policies in order to integrate these new residents into their societies and to adapt their public institutions to this growing sociocultural and linguistic diversity.

Belonging to an immigrant, refugee, indigenous, ethnic or linguistic minority group can be a risk and/or a protective health factor. This is epitomized by the 'healthy im/migrant effect', which describes the phenomenon of how immigration is a protective health factor soon after immigration, but then becomes a risk factor as the health of immigrants deteriorates over time spent in the host society (Gushulak *et al.*, 2011; McDonald & Kennedy, 2004; Newbold, 2005).

This healthy migrant effect may not hold when it comes to mental health, however; the prevalence of depression seems to be lower among several minority ethnic groups in Canada in comparison to the majority ethnic group (White people with English, French or other European ancestors; Wu *et al.*, 2003). Nevertheless, research also indicates that ethnic minorities are less likely to access mental health services than are people belonging to the majority group, and when ethnic minorities do access care, they are more likely to receive lower-quality services (Whitley *et al.*, 2006). In addition, not all minority groups are the same; while some ethnic minority groups have better mental health than the majority group, some are at greater risk of mental health problems. For example, non-English-speaking immigrants are more at risk of emotional problems than English-speaking Canadians and immigrants (Kopec *et al.*, 2001). A similar trend has been observed with immigrants who do not master one of the official languages of Canada (Pottie *et al.*, 2008) as they report lower health status than individuals who master English or French.

Some healthcare professionals have described work with patients with whom no verbal communication is possible as *veterinary medicine* (e.g. Drennan & Swartz, 1999), as a means of drawing attention to the fact that providing care in a language that a patient can understand is critical to human health care. The ethical necessity to address language barriers is obvious: without clear communication, provided through a community interpreter, there cannot be adequate health care (Blake, 2003). Healthcare systems need to ensure equal access to their services and equal quality of services to their nation's inhabitants who speak none of the official languages (Bezuidenhout & Borry, 2009; Bjorn, 2005). Most of the procedures ensuring quality and equality of care (informed consent, diagnostic and treatment explanations, etc.) depend on verbal interactions with patients (Bowen, 2001).

What Exactly are Community Interpreters and What do They do?

Today, interpreting occurs in many fields, such as trade, military, development promotion, research, courts, conferences and community. The last three settings have been the subject of scientific investigations for the past few decades. Conference interpreting, the most known type of interpreting, has been a particular focus of researchers and is considered as the gold standard for all interpreting independently of the field. However, there also exists *community interpreting*. 'In the most general sense, [it] refers to interpreting in institutional settings of a given society in which public service providers and individual clients do not speak the same language' (Pöchhacker, 1999: 126). The community interpreter is sometimes called a *dialogue interpreter* because s/he interprets a discussion between two people. In the French literature, the term *social environment interpreter* [*interprète en milieu social*] is also used (Jiménez-Salcedo, 2014b), and the term *public service interpreters* can be found in some European countries. These designations reflect fundamental differences between community and conference interpreters, who may have access to the text of the talk before it is actually given in front of an audience and for whom there is little or no interaction between the speaker and the audience.

In the mid-1990s, a small group of academics started to investigate the different forms of community interpreting. Their object of study switched from texts, the 'classical' study object of translatology, to spoken discourse and from interpreters as complex translating machines to interpreters as interacting individuals, with an emphasis on their psychosocial roles. These investigators applied sociological and anthropological methods and theories to this work. This change of focus to community interpreting is referred to as the 'cultural turn' in interpreting studies (Pöchhacker, 2004). These new empirical data demonstrated that community interpreters played a very active role during the triadic interaction as opposed to taking a neutral stance. For example, the pioneering work of Cecilia Wadensjö (1998) described how interpreters were not only *translators* (relaying the respective utterances), but also *coordinators* of the flow of speech in the dialogue. Another example is Claudio Baraldi and Laura Gavioli's (2007: 171) description of the *responder* stance in which the interpreter 'gets an access to the emotions of the interlocutors and is thus in a position to provide her/his own understanding, support and confirmation of them'. Beyond the strictly linguistic aspects, different factors will influence the interpreter's position in the interaction, such as one's status (professional or untrained), gender, age and socioeconomic status (Leanza *et al.*, 2014a). All of these factors will organize the relational dynamic in the consultation room. For example, when a child has to interpret for one of his parents, or when a male interpreter has to interpret for a female patient consulting for gynecological issues, the relational dynamic will most probably be affected in a way that is most likely not to the patient's advantage.

In light of these findings, the assumption that interpreters should be totally neutral is unrealistic. Despite these findings, neutrality remains one of the most prevalent imperatives in ethical codes and professional standards of community interpreters around the world (Bancroft, 2005). As interpreters cannot be entirely neutral, they can play a wide range of possible roles. If recognized, these roles could be beneficial to the interpreted interaction. Interpreters' roles have been described in different typologies (see Brisset *et al.*, 2013, for a review) and could be organized

> along a continuum between alliance with and serving the needs of the system (healthcare institutions) and the lifeworld (patient's life context and narrative about health and illness; Brisset *et al.*, 2013). Interpreters' stance oscillates along this continuum, like a pendulum. (Leanza *et al.*, 2015: 354)

Interpreting in Public Institutions in Canada

The Canadian Charter of Rights and Freedoms dictates that an interpreter is necessary when a witness or a party does not understand or speak the language of any legal proceedings (article 14). This principle of facilitated linguistic access has been interpreted to apply to all public services (Jiménez-Salcedo, 2014a). Furthermore, Canada's common law establishes that, in cases where a patient has not mastered the physician's language, the physician is responsible for the patient's understanding of the clinical situation (diagnostic, consent and treatment; Bowen, 2001). In addition, all healthcare practitioners are bound by ethical codes to provide the best quality of care to all patients, making it their duty to overcome potential language barriers (Bowen, 2001).

In Canada, interpreting services are organized at the provincial level, and all but one of the 10 Canadian provinces offer this service.[2] These services are usually maintained by one or more non-governmental or non-profit organizations. Not all provinces have developed policies to regulate interpreting practices in public institutions, including health care. As a consequence, the quality of services across provinces is variable owing to differences in requirements for interpreter training (which are sometimes zero), the range and diversity of available languages, the dissemination of information about the services, the knowledge of the procedures to access linguistic services among healthcare practitioners, etc. In an effort to standardize and professionalize community interpreting, the Language Industry Association of Canada (AILIA[3]) undertook a national initiative to develop standards for interpreting in public institutions in Canada.[4] The result was the National Standard Guide for Community Interpreting Services in 2007. AILIA now provides accreditation to organizations following this guide. However, this accreditation is not mandatory to offer interpreting services in public institutions and very few organizations have been accredited. Most of them are located in the Toronto and Vancouver areas. AILIA also promotes a model in which community interpreter training would be offered at a post-secondary level, with four levels of training. The first level includes 180 hours of training, language interpreter tests, English proficiency test and 200 hours of documented interpreting experience. The final level comprises a specialization in medical, legal or social services interpreting. It includes 1500 hours of documented interpreting experience and a 120 hours medical, legal or social curriculum. According to the AILIA website, only a few colleges in Ontario offer such training.

Research in Healthcare Interpreting in Canada

The first studies about interpreting in health care in Canada were done by the anthropologist Joseph Kaufert and his colleagues in Manitoba (Kaufert & Koolage, 1984; Kaufert *et al.*, 1984; O'Neil, 1989). This work is acknowledged as one of the foundational investigations on healthcare community interpreting. Joseph Kaufert studied First Nation interpreters' role conflict and the sociocultural, ethical and political implications of their presence in health care (Kaufert, 1999; Kaufert et al., 1999). He demonstrated how pressures from the healthcare system, interpreters and patients' communities create role conflict for interpreters which impacts quality of care. He also described how interpreters could act as a mediator in very sensitive or difficult communication, such as in palliative care. Kaufert's colleague, John D. O'Neil (1989), promoted the role of patient advocate for Inuit interpreters as a means of improving patient satisfaction with care in the context of low intercultural understanding between healthcare practitioners and their patients.

There have been surprisingly few studies conducted in the field of healthcare interpreting in Canada since the publication of these seminal works. The most recent studies have been conducted mostly in the French-speaking province of Quebec, which does not yet have a policy to regulate and organize community interpreters' activities. These studies mainly address language barriers in the context of family medicine (Leanza et al., 2010, 2013, 2014b; Rosenberg et al., 2007, 2008, 2011), but also nursing, although to a lesser extent (Labun, 1999; this research is the only study conducted outside of Quebec; Vissandjee et al., 1998). Mental health interpreting was a completely unexplored field before Leanza, Brisset and colleagues' work in Montreal and Quebec City areas (Brisset et al., 2014; Leanza et al., 2015; Leanza et al., 2014a).

Research and Recommendations for (Mental Health) Care Interpreting: Successful Examples of Building a Partnership

Verbal communication is particularly vital in mental health care, even if such care involves non-verbal techniques such as art therapy. Successful communication of complex ideas and feelings is essential in assessment and treatment of mental disorders. Patient and therapist must be able to express and comprehend subtle distinctions and to express and respond to intense emotions. Twenty-five years ago, a US psychiatrist, Joseph Westermeyer, a specialist in refugee health, published one of the first reflective papers offering his view and recommendations relating to working with interpreters in mental health (Westermeyer, 1989, 1990). Since then, many other manuscripts from different locations around the world, including research papers and at least two literature reviews (Bauer & Alegría, 2010; Searight & Armock, 2013), have been made available. As a result of a growing interest in research in the field of community interpreting in mental health, two main questions may now be answered for the Canadian/Quebec context: how did institutional and practice responses to linguistic diversity evolve; and what are the recommendations on how to work with interpreters in mental health that researchers put forward according to their results? Since most Canadian research in this field has been conducted in the province of Quebec, the answers to the previous questions will be provided as a function of the Quebec context.

The province of Quebec has a public healthcare system. The State acts as primary insurer and administrator, and its funding comes through general taxation, thus ensuring accessibility to health care for all, regardless of income level. The public healthcare system provides a range of psychosocial services for both the general population and vulnerable groups, including 'Interpreters' Banks'. Established in 1993, the mission of the Montreal Interregional Interpreters' Bank is to promote access to care for individuals who do not speak any of the official languages of Canada (i.e. who speak neither French nor English), and to facilitate communication, both verbally and culturally. Interpretation services are currently available in more than 50 languages (Agence de la santé et des services sociaux de Montréal, 2014). Interpreters recruited by the Interregional Interpreters' Bank must take a 45 hour course in community interpreting at the University of Montreal and pass a language proficiency test for the language they wish to interpret, as well as French or English. Other interpreter banks are also available outside of Montreal. They are managed by community organizations in collaboration with Health and Social Services Agencies. Interpreters' training modalities are unique to each organization and do not follow particular standards.

To better understand the needs of primary mental health providers and how they provide care to individuals who encounter language barriers in Montreal, we surveyed more than 100 practitioners about available linguistic resources, their views of the roles of interpreters and how they use interpreters in the mental health context (Brisset et al., 2014).

We found these providers have significant unmet needs in addressing language barriers. While practitioners considered the use of professional interpreting services as best practice, none of them were trained on how to work with interpreters or how to access them. They usually did not know whether interpreters they used in consultations were professional or untrained, ad hoc interpreters. When practitioners do know the type of interpreter, it is more frequently a family member, which is consistent with the existing literature (Brisset et al., 2014). The less frequent use of professional interpreters was due to a lack of knowledge about the availability of interpreter services and the complexity of procedures that providers said they had to go through to access them. Also, it is probable that practitioners prefer patients' relatives as they have the advantage of being present at the same time as the patients and at each visit, and a relationship of trust is already established between the patient and the family member (Edwards et al., 2005).

One of our hypotheses was that, the more patients with a language barrier providers saw, the more they would be aware of available linguistic resources. It was not confirmed. We found that only one-third of providers were aware of the available resources, regardless of the number of their patients needing interpreting. The financial cost associated with interpreting service was mentioned as an additional obstacle, which is paradoxical for two reasons. First, such services reduce long-term costs. More precisely, the initial cost certainly appears to be higher but the use of a professional interpreter allows a problem to be targeted faster and unnecessary medical examinations or hospitalizations avoided (Bischoff & Denhaerynck, 2010; Hampers & McNulty, 2002). Second, the cost of interpreters is covered by the healthcare system. However, practitioners might be put under pressure not to use interpreters by team coordinators, who have to manage limited and ever reducing budgets. Also, most family physicians (about half of our respondent) work in clinics outside of institutions, and they are paid a fee for each healthcare service by the Quebec health insurance plan. If they were to hire interpreters, they would pay these costs themselves. The cost of an interpreter is equal to the average cost of most clinic visits.

With regard to interpreting in mental health, access to emotions and transmitting empathy were considered difficult tasks for the practitioners. Continuity, i.e. having the same interpreter with the same patient throughout the care process, appears crucial, just as much as the need for the interpreter to possess basic knowledge in mental health. Based on participants' responses, the ideal interpreter would be a professional interpreter who specializes in mental health, who is familiar with both the patient's and the host society's culture, and who possesses abilities to navigate the different layers of the healthcare system. Practitioners in this study expected interpreters to engage in expanded roles beyond neutral transmission of information from one language to another. They indicated that interpreters should translate everything said with precision, without adding anything, while giving sociocultural information about the patient, and that they should be neutral, while being empathetic. These expectations are contradictory and need to be discussed between interpreters and practitioners to avoid any misunderstanding. Such clarification requires being aware of the different roles that interpreters can play, which is not necessarily the case for practitioners and interpreters themselves.

We also conducted semi-structured interviews with 23 first-line practitioners, mainly social workers, psychologists and physicians, and asked them to describe situations in which they had established an effective collaboration with interpreter. Thirty examples were collected and analyzed so as to be able to describe the characteristics of an effective collaboration. Interestingly, participants viewed the interpreter as a healthcare professional who needs to be included in the team. The healthcare organization should allow such an integration of the interpreter. As a corollary to this integration, collaboration is also more effective when continuity is possible, i.e. when the same interpreter interprets for a patient across appointments. In the same vein, some practitioners thought that interpreters are essential and should be considered as stakeholders in the consultation. They stressed the importance of trust, which develops over time. Practitioners also emphasized the importance of a good spatial organization. The principle is quite simple: regardless of the seat arrangement, no one should be in a position to block the communication or to be excluded from it. The interpreter needs to possess knowledge in mental health, and interpreting, as well as linguistic and cultural specificities relating to the patient's background. The interpreter must also have professional qualities, such as punctuality, and must show humane feelings. In complex situations like major mental health issues or abuse, a strong and trusting collaboration with the interpreter becomes particularly important. An interpreter's help is also very much appreciated with individuals whose immigration status is precarious. Interpreters who have knowledge of the immigration procedures and difficulties may be highly relevant to healthcare practitioners.

Two necessary requirements for the development of a collaborative relationship between interpreters and practitioners have been identified by other studies. Nurses in the US and Canada (Labun, 1999) and psychotherapists in the UK (Raval & Smith, 2003) reported, as did the above-mentioned practitioners in Montreal and Quebec City, that it is necessary to have enough time for interpreters and practitioners to work together (before, during and after an encounter) and to have continuity in the relationship (working with the same interpreter). This is how the interpreter becomes fully part of the interaction, and the practitioners and interpreters can both learn to refine the interpretive process in order to use their shared knowledge and expertise for the benefit of the patient. These conditions are not often encountered. Employing in-house interpreters was suggested as a solution and could facilitate the development of clinical competencies while increasing the continuity of the relationship (Raval & Smith, 2003).

In a context with favorable conditions, working with interpreters is not only essential, but is also conducive to creating better conditions for intercultural care. For example, experienced nurses interviewed by Labun (1999) describe a type of collaboration that the researcher termed 'shared brokering'. This type of collaboration is developed only if three conditions are met: (a) time is allowed to build a trusting relationship between nurses and the interpreters; (b) nurses understand the complexity of interpreters' roles and work; and (c) interpreters understand and are able to work with nurses' values and beliefs and at the same time are seen as knowledgeable in their own community. Interpreters can also play important roles outside the consultations. Chen Wu et al. (2006) organized continuing education (in a US university hospital) for physicians and asked interpreters to offer this training. Interpreters taught basic notions of the Spanish language and sensitized physicians to educational practices and care techniques of Latin-American parents. This resulted in a significant increase in parents' satisfaction with the consultations in this paediatric hospital. This example reveals the great potential to be gained in the collaboration between interpreters (here in the role of culture brokers) and practitioners.

Altogether, it seems that an effective collaboration with an interpreter in mental health (or in any other healthcare specialty) requires a flexible and sensitive system that will acknowledge the necessity of working closely with interpreters. The building of trust between interpreters and practitioners, a fundamental characteristic of interpreted healthcare consultations (Brisset et al., 2013), is also necessary. Building trust nevertheless takes time, and time is a rare commodity in public healthcare systems. Practitioners' representations of the interpreter depict someone who is very humane and who possesses knowledge about culture, migration processes and status, interpreting and mental health, and who is able to navigate the healthcare system. They also need to adjust their practice to situations: the more complex the situation, the more flexible their roles might be. Only highly trained interpreters, with at least a college degree and a mental health expertise, can match this description of a qualified mental health interpreter. Such interpreters are very rare in Canada, and even rarer in the province of Quebec as there are no post-secondary community interpreter training programs.

How to Work with a Community Interpreter in Mental Health

According to the literature, mental health practitioners seem to be more flexible about interpreters' roles than other healthcare practitioners. The addition of text to the dialogue by an interpreter or playing the role of cultural informant and/or co-therapist is accepted in the mental healthcare context more readily and even recommended under certain conditions (Darling, 2004; Hémon, 2001; Loshak, 2003; Mudarikiri, 2002; Rousseau et al., 2011; Westermeyer, 1989). Clinicians from two transcultural mental health clinics in Paris and in Montreal report nuanced interpreter roles and activities which are perceived as more complex (Leanza et al., 2015) than what the overused and inappropriate conduit metaphor suggests (Reddy, 1993). Although mental health practitioners are more open to interpreters' involvement in the therapeutic process, some still exhibit resistance to it, as they view it as an intrusion (Raval & Smith, 2003).

Considering the ethical issues that may arise in psychotherapy with an interpreter, Wright (2014) provides recommendations regarding: (a) psychologist's competencies; (b) delegation of work to others; and (c) multiple roles. For psychologist's competencies, the author suggests, as do many others, including work with interpreters in basic and continuous training and in supervision. This might include the building of a relationship with interpreters in order to enhance the working alliance (Leanza, 2005). Including an interpreter in a psychotherapeutic process is equivalent to delegating a part of this work, and it might entail multiple roles conflict. As such, the psychologist must:

(1) ensure the interpreter has received the proper training to interpret in the mental healthcare context;
(2) abstain from being the interpreter's trainer in order to avoid role conflict with him/her;
(3) arrange a formal written agreement with the interpreter or his/her agency regarding maintaining confidentiality, training and supervision, as well as role boundaries;
(4) obtain informed consent from the patient in order 'to clarify the roles of the interpreter and psychologist, discuss the confidentiality obligations of both the psychologist and the interpreter, explain the circumstances in which the interpreter and psychologist may communicate outside of sessions, and describe the limits to client confidentiality' (Wright, 2014: 225);
(5) prepare the interpreter before consultations, for issues that may arise in the encounter, and debrief with them afterwards to identify issues that they may have missed or to coach the interpreter to refine the partnership.

This last point is probably the most common recommendation found in the literature. There are steps to take before, during and after the consultation (see Leanza *et al.*, 2014a: 98–101, for a detailed description). Before the consultation, it is usually recommended that the interpreter be provided with some information about the patient and about the consultation (what is expected in this particular consultation). It is also highly recommended to ask the interpreter whether s/he has any link with the patient, and whether s/he has received any kind of training to interpret. This information will orient the way the consultation will be directed. The interpreter should also be informed of the style of interpreting the practitioner is at ease with (translation only or possibility of adding text, how and when). Finally, the interpreter must be asked to warn the practitioner when some words or expressions are used that are difficult to translate accurately. During the consultation, the practitioner needs to use simple and short sentences and be aware of his/her communication style (direct or indirect), which will have an effect on the interpreting process. If the patient and the interpreter are having several exchanges in their language, the practitioner could interrupt and ask for the interaction to be translated. After the consultation, it is essential to ask the interpreter how s/he feels and whether s/he has something to add, for example about parts of the consultation that might have been difficult to translate, metaphors that were used by the patient and their possible meanings, or observations about the patient's non-verbal behavior. It is important that practitioners and interpreters also be aware of specificities depending on the psychotherapeutic orientation or setting (psychodynamic, CBT, family or group therapy; Leanza *et al.*, 2014a: 105–109). This last point, combined with assessment challenges, is probably what most distinguishes interpreting in mental health from other specialties in health care.

Assessment is a crucial activity in any mental health process, and assessing patients in the context of a language barrier can be a real challenge. Again, very few recommendations have been provided pertaining to mental health evaluations with the help of an interpreter (Leanza *et al.*, 2014a: 101–104). Practitioners need to attend to both the denotative and connotative meanings of language, styles of emotion expression and linguistic idioms. During the assessment, the interpreter could be of invaluable help to explain the nuances of words and emotions. In order to be effective, interpreters need to be alert to regional accents, dialects and implications of language for social status (both their own and that of the patient). They can provide information on cultural norms of communication that can assist in determining whether specific behaviors or experiences are unusual and if the evaluation context is adequate or unfamiliar for the patient, which will have dramatic consequences on his/her performance. Ideally, interpreters also need to possess observational skills as well as knowledge of psychopathology so that they can help the clinician recognize specific symptoms. During the assessment session, the patient might switch from one language to another. This conveys important information about the emotional meaning of specific memories and experiences as well as about the patient's efforts to position themselves in the clinical interaction.

Of course, these recommendations, aimed at practitioners, are fruitless if there is no supporting context for practitioners to incorporate them into their practice and maintain them over time. Institutions and governments need to promulgate policies that will enforce the use of interpreters. In order to do so, linguistic needs and resources must first be evaluated, and such resources should be reorganized to make them easier to access. Furthermore, a budget must be allocated for training and hiring interpreters. Training, as mentioned previously, should be offered not only to interpreters but also to practitioners and all other institutional staff. Gatekeepers and frontline workers should also receive training since their duty is to evaluate the patient's need for interpreting services. The next important step, at least for Canadian healthcare public institutions, is to recognize interpreters as invaluable professionals and to integrate them in the clinical teams.

In recent decades, research on interpreting has focused on interpreters' roles, communication characteristics and difficulties separately (Brisset *et al.*, 2013). Research projects combining two or three of these themes would help understand in more depth the complexities of interpreted consultation dynamics. The focus has also been on interpreters and practitioners, but rarely on patients. Better understanding patients' perspectives on receiving care through an interpreter would be very useful for drawing fine-tuned recommendations, especially in working with ad hoc interpreters. Moreover, very few international comparative studies have been conducted. Such studies may provide knowledge about what is universal and particular in healthcare interpreting. They also would help in understanding how the sociopolitical context shapes interpreting practices. However, research results from more recent interpreting studies tend to repeat themselves from one study to another. In order to ensure that the field keeps progressing, it would be relevant to experiment with new ways of integrating interpreters in clinical teams. Action research is probably the most promising path for this, as it allows observation of how practice changes affect different outcomes. These types of studies could aim to provide training, supervision and case discussion workshops to clinical teams that integrate interpreters, thus considering interpreters as members of the team. In turn, researchers could measure the impact of this integration on patients' health, on communication dynamics and on practitioners', interpreters' and patients' satisfaction. Such studies would provide valuable data concerning ways to offer appropriate care involving interpreters. After all, considering the worldwide migration phenomenon, interpreted consultations will become, more and more, part of healthcare practitioners' daily routine.

In other words, it is not only about establishing effective, creative and trusting interpersonal collaborations between the interpreter and the practitioner, but it is also about providing each practitioner and interpreter with the necessary conditions to develop innovative practices. It is about transforming the representations of the interpreter and of his/her place in interventions. This change is possible and would also be very satisfying for the different protagonists in the interpreting trio (Miller *et al.*, 2005). This is possible only if all decision-making levels are involved and work toward establishing courageous guidelines that will influence training, practices, institutional and social norms, and research programs.

Notes

(1) This number includes all kind of migrants: internally displaced, refugees, workers with a legal permit, etc.
(2) A list of the main services is provided at http://www.multiculturalmentalhealth.ca/services/find-an-interpreter/
(3) The mission of AILIA is to promote and increase the competitiveness of the Canadian language industry nationally and internationally. As English and French are the two official languages in Canada, AILIA acronym is bilingual and stands for 'Association de l'Industrie de la Langue/Language Industry Association'.
(4) See AILIA website for detailed information and the National Standard Guide for Community Interpreting Services: http://www.ailia.ca/Home

References

Agence de la santé et des services sociaux de Montréal (2014) *La Banque interrégionale d'interprètes: pour comprendre, pour être compris.* Québec: Gouvernement du Québec.

Bancroft, M. (2005) *The Interpreter's World Tour: An Environmental Scan of Standards of Practice for Interpreters* (p. 54). Ellicott City, MD: National Council on Interpreting in Health Care.

Baraldi, C. and Gavioli, L. (2007) Dialogue interpreting as intercultural mediation. An analysis in healthcare multicultural settings. In M. Grein and E. Weigand (eds) *Dialogue and Culture* (pp. 155-175). Amsterdam: John Benjamins.

Bauer, A. and Alegría, M. (2010) Impact of patient language proficiency and interpreter service use on the quality of psychiatric care: A systematic review. *Psychiatric Services* 61 (8), 765-773; doi: 10.1176/appi.ps.61.8.765.

Bezuidenhout, L. and Borry, P. (2009) Examining the role of informal interpretation in medical interviews. *Journal of Medical Ethics* 35 (3), 159-162; doi: 10.1136/jme.2008.026286

Bischoff, A. and Denhaerynck, K. (2010) What do language barriers cost? An exploratory study among asylum seekers in Switzerland. *BMC Health Service Research* 10, 248; doi: 10.1186/1472-6963-10-248

Bjorn, G. (2005) Ethics and interpreting in psychotherapy with refugee children and families. *Nordic Journal of Psychiatry* 59 (6), 516-521; doi: 10.1080/08039480500360740

Blake, C. (2003) Ethical considerations in working with culturally diverse populations: The essential role of professional interpreters. *Bulletin de l'Association des psychiatres du Canada* juin, 21-23.

Bowen, S. (2001) *Barrières linguistiques dans l'accès aux soins de santé* (p. 155). Ottawa: Santé Canada.

Brisset, C., Leanza, Y. and Laforest, K. (2013) Working with interpreters in health care: A systematic review and meta-ethnography of qualitative studies. *Patient Education and Counseling* 91 (2), 131-140; doi: 10.1016/j.pec.2012.11.008

Brisset, C., Leanza, Y., Rosenberg, E., Vissandjee, B., Kirmayer, L.J., Muckle, G., Xenocostas, S. and Laforce, H. (2014) Language barriers in mental health care: A survey of primary care practitioners. *Journal of Immigrant and Minoritty Health* 16 (6), 1238-1246; doi: 10.1007/s10903-013-9971-9

Chen Wu, A., Leventhal, J., Ortiz, J., Gonzalez, E. and Forsyth, B. (2006) The interpreter as cultural educator of residents: Improving communication for Latino parents. *Archives of Pediatric and Adolescent Medicine* 160 (11), 1145-1150.

Darling, L. (2004) Psychoanalytically-informed work with interpreters. *Psychoanalytic Psychotherapy* 18 (3), 255-267.

Drennan, G. and Swartz, L. (1999) A concept over-burdened: Institutional roles for psychiatric interpreters in Post-Apartheid South Africa. *Interpreting* 4 (2), 169-198.

Edwards, R., Temple, B. and Alexander, C. (2005) Users' experiences of interpreters: The critical role of trust. *Interpreting* 7 (1), 77-95.

Gushulak, B.D., Pottie, K., Hatcher Roberts, J., Torres, S., DesMeules, M. and Canadian Collaboration for Immigrant and Refugee Health (2011) Migration and health in Canada: Health in the global village. *Canadian Medical Association Journal* 183 (12), E952-958; doi: 10.1503/cmaj.090287

Hampers, L. and McNulty, J. (2002) Professional interpreters and bilingual physicians in a pediatric emergency department: Effect on resource utilization. *Archives of Pediatrics and Adolescent Medicine* 156 (11), 1108-1113.

Hémon, E. (2001) Le temps des migrants; les temps de l'exil. *Thérapie familiale* 22 (2), 169-186.

Jiménez-Salcedo, J. (2014a) Politiques linguistiques et interprétation en milieu social au Canada: des droits linguistiques aux droits d'accès aux services publics. *Çédille – Revista de estudios franceses, Monografías* 4, 131-147.

Jiménez-Salcedo, J. (2014b) Pour un discours francophone autour de l'interprétation en milieu social. *Çédille – Revista de estudios franceses, Monografías* 4, 5-8.

Kaufert, J. (1999) Cultural mediation in cancer diagnosis and end of life decision-making: The experience of aboriginal patients in Canada. *Anthropology and Medicine* 6 (3), 405–421.

Kaufert, J. and Koolage, W. (1984) Role conflict among 'culture brokers': The experience of native Canadian medical interpreters. *Social Science and Medicine* 18 (3), 283–286.

Kaufert, J., Koolage, W., Kaufert, P. and O'Neil, J. (1984) The use of 'trouble case' examples in teaching the impact of socio-cultural and political factors in clinical communication. *Medical Anthropology* 8, 36–45.

Kaufert, J., Putsch, R. and Lavallee, M. (1999) End-of-life decision making among Aboriginal Canadians: Interpretation, mediation, and discord in the communication of 'bad news'. *Journal of Palliative Care* 15 (1), 31–38.

Kopec, J., Williams, J., To, T. and Austin, P. (2001) Cross-cultural comparisons of health status in Canada using the Health Utilities Index. *Ethnicity and Health* 6 (1), 41–50; doi: 10.1080/13557850125061

Labun, E. (1999) Shared brokering: The development of a nurse/interpreter partnership. *Journal of Immigrant Health* 1 (4), 215–222.

Leanza, Y. (2005) Roles of community interpreters in pediatrics as seen by interpreters, physicians and researchers. *Interpreting* 7 (2), 167–192.

Leanza, Y., Boivin, I. and Rosenberg, E. (2010) Interruptions and resistance: A comparison of medical consultations with family and trained interpreters. *Social Science and Medicine* 70 (12), 1888–1895.

Leanza, Y., Boivin, I. and Rosenberg, E. (2013) Patients' lifeworld: Building meaningful clinical encounters between patients, physicians and interpreters. *Communication and Medicine* 10 (1), 81–93.

Leanza, Y., Miklavcic, A., Boivin, I. and Rosenberg, E. (2014a) Working with interpreters. In L. Kirmayer, C. Rousseau and J. Guzder (eds) *Cultural Consultation: Encountering the Other in Mental Health Care* (pp. 89–114). New York: Springer Science and Business Media.

Leanza, Y., Rizkallah, E. and Michaud Labonté, T. (2014b) Intégrer un interprète dans les consultations de médecine familiale: une analyse de discours assistée par ordinateur. *Çédille – Revista de estudios franceses Monografías* 4, 9–30.

Leanza, Y., Boivin, I., Moro, M.-R., Rousseau, C., Brisset, C., Rosenberg, E. and Hassan, G. (2015) Integration of interpreters in mental health interventions with children and adolescents: The need for a framework. *Transcultural Psychiatry* 52 (3), 353–375; doi: 10.1177/1363461514558137

Loshak, R. (2003) The role of the interpreter in child mental health: The changing landscape. In R. Tribe and H. Raval (eds) *Working with Interpreters in Mental Health* (pp. 151–167). Hove and New York: Brunner–Routledge.

McDonald, J. and Kennedy, S. (2004) Insights into the 'healthy immigrant effect': Health status and health service use of immigrants to Canada. *Social Science and Medicine* 59 (8), 1613–1627.

Miller, K., Martell, Z., Pazdirek, L., Caruth, M. and Lopez, D. (2005) The role of interpreters in psychotherapy with refugees: An exploratory study. *The American Journal of Orthopsychiatry* 75 (1), 27–39.

Mudarikiri, M. (2002) Working with the interpreter in adult mental health. In R. Tribe and H. Raval (eds) *Working with Interpreters in Mental Health* (pp. 182–197). Hove and New York: Brunner–Routledge.

Newbold, K.B. (2005) Self-rated health within the Canadian immigrant population: Risk and the healthy immigrant effect. *Social Science and Medicine* 60 (6), 1359–1370; doi: doi: 10.1016/j.socscimed.2004.06.048

O'Neil, J. (1989) The cultural and political context of patient dissatisfaction in cross-cultural clinical encounters: A Canadian Inuit study. *Medical Anthropology Quarterly* 3 (4), 325–344.

Pöchhacker, F. (1999) 'Getting organized': The evolution of community interpreting. *Interpreting* 4 (1), 125–140.

Pöchhacker, F. (2004) *Introducing Interpreting Studies*. London: Routledge.

Pottie, K., Ng, E., Spitzer, D., Mohammed, A. and Glazier, R. (2008) Language proficiency, gender and self-reported health: An analysis of the first two waves of the longitudinal survey of immigrants to Canada. *Canadian Journal of Public Health* 99 (6), 505–510.

Raval, H. and Smith, J. (2003) Therapists' experiences of working with language interpreters. *International Journal of Mental Health* 32 (2), 6–31.

Reddy, M.J. (1993) The conduit metaphor: A case of frame conflict in our language about language. In A. Ortony (ed.) *Metaphor and Thought* (2nd edn, pp. 164–201). Cambridge: Cambridge University Press.

Rosenberg, E., Leanza, Y. and Seller, R. (2007) Doctor–patient communication in primary care with an interpreter: Physician perceptions of professional and family interpreters. *Patient Education and Counseling* 67 (3), 286–292.

Rosenberg, E., Seller, R. and Leanza, Y. (2008) Through interpreters' eyes: Comparing roles of professional and family interpreters. *Patient Education and Counseling* 70 (1), 87–93.

Rosenberg, E., Richard, C., Lussier, M.-T. and Shuldiner, T. (2011) The content of talk about health conditions and medications during appointments involving interpreters. *Family Practice* 28 (3), 317–322; doi: 10.1093/fampra/cmq094

Rousseau, C., Measham, T. and Moro, M.-R. (2011) Working with interpreters in child mental health. *Child and Adolescent Mental Health* 16 (1), 55–59.

Searight, H. and Armock, J. (2013) Foreign language interpreters in mental health practice: A literature review and research agenda. *North American Journal of Psychology* 15 (1), 17–38.

United Nations Development Programme. (2009) *Human Development Report 2009. Overcoming Barriers: Human Mobility and Development* (p. 217). New York: United Nations Development Programme.

Vissandjee, B., Ntetu, A., Courville, F., Breton, E. and Bourdeau, M. (1998) L'interprete en milieu clinique interculturel. *The Canadian Nurse* 94 (5), 36–42.

Wadensjö, C. (1998) *Interpreting as Interaction*. London: Longman.

Westermeyer, J. (1989) *Psychiatric Care of Migrants: A Clinical Guide*. Washington, DC: American Psychiatric Press.

Westermeyer, J. (1990) Working with an interpreter in psychiatric assessment and treatment. *Journal of Nervous and Mental Disease* 178 (12), 745–749.

Whitley, R., Kirmayer, L. and Groleau, D. (2006) Understanding immigrants' reluctance to use mental health services: A qualitative study from Montreal. *The Canadian Journal of Psychiatry/La Revue canadienne de psychiatrie* 51 (4), 205–209.

Wright, C. (2014) Ethical issues and potential solutions surrounding the use of spoken language interpreters in psychology. *Ethics and Behavior* 24 (3), 215–228; doi: 10.1080/10508422.2013.845532

Wu, Z., Noh, S., Kaspar, V. and Schimmele, C. (2003) Race, ethnicity, and depression in Canadian society. *Journal of Health and Social Behavior* 44 (3), 426–441.

5 Toward a Theoretical Framework of Informal Interpreting in Health Care: Explaining the Effects of Role Conflict on Control, Power and Trust in Interpreter-mediated Encounters

Barbara Schouten

Informal interpreters, such as family members and bilingual healthcare staff, are commonly used to bridge the language barrier between patients with limited language proficiency in the dominant language and their healthcare providers. Despite an increasing body of research on informal interpreting in health care, the research field remains sparse and represents many different approaches owing to a lack of a theory-based framework on how informal interpreters may influence the healthcare interactions in which they participate. Developing such a framework could move the field from a predominantly descriptive one into a more explanatory one. The aim of this chapter is thus to build a theory-based framework of informal interpreting in health care, based on a review of the pertinent empirical and theoretical literature. The literature analysis focuses on discrepancies and commonalities between the perspectives and communicative behaviors of patients, informal interpreters and healthcare providers, and includes a much-needed explication of several theoretical constructs (i.e. interpreter roles, control and power dynamics during the medical encounter, and trust in the informal interpreter) that are known to play a fundamental part in interpreter-mediated health encounters. Based on the literature and issues that have arisen in the field, a theoretical framework of informal interpreting is proposed, which can be used in future research to further our understanding of how to develop effective interventions to improve the quality of health of patients with low language proficiency.

Introduction

> I never know whether these women want their husbands to accompany them or that these men think they ought to come along, to control part of the conversation. Maybe I should ask them at the start of the consultation: are you here just to translate?

These words, voiced by a Dutch female general practitioner who was part of a study on intercultural and bilingual competencies in health and social care (Meeuwesen & Twilt, 2011), reflect some of the fundamental issues that can arise when informal interpreters help low-language-proficient patients to communicate during the medical encounter. First, by stating her doubts about the motives of the husband to be present, the general practitioner hints at a possible lack of trust in informal interpreters. As building a relationship of trust not only plays a central role in fostering a good therapeutic alliance but is also a necessary prerequisite to achieve adequate health-related outcomes (Haes & Bensing, 2009; Pearson & Raeke, 2000; Robb & Greenhalgh, 2006), insufficient levels of trust of healthcare providers toward informal interpreters might seriously compromise the patient's health. Second, by stating that the husband might be present to 'control part of the conversation', she indirectly refers to a possible loss of control over the conversational content and flow for the patient (and possibly for herself as well). While issues of control and power asymmetry are a concern in all patient–doctor relationships (e.g. Stewart, 1995), the presence of an informal interpreter often changes the power balance between the interlocutors in favor of the patient, leaving the healthcare provider feeling powerless to deliver what they perceive to be good-quality health care (e.g. Greenhalgh et al., 2006; Rosenberg et al., 2007). Last, by asking herself whether the husband is there 'just to translate', the general practitioner implicitly voices an expectation that the interpreter embody the so-called conduit role, rendering literal translations and taking a neutral stance, which is based on an outdated and simplistic conceptualization of the communication process as purely transmitting information (Shannon & Weaver, 1964), but hardly descriptive of the actual work interpreters do in practice (e.g. Dysart-Gale, 2005). In fact, informal interpreters (as well as their professional counterparts) are known to perform a wide variety of roles besides 'just' translating (e.g. Hilfinger Messias et al., 2009; Leanza, 2005), which could be placed on a continuum ranging from roles that are more in alignment with the patient's lifeworld on the one hand (e.g. patient advocate) to roles that are more in alignment with the biomedical system on the other hand (e.g. institutional gatekeeper; Brisset et al., 2013a).

The constructs of interpreters' roles, power and control, and trust are fundamental elements of interpreter-mediated health encounters, and as such have been central topics of previous studies within the field (albeit less frequently in the context of informal interpreting). However, although much valuable knowledge has already been gained, the research field remains fairly fragmented owing to the lack of a theory-based framework; such a framework would help to synthesize previous research findings and move the field from a predominantly descriptive one to a more explanatory one. As it is known that interventions that are based on a sound theoretical base are more effective compared with interventions that are not (e.g. Glanz & Bishop, 2010; Li et al., 2010), it is thus essential to start building a theory-based framework in order to be able to design and implement effective interventions to improve the quality of healthcare delivery for patients who make use of informal interpreters to communicate with their healthcare providers. Therefore, a theory-based framework of informal interpreting in health care is proposed, based on an overview of the pertinent empirical and theoretical literature on patients', interpreters' and healthcare providers' perspectives on informal interpreting and actual communicative discourses in medical consultations with informal interpreters. Before turning to the proposed framework, I provide a rationale for focusing on informal interpreters.

Why is There a Need to Conduct Research on Informal Interpreters?

Officially, the European Union has 24 languages. Unofficially, the number of languages spoken in Europe far exceeds this number. For instance, in London alone over 300 different languages are spoken (Baker & Eversley, 2000), and the Dutch Interpreter and Translator Service provides interpreting services in approximately 130 languages. Hence, a significant proportion of European healthcare encounters involve patients and providers who do not share a common language. Regarding the Netherlands, 21% of the population consists of first- or second-generation migrants (Statistics Netherlands, 2014), of whom about half come from non-Western countries. The largest non-Western immigrant groups in the Netherlands originate from Turkey, Morocco, Surinam and the Antilles, and China. It has been estimated that at least half of all non-Western immigrants do not have sufficient Dutch language proficiency to communicate adequately with their healthcare provider without some form of interpretation service (Meeuwesen & Twilt, 2011), with Dutch language proficiency being lowest among Turkish migrants, the largest ethnic minority group in the

Netherlands; over 50% of them indicate having trouble speaking Dutch (Turkenburg & Gijsberts, 2007).

To bridge the language barrier between patients with insufficient Dutch language proficiency and their healthcare providers, the Dutch healthcare inspectorate regards the use of professional interpreters as the gold standard and recommends avoiding using untrained, informal interpreters, such as family members, friends or bilingual healthcare staff. The onus of arranging for a professional interpreter is placed on the healthcare provider, because they are, according to the Dutch Law on Medical Treatment which was passed in 1995, legally responsible to inform their patients in a clear and understandable way about the proposed treatment and to obtain the patient's informed consent before carrying out a treatment plan. However, no mention whatsoever is made in Dutch law about the patient's right to a professional interpreter, a situation comparable to that in most other European countries. In fact, there is not only an absence of European law securing patients' right to professional interpreting services when facing language barriers in health care (Phelan, 2012), but national laws to ensure patients' right to professional interpreters during medical encounters are also practically non-existent as well.

The lack of legislation has probably contributed to the common practice of using informal interpreters in medical consultations. For instance, in the Netherlands about two-thirds of Turkish and Moroccan migrant patients regularly make use of informal interpreters when visiting healthcare facilities, with percentages increasing to over 80% among women (Schaafsma *et al.*, 2003). In addition, the absence of legislation on patients' right to professional interpreters has made it possible for the Dutch government to withdraw the provision of free interpreting services in health care since 2012, justifying these budget cuts by stating that 'patients/clients (or their representatives) are responsible for their own command of the Dutch language' (Schippers & Veldhuijzen van Zanten-Hyllner, 2011: 4). Hence, the use of informal interpreters in the Netherlands is likely to persist and even increase in the near future.

Although the lack of legislation in Europe clearly hinders the use of professional interpreting services in health care, previous research has shown that, even when professional interpreting services are (to some extent) available, healthcare providers in a wide variety of settings continue to use informal interpreters instead of professional ones (e.g. Bischoff & Hudelson, 2010a, 2010b; Gerrish *et al.*, 2004; Kale & Syed, 2010; MacFarlane *et al.*, 2008; Pöchhacker, 2000). Factors commonly reported as barriers to working with professional interpreters are poor access to interpreting services, a lack of awareness among healthcare staff of existing interpreting services, lack of availability of professional interpreters on short notice, and organizational pressures to keep costs down. In addition, a few studies have reported that healthcare providers might actually prefer working with informal interpreters (e.g. Hudelson & Vilpert, 2009) because, for instance, they know the patient firsthand and might therefore be more readily accepted by patients in comparison to professional interpreters (e.g. Gerrish *et al.*, 2004; MacFarlane *et al.*, 2008). Although there are some fundamental differences between the healthcare and legal systems in the US and Europe and US healthcare providers can be and have been held liable for not communicating properly with low-language-proficient patients through the use of professional interpreters (e.g. Kempen, 2007), the same situation prevails there too. That is, a high use of informal interpreters has been reported in various healthcare settings in the US (and Canada), ranging from primary care (Gadon *et al.*, 2007; Hornberger *et al.*, 1997; Papic *et al.*, 2012) and emergency care (Ramirez *et al.*, 2008) to hospital care (Lee *et al.*, 2006; Schenker *et al.*, 2011; Tschurtz *et al.*, 2010), for the same reasons as mentioned in the European studies.

Hence, owing to international, national, organizational, social and individual factors, healthcare practitioners in a wide variety of settings worldwide continue to work with informal interpreters on a frequent basis. This situation is unlikely to change in the near future and might even become more pronounced owing to the ongoing global economic downturn and its corresponding budget cuts in health care. Instead of condemning the use of informal interpreters as morally wrong and below standard, a more fruitful approach would be to investigate the conditions under which working with informal interpreters is 'good enough' or even warranted and to implement guidelines that help healthcare providers decide which type of interpreter to use in a specific situation (see for a similar view Gray *et al.*, 2012). A theory-based approach to investigating the potentially role that informal interpreters can play in health care could go a long way toward developing guidelines as to if and when they can be effectively used.

Informal interpreters and role conflict

To theoretically explain informal interpreting in health care, it is necessary to relate several central concepts. As has been described, interpreters' roles, power and control dynamics during the encounter and trust all play a fundamental part in the communication process and its outcomes, with interpreters' roles being investigated most extensively. Roles have been defined as 'behaviours and skills associated with being an interpreter as expected by institutions, practitioners and patients' (Brisset *et al.*, 2013a: 135). Although dozens of specific roles have been identified in the literature, they have been grouped into a handful of key categories (e.g. Leanza, 2005), based partly on Habermas's theoretical distinction between the *lifeworld* and the *system* (Habermas, 1991). That is, some interpreter roles can be conceptualized as predominantly reflecting the voice of the system, because they entail performing strategic communicative actions that strive toward efficiency and ensuring certain outcomes, while other roles are primarily concerned with reflecting the voice of the lifeworld, because they entail communicative actions that are meant to build meaningful relationships and to come to a mutual understanding and consensus in a given situation (see also Mishler, 1984).

According to the proposed framework, patients', healthcare providers' and informal interpreters' expectations about the role(s) the informal interpreter is supposed to perform during the medical encounter are shaped by individual, social and system level factors (see Figure 5.1). Individual factors refer to the personal characteristics of each interlocutor, such as their gender, age, ethnic background and language proficiency. For instance, the extent to which a family interpreter[1] is bilingual, how proficient they are in both languages and in what way they acquired these languages, influence how they construct their roles (Angelelli, 2010). An informal interpreter who is fluent in both languages can more easily perform the role of linguistic agent and might be more strongly expected by patients and healthcare providers to perform this role than one who is less bilingually fluent. In the same vein, a family interpreter's gender not only influences what topics they feel comfortable discussing (e.g. Green et al., 2005), but also the type of interpreter role they more readily identify with (i.e. a caretaking role for females versus an advocating role for males; Garabetian, 2014). Social factors refer for instance to the interpersonal relationships between the interlocutor and others, such as family, friends and other reference groups, with the most important relations influencing the interpreter-mediated encounter being between patient, interpreter and healthcare provider. Lastly, system-level factors refer to the contexts in which the medical encounter takes place, such as the type of healthcare setting and the sociopolitical and cultural contexts in which the interpreter performs his or her task. That is, different medical disciplines have, to a certain extent, dissimilar communicative and relational goals, which influence the importance that healthcare providers from different disciplines place on the various interpreter roles (Diamond et al., 2012; Hsieh et al., 2013). In addition, it has been shown that the sociopolitical and cultural contexts in which informal interpreters carry out their task influence how they construct their roles as well (Schouten et al., 2012).

Although research directly comparing healthcare practitioners', patients' and informal interpreters' perspectives on their roles is scarce (but see for an exception Greenhalgh et al., 2006), previous findings show some notable discrepancies in the role expectations among the three interlocutors in the triad. Healthcare practitioners often expect informal interpreters (in particular family interpreters) to take on a caretaker role by, for instance, assisting the patient outside the consultation with their health-related activities (e.g. Brisset et al., 2013b), a role obviously not expected from professional interpreters. In addition, they mainly expect informal interpreters to perform according to professional guidelines that emphasize neutrality and

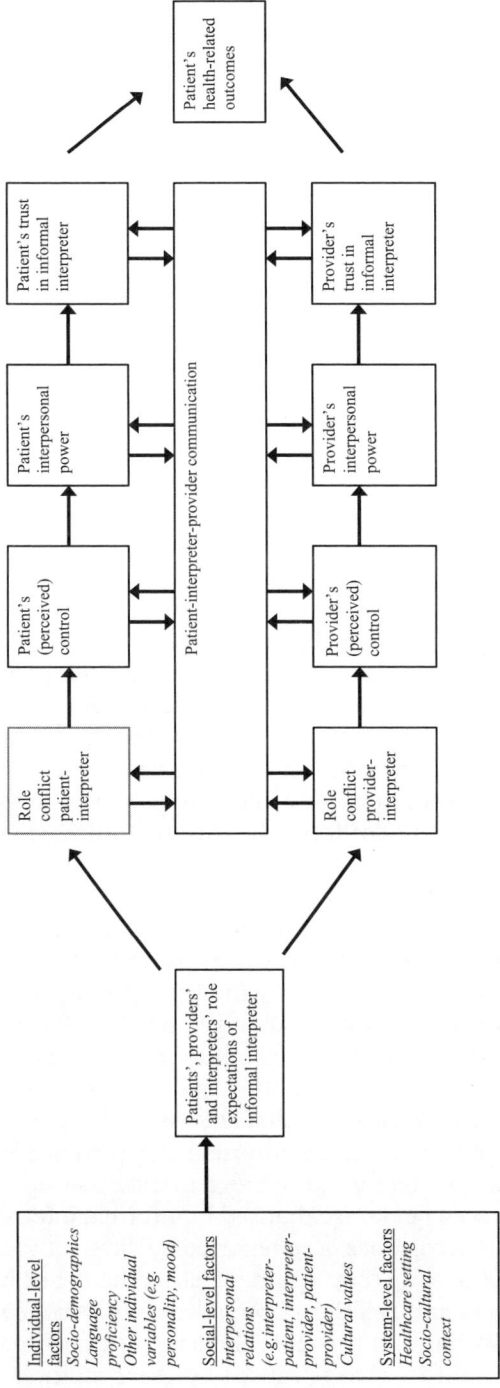

Figure 5.1 Theoretical framework of informal interpreting in health care

interpreting accuracy (Fatahi *et al.*, 2010; Kale & Syed, 2010) and place most importance on the role of linguistic agent (Brisset *et al.*, 2013b), while – paradoxically – at the same time realizing that their linguistic competencies are often insufficient to ensure accurate translations (e.g. Rosenberg *et al.*, 2007). Indeed, previous research has abundantly shown that both family interpreters and bilingual healthcare staff commonly make interpreting errors (e.g. Aranguri *et al.*, 2006; Bührig & Meyer, 2004; Cambridge, 1999; Ebden *et al.*, 1988; Hagan *et al.*, 2013), although the extent to which these errors are clinically significant is still unclear. Some researchers have found evidence for negative effects of communicative errors on quality of care (Flores, 2005; Jacobs *et al.*, 2006; Killian *et al.*, 2014), while others could not establish effects of communication errors on (clinical) outcomes (Karliner *et al.*, 2007) or have even shown that changes in translations might have potentially positive effects, such as increased clarification and simplification of information for patients (Butow *et al.*, 2011). Owing to these mixed results, the effects of the type of translation and communication errors on the communication process and its outcomes remain an important topic for future research.

Although there is a dearth of research investigating the perspectives of patients, the few studies that have been carried out indicate that, besides having adequate linguistic skills to communicate their needs to the healthcare provider (Larrison *et al.*, 2010; Zendedel *et al.*, 2016), patients mainly expect the family interpreter to protect their interests, provide emotional support and act as their advocate during the medical encounter, for instance by helping them to receive adequate treatment for their health complaints (Edwards *et al.*, 2005; Hadziabdic *et al.*, 2009; Zendedel *et al.*, 2016).

The conflicting expectations of healthcare providers and patients about the informal interpreter's roles force the informal interpreter to perform a delicate balancing act between the two parties, which could easily lead to role overload and conflicted feelings about how to perform their interpreting task. In their work on professional interpreters in mental health care, Drennan and Schwartz (1999) warn against placing too many expectations on the interpreter, because performing multiple roles at the same time (in their case being both a linguistic agent and an advocate) requires high levels of skills and self-confidence that might not be reasonably expected from most interpreters and 'may risk the integrity of both [roles]' (Drennan & Schwartz, 1999: 191). Given the fact that at least the level of skill, if not their self-confidence as well, of untrained, informal interpreters is lower than that of their professional counterparts, the problematic situation of role overload and conflict might even be more enhanced in informal interpreter-mediated health encounters. Indeed, it has been reported by different types of informal interpreters that not only do they at times feel overburdened by the expectations of both patients and healthcare providers (e.g. Matthews *et al.*, 2000; Schouten *et al.* 2012), but that the most challenging aspect of their task is to cope with the role conflict that is caused by these multiple and divergent expectations (Green et al., 2005; Hilfinger Messias et al., 2009). As a consequence, one solution they might use to navigate these encounters is to enact a wide variety of roles, ranging from being the patient's caretaker and advocate (Angelelli, 2010; Gerrish et al., 2004; Green et al., 2005; Rosenberg et al., 2008; Yang & Gray, 2008) to being a system agent and acting as a co-healthcare practitioner (Matthews et al., 2000). It should be noted though that many studies point out that family interpreters conceptualize their role primarily as an extension of their social responsibilities of being a family member (e.g. Angelelli, 2010; Rosenberg et al., 2008). Hence, family interpreters often 'solve' the problem of role conflict by taking the side of the patient.

In sum, patients and healthcare providers tend to have dissimilar and often conflicting expectations about the roles that the informal interpreter is supposed to perform during the medical encounter. As a consequence, informal interpreters might try to take on a wide variety of roles within the medical encounter as a way to cope with the demands of both parties. The roles the interpreter takes upon him- or herself in a specific situation will be shaped by his or her own role expectations, which, in turn, are dependent on a combination of individual, social and system-level factors. For instance, the existing relations between the informal interpreter and patient or healthcare provider might shift the choice more toward roles in favor of the patient or more toward roles in favor of the healthcare provider. Family members who act as informal interpreters more frequently take on roles that are in alignment with the patient's needs, because of feelings of social responsibility and strong ties of kinship, and might resist attempts of the healthcare provider to put them in a role that is more in favor of the system (e.g. Green et al., 2005). On the other hand, bilingual healthcare staff who act as informal interpreters will probably align more often with the needs of the healthcare provider, because they are themselves part of the biomedical system and might feel pressured to conform to its expectations (e.g. Davidson, 2000). As a consequence, they will more readily resist taking on roles that patients expect of them, such as advocating (e.g. Matthews et al., 2000). In either case, role conflicts will emerge within the triad, which can be described as 'the simultaneous occurrence of two (or more) sets of pressures; compliance with one would make it difficult to comply with the other' (Steers, 1991: 551).

Control and Power in Informal Interpreter-mediated Health Encounters

The framework proposes next that the more severe the role conflict between informal interpreter and healthcare provider, the lower the physician's perceived and/or actual control during the communication process, which, in turn, results in a loss of his or her interpersonal power. In the same vein, the stronger the role conflict between informal interpreter and patient, the lower the patient's perceived or actual control during the communication process, resulting in a loss of the patient's interpersonal power (see Figure 5.1). Thus, although the constructs of control and power in medical encounters are closely related, they are distinct and should be treated as such in order to get a clearer picture of their respective influence during the medical communication process.

Perceived (and actual) behavioral control is a central component of the Theory of Planned Behavior (Ajzen, 1991) and similar to Social Cognitive Theory's construct of self-efficacy, which can be defined as 'the conviction that one can successfully execute the behavior required to produce the [desired] outcomes' (Bandura, 1977: 193). Judgments of one's perceived behavioral control are based on both internal (e.g. skills and abilities) and external factors (e.g. barriers, resources, dependency on others; Ajzen, 1991). In the context of health communication, it thus refers to the extent to which the patient and healthcare provider perceive themselves to be able, or are actually able, to have control over the course and content of the communication process (see for a similar definition Brisset et al., 2013a), in order to achieve relational and strategic outcomes. Internal factors influencing healthcare providers' and patients' level of control are, for instance, their linguistic and communicative skills, while the informal interpreter, as an external factor, can be seen as both an impediment or resource for their respective control. Previous research has shown that a strong sense of control is an important determinant of the attainment of goals (e.g. Bandura, 2004; Conner & Sparks, 2005). Extrapolating from these findings to the medical communication process, patients and healthcare providers need to have sufficient levels of (perceived) control during the encounter to ensure both relational and strategic goals.

In medical encounters with low levels of role conflict between the informal interpreter and either the healthcare provider or patient, the interpreter thus functions as an external resource for increasing the amount of control over the communication process for patient and healthcare provider. For instance, when all three interlocutors in the triad agree that the dominant role of the interpreter should be to transmit information and perform the role of linguistic agent, levels of control over the communication process for both patient and physician are assumed to be high. As stated above though, owing to possible conflicting role expectations of patients and healthcare providers, the informal interpreter faces the complicated task to simultaneously comply with the demands of both parties, which entails the ability to effectively switch roles during one encounter to bridge this gap in patients' and healthcare providers' expectations. More often than not, informal interpreters do not have sufficient skills and abilities to be this bridge and tend to 'resolve' the ensuing role conflicts by either siding more with the patient or the healthcare provider, depending on their own role expectations. As a result, the informal interpreter then becomes an impediment instead of a resource for the healthcare provider's or patient's level of (perceived) control.

Indeed, observational and self-report studies alike have indicated that in particular healthcare providers have a diminished sense of control over the medical communication process when working with informal interpreters. For instance, in Rosenberg *et al.*'s (2007) study, physicians reported feeling more in control over the communication process when working with professional interpreters as compared with family interpreters, because the former ones adhere more strongly to their (expected) conduit role of transmitting information. Family interpreters, on the other hand, are unlikely to perform a neutral conduit role, because of their emotional involvement with the patient, cultural norms or expectations, and possible inadequate linguistic skills. For instance, they often act as the primary interlocutor by speaking on behalf of the patient, engage in side-talk activities and do not translate everything that is being communicated (e.g. Aranguri *et al.*, 2006; Fatahi *et al.*, 2010; Hasselkus, 1992; Hudelson *et al.*, 2013; Meeuwesen *et al.*, 2010). Hence, as a result of the interpreter's divergence from the role expectations of the healthcare provider, role conflict between the two emerges during the encounter, resulting in healthcare providers' perceptions of or actual loss of control over the communication process.

With regard to the patient's level of control during the medical communication process, results of previous empirical work show two slightly opposing trends. The bulk of research indicates that family interpreters tend to exclude the patient from taking part in the communication process (e.g. Aranguri *et al.*, 2006; Hasselkus, 1992; Hudelson *et al.*, 2013; Leanza *et al.*, 2010; Rosenberg *et al.*, 2011; Schouten & Schinkel, 2014), in particular when it comes to affective communication. That is, they frequently block patients' expression of emotions and psychosocial aspects of their health complaint, either because the mere presence of the family interpreter inhibits patients' expression of emotions, possibly out of feelings of embarrassment to discuss sensitive topics in the presence of a close relative (Rosenberg *et al.*, 2011), or because the interpreter ignores or does not translate patients' affective utterances (Leanza *et al.*, 2010; Schouten & Schinkel, 2014), seeing them as irrelevant for the medical communication process. This blocking of patients' affective utterances by family interpreters reflects a role conflict with the patient (e.g. between being an agent for the patient's lifeworld versus being, for instance, an agent for the medical system), resulting in a diminished level of control among patients over the (affective) communication process.

However, although the above-mentioned communicative behaviors of the family interpreter make it indeed difficult to achieve relational goals, such as the establishment of rapport (Fernández, 2010), it is unclear whether patients themselves perceive these communicate acts as an impediment for their level of control. The few studies that have addressed this issue have yielded mixed results. On the one hand, patients themselves have indeed indicated that they experience difficulties conveying emotions in the presence of family interpreters (e.g. Hadziabdic *et al.*, 2009) and do feel inhibited from discussing sensitive topics (Bauer & Alegría, 2010), in particular when children are being used to interpret (MacFarlane et al., 2009; Rhodes et al., 2003), because discussion of such topics could potentially lead to role reversals between parents and children (e.g. Ngo-Metzger et al., 2003). According to the Western construction of childhood, there is a moral obligation to protect children from and raise them without burdening them with adult responsibilities, such as having to interpret for their relatives, and healthcare providers are indeed known to struggle with the ethical ramifications of accepting minors as family interpreters in the healthcare consultation (e.g. Cohen et al., 1999).

On the other hand, Greenhalgh et al.'s (2006) study found the opposite. Patients who used family or friends as informal interpreters reportedly felt they had more control over what was being discussed compared with being in medical encounters with professional interpreters, a finding corroborated in our own research among Turkish migrant patients (Zendedel et al., 2016). The mixed results might partly be explained by distinguishing between patients' relational and strategic goals. That is, patients may have diminished control over the affective part of the communication process, because of their own inhibitions as well as the interpreter's tendency to filter 'irrelevant non-medical' information, possibly in an attempt to adhere to a more neutral conduit or system agent role – thereby hindering the building of a good relation between the interlocutors. On the other hand, strategic goals, such as obtaining the treatment the patient wants, may be more likely to be attained because of the informal interpreter's tendency to act as the patient's advocate. Clearly, more research is needed to verify the differential effects of the informal interpreter on patients' level of control over the affective versus instrumental communication process.

In the next step of the framework, it is proposed that patients' and healthcare providers' level of control over the communication process subsequently determines the amount of interpersonal power one has during the medical encounter. Much research on power in interpersonal relations can be traced back to French and Raven's seminal work on the bases of social power,[2] which is defined as the potential to influence beliefs or behaviors of a person, resulting from the actions or presence of another person (French & Raven, 1959). Thus, the main perspective on power taken here is in accordance with Hanna Arendt's theorizing on the construct of power, which

> is never the property of an individual; it belongs to a group and remains in existence only so long as the group keeps together. When we say of somebody that he is 'in power' we actually refer to his being empowered by a certain number of people to act in their name. (Arendt, 1970: 44)

Hence, the healthcare provider's and patient's level of interpersonal power is assumed to be determined by the informal interpreter's presence and actions, through his/her influence on the amount of control both have during the medical encounter.

A central premise of French and Raven's model is that the potential influence over others is derived from six different bases of power.[3] Within the patient–interpreter–doctor triad, *expert power* and *legitimate power* are the two most relevant power bases. *Expert power* is based on having expertise or knowledge that is needed by another, such as healthcare providers having medical skills and expertise, or informal interpreters having bilingual skills. The often-noted power asymmetry in doctor–patient relations (e.g. Stewart, 1995) primarily refers to a difference in the level of expert power between doctor and patient. However, this does not mean that patients are powerless parties in the medical interaction. Their potential influence is derived from a different base though, so-called *legitimate power*, which is based on feeling entitled to exert power over another because of existing cultural norms and values. For instance, patients may make use of the norm of equity when they enlist the help of their relatives to communicate with the healthcare provider or use the social norm that one should help people who cannot help themselves, which has also been referred to as the 'power of the powerless' (Raven, 1992). Thus, patients who bring along a family interpreter to the medical encounter essentially make an appeal to their legitimate power by involving the help of a third party.

Owing to a (perceived) loss of control over the communication process, both patient and healthcare provider might feel that they cannot influence the other sufficiently enough to get or deliver adequate care, but the power base that is threatened is different for both interlocutors. That is, healthcare providers predominantly experience a loss of expert power, because the medical skills and expertise they normally rely on to influence patients become less available as a power base, as the provider struggles to keep track of everything that is being discussed during the interpreted medical encounter (e.g. Greenhalgh *et al.*, 2006; Rosenberg *et al.*, 2007). Hence, they have diminished influence to achieve strategic and relational goals, such as obtaining the patient's voice (e.g. Fernández, 2010; Kai *et al.*, 2011). Note though that their interpretations of the consequences of losing control over the communication process might not always be correct. For instance, in a study by Free *et al.* (2003) among bilingual adolescents in London who regularly perform interpreting work for their relatives, the interpreters reported that the healthcare provider sometimes erroneously attributed disagreements of the patient with their medical advice to interpreting errors in translation instead of to genuine disagreements. Hence, in this case the patient's voice is being communicated by the interpreter, but not accepted as such. The same process is hypothesized to occur among patients, but owing to the lack of empirical research and the tendency of researchers to collapse control and power into one construct, more empirical research is needed to be able to draw any conclusions. In our own work among Turkish migrant patients in general practice, patients indicated feeling empowered by the presence of a family interpreter, because he or she made it possible to discuss the patient's needs (Zendedel et al., 2016), lending some support for the proposed relation between patients' level of control over the communication process and enhanced legitimate power.

Trust and Distrust in the Informal Interpreter

The last step of the model proposes that the amount of interpersonal power determines the extent to which patient and healthcare provider have trust in the informal interpreter. Thus, the more influence either patient or healthcare provider has on the behavior of the other, the more they will trust the informal interpreter. Trust can be defined as 'the optimistic acceptance of a vulnerable situation in which a truster believes the trustee to care for the truster's interests' (Hall et al., 2001: 615), and is an important determinant of achieving good health-related outcomes (e.g. Haes & Bensing, 2009; Hall et al., 2001). Hence, both patients and healthcare providers (i.e. the 'trusters') should have sufficient trust in the informal interpreter (i.e. the 'trustee') to optimize the quality of care the patient receives.

Trust is a multidimensional construct, with several researchers proposing somewhat different dimensions (e.g. Hall et al., 2001; Robb & Greenhalgh, 2006). Here, the five dimensions of trust as proposed by Hall et al. (2001) will be used – *fidelity, competence, honesty, confidentiality* and *global trust* – because they share many commonalities with other trust dimensions and are useful in assessing trust in the different aspects of interpreters' role performances. *Fidelity* entails 'pursuing another's best interests and not taking advantage of his or her vulnerability' (p. 621), *competence* refers to 'avoiding mistakes and producing the best achievable results' (p. 621), *honesty* entails 'telling the truth and avoiding intentional falsehoods' (p. 622), *confidentiality* refers to the 'protection and proper use of sensitive or private information' (p. 622) and *global trust* is the irreducible, holistic, component of trust, also referred to as 'the soul of trust' (p. 623).

Previous research findings indicate that healthcare providers do not have a lot of trust in informal interpreters, in particular when it comes to family interpreters (Fatahi et al., 2010; Gadon et al., 2007; Gerrish et al., 2004; Hsieh, 2006; Kai et al., 2011; Pöchhacker, 2000; Robb & Greenhalgh, 2006). Their distrust can mostly be traced back to concerns over the family interpreter's lack of linguistic competence and possible honesty during the medical consultation. Hence, healthcare providers' lack of trust is based on both concerns about the reliability and accuracy of family interpreters' translations and worries about their tendency to filter and omit information and possibly pursue their own agenda instead of the patient's. Their concerns about the family interpreter's honesty are corroborated by empirical findings showing that they might indeed control the patient's agenda in some instances by failing to translate the patient's utterances when these are in disagreement with the family interpreter's views (Leanza et al., 2010). In addition, some concern over a potential loss of confidentiality when working with family members or friends as interpreters has been reported as well (Diamond et al., 2009; Gadon et al., 2007; Gerrish et al., 2004; Hsieh, 2006; MacFarlane et al., 2008). Family interpreters themselves do seem to pick up the healthcare providers' distrust about their competencies during the consultation (e.g. Free et al., 2003), which might have a detrimental impact on their task performances and, as a consequence, limit the healthcare providers' influence on the patient's care, thereby further eroding their trust in the family interpreter.

In contrast, family interpreters do feel that patients have more trust in them as compared with professional interpreters (Free et al., 2003; Rosenberg et al., 2008), because they have a better understanding of the patient's health complaints and lifeworld (Hsieh, 2006). These feelings have indeed been supported in a few studies among patients themselves (e.g. Edwards et al. 2005; Robb & Greenhalgh, 2006). Because of the shared history of understanding and kinship obligations between patient and family interpreter, and in some contexts a reluctance to talk about personal issues in the presence of someone belonging to the wider community to which they belong (e.g. Rhodes et al., 2003), family members are often preferred over professional interpreters. In addition, patients perceive professional interpreters as someone who might be more engaged in serving the provider's agenda than in serving their agenda (Edwards et al., 2005), thereby limiting their influence during the healthcare encounter. However, in a few other studies opposing results have emerged (Hadziabdic et al., 2009; MacFarlane et al., 2009), with the patient preferring professional interpreters. Reasons for those patients' preferences are related to having more confidence in the professional interpreters' linguistic skills and having more guarantees of confidentiality as compared with using family members or friends as interpreters. Hence, these partly opposing findings on patients' preferences for either professional or informal interpreters can be explained by the fact that patients use different dimensions of trust to evaluate them. That is, while family interpreters are preferred because they are trusted to act in the best interests of the patient and protect the privacy of the family (i.e. *fidelity, global trust*), professional interpreters are preferred when patients attach more importance to having confidence in the interpreters' linguistic competencies and professional confidentiality (i.e. *competence, confidentiality*).

Conclusion

Because low-language-proficient patients' health often depends on the presence and actions of informal interpreters in a wide variety of healthcare settings across the globe, it is important to understand how these interpreters might impact the medical communication encounter and its outcomes. The proposed theoretical framework provides a first step in explaining how interpreter-mediated encounters are shaped by each interlocutor's role expectations of the informal interpreter and their subsequent influence on control and power dynamics and, ultimately, trust in the informal interpreter. Individual, social and system-level factors all contribute to how the informal interpreter is expected to behave during the medical encounter and, consequently, influence the extent to which role conflicts might arise between the interlocutors. Hence, the often remarked upon struggles over control and power in triadic medical encounters unfold because of those, often unconscious, conflicting expectations of the informal interpreter's roles. A loss of power among healthcare providers or patients will to a large extent be attributed, justifiable or not, to the interpreter deviating from their role expectations, and consequently diminish the trust the provider and/or patient has in the informal interpreter. For example, a deviation by the interpreter from his or her often-expected linguistic role might diminish the influence that the provider can exert on the patient and will probably be more readily attributed to the interpreter's lack of bilingual language skills, instead of to possible genuine disagreements between provider and patient over the course of action to be taken (e.g. Free *et al.*, 2003), leading to a loss of trust in the interpreter's competencies. As the establishment of sufficient levels of trust in the interpreter from both the side of the patient and that of the healthcare provider is a necessary condition to achieve good health-related outcomes, it is easy to see how detrimental miscommunication and misattributions in triadic encounters with informal interpreters might be to the patient's health.

Owing to the lack of empirical work on the interrelationships between informal interpreters' roles, control and power, and trust, it is obvious that first and foremost more research is needed on this topic. Furthermore, the effect of the informal interpreter-mediated encounter on clinical outcomes has been a neglected research domain so far. More knowledge on which elements of the communication process and which dimensions of trust are related to enhanced health-related outcomes for the patient is critical to be able to improve upon the health of patients with limited language proficiency. Last, as most research on interpreter-mediated communication itself has taken a discourse-based approach, remarkably little is known about non-verbal communication in interpreter-mediated interactions. The importance of non-verbal communication, such as body orientation, posture, gaze, facial expressions, gesturing and tone of voice in the medical interaction for the establishment of rapport and trust during medical interactions has been acknowledged and studied over decades (see for a review Hall *et al.*, 1995), but has hardly been taken up by scholars in the medical interpretation field (but see for a recent exception Krystallidou, 2014). Because of the increased ambiguity of verbal utterances in interpreter-mediated consultations, interlocutors' alertness to non-verbal cues in order to gain a sense of control and clarity over 'what is going on' is in all probability quite pronounced, thereby making non-verbal communication an even more important tool to build trust compared with dyadic medical interactions. Hence, more observational research should be carried out to investigate non-verbal communication patterns in interpreter-mediated health encounters. To account for possible cultural differences in the use of non-verbal cues, coders of different cultural and ethnic backgrounds should be used in such studies.

Notwithstanding the necessity for more research, sufficient evidence has already been gathered that can be used as a base for improving the quality of low-language-proficient patients' health and well-being. One method that might be suitable in light of the proposed framework is the three-step method developed by Pinto (2000), which has already been used with some success in improving communication (outcomes) between patients and healthcare providers from different cultural backgrounds (e.g. Harmsen et al., 2005). According to this method, interventions to improve interpreter-mediated communication should focus on raising awareness about one's own often-unconscious culture-related values and their influence on thinking and behavior, raising awareness about the fact that these values and the subsequent influence on thinking and behavior might be different for others, and learning skills to deal with the identified differences in such a way that everyone's core values are respected and preserved. To be specific, providers need to develop an awareness of their expectations of the role of the informal interpreter and the expectations that patients and interpreters themselves have of the informal interpreter's role, as well as skills for effectively and respectfully addressing potential role discrepancies. This awareness and skill development could go a long way in preventing role conflicts from escalating into problems and, instead, establishing a mutually trusting relationship. This task obviously requires an immense effort from scientists, practitioners and other stakeholders alike or, as has been written in such moving words by one of the pioneering social action researchers of minority problems: 'It needs the best of what the best among us can give, and the help of everybody' (Lewin, 1948: 216). These words remain as true today as they were in his era.

Notes

(1) Because different types of (informal) interpreters are known to have a differential influence on interpreter-mediated encounters (e.g. Hsieh, 2006), the type of informal interpreter is reported in refering to the literature if the research has explicitly specified their study sample. The proposed framework takes into account the type of informal interpreter under social level factors.
(2) Note that social power is but one of the various types and levels of power influencing the medical communication process. Other conceptualizations of power, such as institutional and covert power, are important to take into account as well (see for

instance Lukes's (1974) three-dimensional approach to power), but fall beyond the scope of this interpersonal theoretical framework.
(3) Besides expert power and legitimate power, the following four power bases are distinguished in French and Raven's typology: reward power, coercive power, referent power and information power. Threats to one of those power bases might be followed by subsequent switches to other power bases in an attempt to restore one's power. For example, healthcare practitioners who cannot fully exert their expert power might resort to coercive power (i.e. administer negative consequences or refrain from giving positive consequences), by ending a consultation abruptly or not giving the patient a needed referral.

References

Ajzen, I. (1991) The theory of planned behavior. *Organizational Behavior and Human Decision Processes* 50, 179–211.

Angelelli, C.V. (2010) A professional ideology in the making: Bilingual youngsters interpreting for their communities and the notion of (no) choice. *Translation and Interpreting Studies* 5, 94–108.

Aranguri, C., Davidson, B. and Ramirez R. (2006) Patterns of communication through interpreters. A detailed sociolinguistic analysis. *Journal of General and Internal Medicine* 21, 623–629.

Arendt, H. (1970) *On Violence*. New York: Harcourt Brace.

Baker, P. and Eversley, J. (2000) *Multilingual Capital: The Languages of London's Schoolchildren and their Relevance to Economic, Social and Educational Policies*. London: Battlebridge.

Bandura, A. (1977) Self-efficacy: Toward a unifying theory of behavioral change. *Psychological Review* 84, 191–215.

Bandura, A. (2004) Health promotion by social cognitive means. *Health Education and Behavior* 31, 143–164.

Bauer, A.M. and Alegría, M. (2010) The impact of patient language proficiency and interpreter service use on the quality of psychiatric care: A systematic review. *Psychiatric Services* 61, 765–773.

Bischoff, A. and Hudelson, P. (2010a) Communicating with foreign language-speaking patients: Is access to professional interpreters enough? *Journal of Travel Medicine* 17, 15–20.

Bischoff, A. and Hudelson, P. (2010b) Access to healthcare interpreter services: Where are we and where do we need to go? *International Journal of Environmental Research and Public Health* 7, 2838–2844.

Brisset C., Leanza Y. and Laforest, K. (2013a) Working with interpreters in health care: A systematic review and meta-ethnography of qualitative studies. *Patient Education and Counseling* 91, 131–140.

Brisset C., Leanza, Y., Rosenberg, E., Vissandjée B., Kirmayer, L.J., Muckle, G., Xenocostas, S. and Laforce, H. (2013b) Language barriers in mental health care: A survey of primary care practitioners. *Journal of Immigrant and Minority Health* 16, 1238–1246.

Bührig, K. and Meyer, B. (2004) Ad hoc interpreting and the achievement of communicative purposes in doctor–patient communication. In J. House and J. Rehbein (eds) *Multilingual Communication*. Amsterdam: John Benjamins.

Butow, P.N., Goldstein, D., Bell, M.L., Sze, M., Aldridge, L.J., Abdo, S., Tanious, M., Dong, S., Iedema, R., Vardy, J., Ashgari, R., Hui, R. and Eisenbruch, M. (2011) Interpretation in consultations with immigrant patients with cancer: How accurate is it? *Journal of Clinical Oncology* 29, 2801–2807.

Cambridge, J. (1999) Information loss in bilingual medical interviews through an untrained interpreter. *The Translator* 5, 201–219.

Cohen, S., Moran-Ellis, J. and Smaje, C. (1999) Children as informal interpreters in GP consultations: pragmatics and ideology. *Sociology of Health and Illness* 21, 163–186.

Conner, M. and Sparks, P. (2005) Theory of planned behavior and health behavior. In M. Conner and P. Norman (eds) *Predicting Health Behaviour: Research and Practice with Social Cognition Models* (2nd edn, pp. 170–222). Maidenhead: Open University Press.

Davidson, B. (2000) The interpreter as institutional gatekeeper: The social-linguistic role of interpreters in Spanish–English medical discourse. *Journal of Sociolinguistics* 4 (3), 379–405.

Diamond, L.C., Schenker, Y., Curry, L., Bradley, E.H. and Fernandez, A. (2009) Getting by: Underuse of interpreters by resident physicians. *Journal of General Internal Medicine* 24, 256–262.

Diamond, L.C., Tuot, D.S. and Karliner, L.S. (2012) The use of Spanish language skills by physicians and nurses: Policy implications for teaching and testing. *Journal of General Internal Medicine* 27, 117–123.

Drennan, G. and Schwartz, L. (1999) A concept over-burdened: Institutional roles for psychiatric interpreters in post-apartheid South Africa. *Interpreting* 4, 169–198.

Dysart-Gale, D. (2005) Communication models, professionalization, and the work of medical interpreters. *Health Communication* 17, 91–103.

Ebden P., Carey, O.J., Bhatt A. and Harrison, B. (1988) The bilingual consultation. *The Lancet* 331, 347.

Edwards, R., Temple, B. and Alexander, C. (2005) Users' experiences of interpreters: The critical role of trust. *Interpreting* 7, 77–95.

Fatahi, N., Mattsson, B., Lundgren, S.M. and Hellström, M. (2010) Nurse radiographers' experiences of communication with patients who do not speak the native language. *Journal of Advanced Nursing* 66, 774–783.

Fernández, E.I. (2010) Verbal and nonverbal concomitants of rapport in health care encounters: Implications for interpreters. *The Journal of Specialized Translation* 14, 216–228.

Flores, G. (2005) The impact of medical interpreter services on the quality of health care: A systematic review. *Medical Care Research and Review* 62, 255–299.

Free, C., Green, J., Bhavnani, V. and Newman, A. (2003) Bilingual young people's experiences of interpreting in primary care: A qualitative study. *The British Journal of General Practice* 53, 530–535.

French, J.R.P and Raven, B. (1959) The bases of social power. In D. Cartwright (ed.) *Studies in Social Power*. Ann Arbor, MI: Institute for Social Research.

Gadon, M., Balch, G.I. and Jacobs, E.A. (2007) Caring for patients with limited English proficiency: The perspectives of small group practitioners. *Journal of General Internal Medicine* 22, 341–346.

Garabetian, S. (2014) A qualitative study on gender differences in interpreter-mediated communication in general practice. Unpublished master's thesis, University of Amsterdam.

Gerrish, K., Chau, R., Sobowale, A. and Birks, E. (2004) Bridging the language barrier: The use of interpreters in primary care nursing. *Health and Social Care in the Community* 12, 407–413.

Glanz, K. and Bishop, D.B. (2010) The role of behavioral science theory in development and implementation of public health interventions. *Annual Review of Public Health* 31, 399–418.

Gray, B., Hilder, J. and Stubbe, M. (2012) How to use interpreters in general practice: The development of a New Zealand toolkit. *Journal of Primary Health Care* 4, 52–61.

Green, J., Free, C., Bhavani, V. and Newman, T. (2005) Translators and mediators: Bilingual young people's accounts of their interpreting work in health care. *Social Science and Medicine* 60, 2097–2110.

Greenhalgh, T., Robb, N. and Scambler, G. (2006) Communicative and strategic action in interpreted consultations in primary health care: A Habermasian perspective. *Social Science and Medicine* 63, 1170–1187.

Habermas, J. (1991) *The Theory of Communicative Action*. Oxford: Polity Press.

Hadziabdic, E., Heikkilä, K., Albin, B. and Hjelm, K. (2009) Migrants' perceptions of using interpreters in health care. *International Nursing Review* 56, 461–469.

Haes de, H. and Bensing, J. (2009) Endpoints in medical communication research, proposing a framework of functions and outcomes. *Patient Education and Counseling* 74, 287–294.

Hagan, S., Swartz, L., Kilian, S., Chiliza, B., Bisogno, P. and Joska, J. (2013) The accuracy of interpreting key psychiatric terms by ad hoc interpreters at a South African psychiatric hospital. *African Journal of Psychiatry* 16, 424–429.

Hall, J.A., Harrigan, J.A. and Rosenthal, R. (1995) Nonverbal behavior in clinician–patient interaction. *Applied and Preventive Psychology* 4, 21–37.

Hall, M.A., Dugan, E., Zheng, B. and Mishra, A.K. (2001) Trust in physicians and medical institutions: What is it, can it be measured, and does it matter? *Milbank Quarterly* 79, 613–639.

Harmsen, H. Bernsen, R., Meeuwesen, L., Thomas, S., Dorrenboom, G., Pinto, D. and Bruijnzeels, M. (2005) The effect of educational intervention on intercultural communication: Results of a randomized controlled trial. *British Journal of General Practice* 55, 343–350.

Hasselkus, B.R. (1992) The family caregiver as interpreter in the geriatric medical interview. *Medical Anthropology Quarterly* 6, 288–304.

Hilfinger Messias, D.K., McDowell, L. and Estrada, R.D. (2009) Language interpreting as social justice work: Perspectives of formal and informal healthcare interpreters. *Advances in Nursing Science* 32, 128–143.

Hornberger J., Itakura H. and Wilson, S.R. (1997) Bridging language and cultural barriers between physicians and patients. *Public Health Reports* 112, 410–417.

Hsieh, E. (2006) Understanding medical interpreters: Reconceptualizing bilingual health communication. *Health Communication* 20, 177–186.

Hsieh, E., Pitaloka, D. and Johnson, A.J. (2013) Bilingual health communication: Distinctive needs of providers from five specialties. *Health Communication* 28, 557–567.

Hudelson, P. and Vilpert, S. (2009) Overcoming language barriers with foreign-language speaking patients: A survey to investigate intra-hospital variation in attitudes and practices. *BMC Health Services Research* 9, 187.

Hudelson, P., Dao M.D., Perron, N.J. and Bischoff, A. (2013) Interpreter-mediated diabetes consultations: A qualitative analysis of physician communication practices. *BMC Family Practice* 14, 1–9.

Jacobs, E., Chen, A.H., Karliner, L.S., Agger-Gupta, N. and Murtha. S. (2006) The need for more research on language barriers in health care: A proposed research agenda. *The Milbank Quarterly* 84, 111–133.

Kai, J., Beavan, J. and Faull, C. (2011) Challenges of mediated communication, disclosure and patient autonomy in cross-cultural cancer care. *British Journal of Cancer* 105, 918–924.

Kale, E. and Syed, H.R. (2010) Language barriers and the use of interpreters in the public health services. A questionnaire-based survey. *Patient Education and Counseling* 81, 187–191.

Karliner, L.S., Jacobs, E.A., Chen, A.H. and Mutha, S. (2007) Do professional interpreters improve clinical care for patients with limited English proficiency? A systematic review of the literature. *Health Services Research* 42, 727–754.

Kempen van, A. (2007) Legal risks of ineffective communication. *Virtual Mentor* 9, 555–558.

Kilian, S., Swartz, L., Dowling, T., Dlali, M. and Chiliza, B. (2014) The potential consequences of informal interpreting practices for assessment of patients in a South African psychiatric hospital. *Social Science and Medicine* 106, 159–167.

Krystallidou, D. (2014) Gaze and body orientation as an apparatus for patient inclusion into/exclusion from a patient-centred framework of communication. *The Interpreter and Translator Trainer* 8, 399–417.
Larrison, C.R., Velez-Ortis D., Hernandez, P.M., Piedra, L.M. and Goldberg, A. (2010) Brokering language and culture: Can ad hoc interpreters fill the language service gap at community health centers? *Social Work in Public Health* 25, 387–407.
Leanza, Y. (2005) Roles of community interpreters in pediatrics as seen by interpreters, physicians and researchers. *Interpreting* 7, 167–192.
Leanza, Y., Boivin, I. and Rosenberg, E. (2010) Interruptions and resistance: A comparison of medical consultations with family and trained interpreters. *Social Science and Medicine* 70, 1888–1895.
Lee, K.C., Winickoff, J.P., Kim, M.K., Campbell, E.G., Betancourt, J.R., Park, E.R., Maina, A.W. and Weissman, J.S. (2006) Resident physicians' use of professional and nonprofessional interpreters: A national survey. *Journal of the American Medical Association* 296, 1049–1054.
Lewin, K. (1948) *Resolving Social Conflicts*. New York: Harper & Row.
Li, S., Pearson, D. and Escott, S. (2010) Language barriers within primary care consultations: An increasing challenge needing new solutions. *Education for Primary Care* 21, 385–391.
Lukes, S. (1974) *Power: A Radical View* (Vol. 1). London: Macmillan.
MacFarlane, A., Glynn, L.G., Mosinkie, P.I. and Murphy, A.W. (2008) Responses to language barriers in consultations with refugees and asylum seekers: A telephone survey of Irish general practitioners. *BMC Family Practice* 9, 68.
MacFarlane, A., Dzebisova, Z., Karapish, D., Kovacevic B., Ogbebor, F. and Okonkwo, E. (2009) Arranging and negotiating the use of informal interpreters in general practice consultations: Experiences of refugees and asylum seekers in the west of Ireland. *Social Science and Medicine* 69, 210–214.
Matthews, C., Johnson M. and Noble C. (2000) Bilingual health communicators: Role delineation issues. *Australian Health Review* 23, 104–112.
Meeuwesen, L. and Twilt, S. (2011) 'If you don't understand what I mean ...' Interpreting in health and social care. Utrecht: Centre for Social Policy and Intervention Studies.
Meeuwesen, L., Twilt, S., ten Thije J.D. and Harmsen, H. (2010) 'Ne diyor?' (What does she say?): Informal interpreting in general practice. *Patient Education and Counseling* 81, 198–203.
Mishler, E.G. (1984) *The Discourse of Medicine: Dialectics of Medical Interviews*. Norwood, NJ: Ablex.
Ngo-Metzger Q., Massagli, M.P., Clarridge, B.R., Manocchia, M., Davis, R.B., Iezzoni, L.I. and Phillips, R.S. (2003) Linguistic and cultural barriers to care. Perspectives of Chinese and Vietnamese immigrants. *Journal of General and Internal Medicine* 18, 44–52.
Papic, O., Malak, Z. and Rosenberg, E. (2012) Survey on family physicians' perspectives on management of immigrant patients: Attitudes, barriers, strategies and training needs. *Patient Education and Counseling* 86, 205–209.
Pearson, S.D. and Raeke, L.H. (2000) Patients' trust in physicians: Many theories, few measures, and little data. *Journal of General Internal Medicine* 15, 509–513.
Phelan, M. (2012) Medical interpreting and the law in the European Union. *European Journal of Health Law* 19, 333–353.
Pinto, D. (2000) *Intercultural Communication: A Three-step Method for Dealing with Differences*. Leuven: Garant.
Pöchhacker, F. (2000) Language barriers in Vienna hospitals. *Ethnicity and Health* 5, 113–119.
Ramirez, D., Engel, K.G. and Tang, T.S. (2008) Language interpreter utilization in the emergency department setting: A clinical review. *Journal of Health Care for the Poor and Underserved* 19, 352–362.

Raven, B.H. (1992) A power/interaction model of interpersonal influence: French and Raven 30 years later. *Journal of Social Behavior and Personality* 7, 217–244.

Rhodes, P., Nocon, A. and Wright, J. (2003) Access to diabetes services: The experiences of Bangladeshi people in Bradford, UK. *Ethnicity and Health* 8, 171–188.

Robb, N. and Greenhalgh, T. (2006) 'You have to cover up the words of the doctor.' The mediation of trust in interpreted consultations in primary care. *Journal of Health Organization and Management* 20, 434–455.

Rosenberg, E., Leanza, Y. and Seller, R. (2007) Doctor–patient communication in primary care with an interpreter: Physician perceptions of professional and family interpreters. *Patient Education and Counseling* 67, 286–292.

Rosenberg, E., Seller, R. and Leanza, Y. (2008) Through interpreters' eyes: Comparing roles of professional and family interpreters. *Patient Education and Counseling* 70, 87–93.

Rosenberg, E., Richard C., Lussier M. and Shuldiner, T. (2011) The content of talk about health conditions and medications during appointments involving interpreters. *Family Practice* 28, 317–322.

Schaafsma, E.S., Raynor, T.D.K. and de Jong-van den Berg, L.T.W. (2003) Accessing medication information by ethnic minorities: Barriers and possible solutions. *Pharmacy World and Science* 25, 185–190.

Schenker, Y., Pérez-Stable, E.J., Nickleach, D. and Karliner, L.S. (2011) Patterns of interpreter use for hospitalized patients with limited English proficiency. *Journal of General Internal Medicine* 26, 712–717.

Schippers, E. and Veldhuijzen van Zanten-Hyllner, M. (2011) Letter from the Dutch Minister and Secretary of Health to the Lower House. The Hague, 25 May.

Schouten, B.C. and Schinkel, S. (2014) Turkish migrant GP patients' expression of emotional cues and concerns in encounters with and without informal interpreters. *Patient Education and Counseling* 97, 23–29.

Schouten, B.C., Ross, J., Zendedel R. and Meeuwesen, L. (2012) Informal interpreters in medical settings. A comparative socio-cultural study of the Netherlands and Turkey. *The Translator* 18, 311–338.

Shannon, C.E. and Weaver, W. (1964) *The Mathematical Model of Communication.* Urbana, IL: The University of Illinois Press.

Statistics Netherlands (2014) *Bevolking; Generatie, Geslacht, Leeftijd en Herkomstgroepering* [Population; generation, sex, age and ethnic origin]. See http://statline.cbs.nl/StatWeb/

Steers, R.M. (1991) *Introduction to Organizational Behavior* (4th edn). New York: HarperCollins.

Stewart, M.A. (1995) Effective physician–patient communication and health outcomes: A review. *Canadian Medical Association Journal* 152, 1423–1433.

Tschurtz, B.A., Koss, R.G., Kupka, N.J. and Williams, S.C. (2010) Language services in hospitals: Discordance in availability and staff use. *Journal of Healthcare Management/American College of Healthcare Executives* 56, 403–417.

Turkenburg, M. and Gijsberts, M. (2007) Opleidingsniveau en beheersing van de Nederlandse taal [Educational level and Dutch language proficiency]. In J. Dagevos and M. Gijsberts (eds) *Jaarrapport Integratie 2007* [Year report Integration 2007]. Den Haag: Sociaal en Cultureel Planbureau.

Yang, C.F. and Gray, B. (2008) Bilingual medical students as interpreters: What are the benefits and risks. *The New Zealand Medical Journal* 121,15–28.

Zendedel, R., Schouten, B.C., van Weert, J.C.M. and van den Putte, B. (2016) Informal interpreting in general practice: The migrant patient's voice. *Ethnicity & Health*, advance online publication.

6 Understanding the Advantages and Disadvantages of the Diversity of Approaches to Overcoming Language Barriers in Medical Encounters

Rebecca Schwei, Mary Rhodes and Elizabeth A. Jacobs

The number of healthcare encounters in which patients and their providers do not speak the same language is increasing worldwide. Approaches to addressing language barriers in health care vary internationally from providing professionally trained interpreters within healthcare systems to utilizing friends and family to help communicate with patients. Each of these approaches has strengths and weaknesses and the best approach may vary across nations and cultural groups.

This choice can be informed by the substantial body of research investigating the quality and acceptability of different methods and modes of providing linguistic access services. In this chapter, we summarize the international literature focusing on comparing different methods of overcoming language barriers in health care in order to provide some guidance as to how to effectively reduce language barriers in health care. Specifically we review the literature on the accuracy of different methods of providing interpretation, what we know about the impact of different types of interpreters on clinical healthcare outcomes, users' satisfaction with different methods of providing linguistic access services and how 'who' is delivering them might impact a patient and/or client's willingness to disclose important healthcare information. As will be clear, the overwhelming preponderance of evidence supports the provision of a professionally trained means of linguistic access, in the form of either a bilingual physician or a trained interpreter.

Interpreter Accuracy

The quantity of literature investigating the accuracy of communication in interpreted medical encounters generally or across different interpreter modalities is somewhat limited (Butow et al., 2011; Elderkin-Thompson et al., 2001; Farooq et al., 1997; Flores, 2005; Flores et al., 2003, 2012; Gany et al., 2010; Hornberger et al., 1996; Karliner et al., 2007; Lee et al., 2002; Prince & Nelson, 1995). Studies about the accuracy of interpretation occurred in the US (seven), Australia (two), New Guinea, Nigeria and the UK. Of the studies that do exist, many are limited by their small sample size (Elderkin-Thompson et al., 2001; Farooq et al., 1997; Flores et al., 2012; Lee et al., 2002; Prince & Nelson, 1995). Nevertheless there are several studies with larger sample sizes that provide insight into how the accuracy of the interpreter type varies (Butow et al., 2011; Flores, 2005; Flores et al., 2003; Gany et al., 2010; Hornberger et al., 1996; Karliner et al., 2007). This literature demonstrates that all types of interpreters make errors in interpretation during medical encounters (Butow et al., 2011; Elderkin-Thompson et al., 2001; Flores et al., 2003; Gany et al., 2010; Hornberger et al., 1996), but that clinically significant errors were much less likely to occur when trained interpreters were compared with untrained or ad hoc interpreters such as non-clinical hospital staff, clinical hospital staff or family members (Flores et al., 2003; Gany et al., 2010). By clinically significant errors, we mean errors that altered or potentially altered the history of present illness, medical history, diagnostic or therapeutic interventions, understanding of the medical condition and/or plans for future medical visits (including follow-up visits and specialty referrals; Flores et al., 2012). In one study, untrained interpreters were over nine times as likely to make clinically significant errors in interpreted concepts compared with professionally trained interpreters (Gany et al., 2010). However, another study did not document differences in clinically significant errors between trained and untrained interpreters (Butow et al., 2011). Another investigated differences in accuracy between remote-simultaneous medical interpretation and in-person interpretation and demonstrated that the remote-simultaneous method had a higher rate of accurately interpreted utterances than the in-person method (Hornberger et al., 1996). With the explosion of technology designed to address language barriers, several investigators have studied the accuracy of using online translation tools such as Google Translate in medical encounters and shown them to have unacceptably low rates of accuracy (Borner et al., 2013; Patil & Davis, 2014). These studies from the UK and Germany suggest that the risks associated with using these online translation tools as a way to communicate verbally with patients far outweigh their convenience (Borner et al., 2013; Patil & Davis, 2014). Although the literature is not entirely consistent, the balance of the evidence suggests that utilization of trained interpreters results in communication that is more accurate than using untrained methods of interpretation, especially when considering clinically significant errors in communication (Flores, 2005; Karliner et al., 2007).

Interpretation Type and Clinical Outcomes

We reviewed the literature to understand the impact that bilingual providers and trained interpreters have on clinical outcomes compared with untrained or ad hoc interpreters, family members or no interpreters. In the overview of the literature, we included systematic reviews and research articles that had large sample sizes ranging from 306 participants (Eamranond et al., 2009) to 6738 participants (Fernandez et al., 2011). Of the studies reviewed 17 were conducted in the US and one was conducted in Australia. Additionally, all of the studies explicitly compared clinical outcomes across patient groups that received different types of language services (bilingual provider, trained interpreter, untrained or ad hoc interpreter, family interpreter or no language service).

Across nations, clinical setting and language group, research consistently demonstrates that patients who experience language barriers in health care have improved clinical outcomes when working with a bilingual provider or a trained interpreter as compared with untrained interpreters, family members or no interpreters at all (Flores, 2005; Karliner et al., 2007; Baker et al., 1996). Patients with language-concordant physicians report asking more questions (Flores, 2005; Green et al., 2005), demonstrate a better understanding of their diagnosis and treatment plans (Baker et al., 1996), have increased documentation of dietary and physical activity counseling (Eamranond et al., 2009), receive more equitable testing in the emergency department (Hampers & McNulty, 2002), have improved glycemic control (in diabetic patients; Fernandez et al., 2011), have increased, appropriate utilization of mental health services (Ziguras et al., 2003) and significantly better information recall after a visit (Flores, 2005). Similarly, patients who use professionally trained interpreters have better clinical outcomes than patients using untrained interpreters, family members or no interpreters. They experience fewer disparities in healthcare utilization in outpatient preventive services (Jacobs et al., 2001) and intensity of emergency department services (Bernstein et al., 2001); lower rates of obstetric interventions (Parsons & Day, 1992); increased provision of health education (Ngo-Metzger et al., 2007), number of office visits (Jacobs et al., 2001), and number of prescriptions written and filled (Jacobs et al., 2001). In addition, pediatric patients receive more equitable treatment of pain (Jimenez et al., 2014) and women who are eligible for screening have increased rates of mammography (Dang et al., 2010). In one study, patients who used a trained interpreter reported having questions they did not ask about their health care and about their mental health more often than patients who had language-concordant clinicians, defined as a clinician who is fluent in the patient's language (Green et al., 2005). Therefore, when only considering optimizing clinical outcomes, language concordant care is the best (described in greater detail in Chapter 7; Fernandez et al., 2011; Baker et al., 1996).

It is clear that trained medical interpreters improve clinical care more than untrained interpreters and can raise the quality of care for patients who experience language barriers to in some cases match or approach that for patients without a language barrier (Flores, 2005; Karliner et al., 2007; Baker et al., 1996).

Satisfaction with Different Types of Interpreters

The literature exploring satisfaction across different interpreting modalities is quite extensive and covers patient, provider and interpreter satisfaction using bilingual providers, trained in-person interpreters, trained video interpreters, trained telephone interpreters, untrained bilingual healthcare workers and family members or friends. However, 16 of the studies we reviewed were conducted in the US with one study being conducted in Switzerland.

This research documents that the use of trained interpreters (in-person, telephonic and video) results in increased patient, provider and interpreter satisfaction in comparison with untrained interpreters, such as bilingual healthcare workers with no formal interpreter training or family members (Flores, 2005; Karliner et al., 2007; Hornberger et al., 1996; Lee et al., 2002; Azarmina & Wallace, 2005; Kuo & Fagan, 1999). Several studies have reported that bilingual providers result in the highest levels of patient satisfaction (Gany et al., 2007; Jacobs et al., 2007) compared with trained interpreters; however, other studies have found no difference in patient satisfaction when using trained interpreters or bilingual providers (Flores, 2005; Lee et al., 2002). One study even found that the participants who had a bilingual provider, documented by interpreter audit, were less satisfied than the participants who received an in-person trained interpreter or a trained telephonic interpreter (Crossman et al., 2010).

When trying to understand which type of trained interpreter – in-person, telephonic or video – results in the highest level of satisfaction, the literature is less clear. Several studies have found that patients, providers and interpreters are more satisfied with in-person interpreters compared with telephonic interpreters (Kuo & Fagan, 1999; Garcia et al., 2004; Locatis et al., 2010; Wu et al., 2006; Price et al., 2012), especially when the interpreter does more than transfer information, helping the provider establish rapport and understand a patient's sociocultural background (Price et al., 2012). One study found the use of remote simultaneous medical interpretation to be significantly associated with increased satisfaction compared with usual customary care of trained interpreters which included both trained and untrained interpreters (Gany et al., 2007). However, other studies reported no difference in satisfaction across telephonic, video and in-person interpreter modes (Lee et al., 2002; Crossman et al., 2010; Price et al., 2012; Napoles et al., 2010). These studies highlight the fact that the type of trained interpreter utilized may not be as important as the fact that one was actually used.

A few studies have reported on patient and provider preferences for different interpreting modalities. In one study a majority of providers reported preferring in-person trained interpreters over telephone interpreters or friends while the patients were more comfortable and preferred working with family members or friends (Ramsey et al., 2012). In a second study, providers and patients preferred remote-simultaneous medical interpreter services to in-person interpreter services (Hornberger et al., 1996). In another study 66% of doctors and nurses preferred to work with untrained interpreters owing to convenience (Hudelson & Vilpert, 2009). Notably, in this study only 9% of those surveyed had any training in working with interpreters and only 23% had been encouraged by their institutions to use trained interpreters (Hudelson & Vilpert, 2009). Rather than supporting the use of untrained interpreters, this study raises the question of whether providers lacking experience and training in the use of trained interpreters underestimate their value. Interestingly, this literature regarding interpreter preference is not consistent with the satisfaction literature, which clearly documents higher satisfaction with utilization of trained interpreters or bilingual providers. This suggests that the patients and providers included in interpreter preference studies are different from the patients and providers studied in the satisfaction literature or that questions regarding interpreter preference and interpreter satisfaction are being asked in ways that generate different answers.

Patients' Willingness to Disclose

Several different studies from the US (two) and Switzerland (two) have explored whether a patient's willingness to disclose sensitive information is influenced by interpreter mode. In one study, 51% of patients using remote simultaneous medical interpreting stated that they thought their interpreter protected their privacy very well compared with only 38% of patients who received either trained in-person, trained telephonic or untrained interpreters ($p < 0.05$; Gany et al., 2007). However, in another study, patient comfort with discussing sensitive issues did not differ by interpreter type (Kuo & Fagan, 1999). Etyan and Bischoff have looked at willingness to disclose in the highly sensitive context of the mental health consultation, specifically the impact of patient–nurse language concordance and the presence of trained interpreters on disclosure of psychological symptoms by refugees arriving in Switzerland (Bischoff et al., 2003; Eytan et al., 2002). When the patient and screening nurse had adequate language concordance (there was either a trained interpreter or the nurse was fluent in language of interview), patients were significantly more likely to report both physical symptoms and psychological symptoms compared with patients who had untrained interpreters or no interpreter at all (Bischoff et al., 2003). There were differences in reporting of traumatic events by patients receiving a trained interpreter versus relative as interpreter versus no interpreter (77 vs 46 vs 55%, p-value = 0.003; Bischoff et al., 2003). Reporting of traumatic events was significantly increased among those using a trained interpreter compared with those using a relative or no interpreter (Eytan et al., 2002). Discrepancies in reporting of psychological symptoms were even greater between patients receiving a trained interpreter, relative as interpreter and no interpreter (33 vs 14 vs 12% respectively, $p = 0.001$). Use of trained interpreters was also associated with increased referral for mental health services compared with using a relative as an interpreter or having no interpreter (15 vs 3 vs 4%, $p = 0.007$).

Taken together, these articles indicate that patients are more likely to disclose sensitive psychological symptoms and traumatic events to providers when language concordance exists or a trained interpreter is used than when untrained interpreter or family members are used. This further supports prior suggestions that trained interpreters are essential to the care of patients at psychological risk or when information is sensitive.

What does this literature tell us?

The preponderance of evidence supports the importance of providing linguistic access in the form of either a truly bilingual physician or a trained interpreter. Not surprisingly, communication using one of these two methods was more accurate, and led to better clinical outcomes, higher satisfaction and greater willingness to disclose in patients who required linguistic access services. There is less evidence for what is the best mode for delivering professionally trained interpretation: in-person, over the telephone or via video. What is encouraging is that, when in-person trained interpretation is not available, telephonic or video interpreting using a trained interpreter probably works just as well.

Clearly more research is needed into how different modes of interpreter service delivery might impact outcomes as well as more international research. The vast majority of the research we identified was conducted in the US and, as our colleagues have pointed out in several other chapters in this book, the use of untrained interpreters is more commonly used and viewed as valuable in other countries and in different cultural contexts. While we believe that accuracy and outcomes will be better in any country and culture where bilingual physicians or trained interpreters are used, this assertion needs more extensive investigation. In the meantime, trained interpreters and truly bilingual physicians should be used in all countries in all contexts, whenever possible, to assure that patients at risk of experiencing disparities owing to language barriers receive the highest quality care possible.

References

Azarmina, P. and Wallace, P. (2005) Remote interpretation in medical encounters: A systematic review. *Journal of Telemedicine and Telecare* 11 (3), 140–145.
Baker, D.W., Parker, R.M., Williams, M.V., Coates, W.C. and Pitkin, K. (1996) Use and effectiveness of interpreters in an emergency department. *JAMA* 275, 783–788.
Bernstein, J., Bernstein, E., Dave, A., Hardt, E., James, T., Linden, J. *et al.* (2002) Trained medical interpreters in the emergency department: Effects on services, subsequent charges, and follow-up. *Journal of Immigrant Health* 4 (4), 171–176.
Bischoff, A., Bovier, P.A., Rrustemi, I., Gariazzo, F., Eytan, A. and Loutan, L. (2003) Language barriers between nurses and asylum seekers: Their impact on symptom reporting and referral. *Social Science and Medicine* 57 (3), 503–512.
Borner, N., Sponholz, S., Konig, K., Brodkorb, S., Buhrer, C. and Roehr, C.C. (2013) [Google translate is not sufficient to overcome language barriers in neonatal medicine]. *Klinische Pädiatrie* 225 (7), 413–417.
Butow, P.N., Goldstein, D., Bell, M.L., Sze, M., Aldridge, L.J., Abdo, S. *et al.* (2011) Interpretation in consultations with immigrant patients with cancer: How accurate is it? *Journal of Clinical Oncology* 29 (20), 2801–2807.
Crossman, K.L., Wiener, E., Roosevelt, G., Bajaj, L. and Hampers, L.C. (2010) Interpreters: Telephonic, in-person interpretation and bilingual providers. *Pediatrics* 125 (3), e631–638.
Dang, J., Lee, J., Tran, J.H., Kagawa-Singer, M.A., Foo, M., Nguyen, T.N. *et al.* (2010) The role of medical interpretation on breast and cervical cancer screening among Asian American and Pacific Islander women. *Journal of Cancer Education* 25 (2), 253–262.
Eamranond, P.P., Davis, R.B., Phillips, R.S. and Wee, C.C. (2009) Patient–physician language concordance and lifestyle counseling among Spanish-speaking patients. *Journal of Immigrant and Minority Health* 11 (6), 494–498.
Elderkin-Thompson, V., Silver, R.C. and Waitzkin, H. (2001) When nurses double as interpreters: A study of Spanish-speaking patients in a US primary care setting. *Social Science and Medicine* 52 (9), 1343–1358.
Eytan, A., Bischoff, A., Rrustemi, I., Durieux, S., Loutan, L., Gilbert, M. *et al.* (2002) Screening of mental disorders in asylum-seekers from Kosovo. *Australian and New Zealand Journal of Psychiatry* 36 (4), 499–503.
Farooq, S., Fear, C. and Oyebode, F. (1997) An investigation of the adequacy of psychiatric interviews conducted through an interpreter. *Psychiatric Bulletin* 21, 209–213.
Fernandez, A., Schillinger, D., Warton, E.M., Adler, N., Moffet, H.H., Schenker, Y. *et al.* (2011) Language barriers, physician–patient language concordance, and glycemic control among insured Latinos with diabetes: The Diabetes Study of Northern California (DISTANCE). *Journal of General Internal Medicine* 26 (2), 170–176.
Flores, G., Abreu, M., Barone, C.P., Bachur, R. and Lin, H. (2012) Errors of medical interpretation and their potential clinical consequences: A comparison of professional versus ad hoc versus no interpreters. *Annals of Emergency Medicine* 60 (5), 545–553.
Flores, G., Laws, M.B., Mayo, S.J., Zuckerman, B., Abreu, M., Medina, L. *et al.* (2003) Errors in medical interpretation and their potential clinical consequences in pediatric encounters. *Pediatrics* 111 (1), 6–14.
Flores, G. (2005) The impact of medical interpreter services on the quality of health care: A systematic review. *Medical Care Research Review* 62 (3), 255–299.

Gany, F., Leng, J., Shapiro, E., Abramson, D., Motola, I., Shield, D.C. et al. (2007) Patient satisfaction with different interpreting methods: A randomized controlled trial. *Journal of General Internal Medicine* 22 Suppl 2, 312–318. PMCID: 2078551.

Gany, F.M., Gonzalez, C.J., Basu, G., Hasan, A., Mukherjee, D., Datta, M. et al. (2010) Reducing clinical errors in cancer education: Interpreter training. *Journal of Cancer Education* 25 (4), 560–564.

Garcia, E.A., Roy, L.C., Okada, P.J., Perkins, S.D. and Wiebe, R.A. (2004) A comparison of the influence of hospital-trained, ad hoc, and telephone interpreters on perceived satisfaction of limited English-proficient parents presenting to a pediatric emergency department. *Pediatric Emergency Care* 20 (6), 373–378.

Green, A.R., Ngo-Metzger, Q., Legedza, A.T., Massagli, M.P., Phillips, R.S. and Iezzoni, L.I. (2005) Interpreter services, language concordance, and health care quality. Experiences of Asian Americans with limited English proficiency. *Journal of General Internal Medicine* 20 (11), 1050–1056. PMCID: 1490255.

Hampers, L.C. and McNulty, J.E. (2002) Professional interpreters and bilingual physicians in a pediatric emergency department: Effect on resource utilization. *Archives of Pediatric and Adolescent Medicine* 156 (11), 1108–1113.

Hornberger, J.C., Gibson, C.D., Jr, Wood, W., Dequeldre, C., Corso, I., Palla, B. et al. (1996) Eliminating language barriers for non-English-speaking patients. *Medical Care* 34 (8), 845–856.

Hudelson, P. and Vilpert, S. (2009) Overcoming language barriers with foreign-language speaking patients: A survey to investigate intra-hospital variation in attitudes and practices. *BMC Health Services Research* 9, 187. PMCID: 2770464.

Jacobs, E.A., Lauderdale, D.S., Meltzer, D., Shorey, J.M., Levinson, W. and Thisted, R.A. (2001) Impact of interpreter services on delivery of health care to limited-English-proficient patients. *Journal of General Internal Medicine* 16 (7), 468–474. PMCID: 1495243.

Jacobs, E.A., Sadowski, L.S. and Rathouz, P.J. (2007) The impact of an enhanced interpreter service intervention on hospital costs and patient satisfaction. *Journal of General Internal Medicine* 22 (Suppl 2), 306–311. PMCID: 2078550.

Jimenez, N., Jackson, D.L., Zhou, C., Ayala, N.C. and Ebel, B.E. (2014) Postoperative pain management in children, parental English proficiency, and access to interpretation. *Hospital Pediatrics* 4 (1), 23–30. PMCID: 4231782.

Karliner, L.S., Jacobs, E.A., Chen, A.H. and Mutha, S. (2007) Do professional interpreters improve clinical care for patients with limited English proficiency? A systematic review of the literature. *Health Services Research* 42 (2), 727–754. PMCID: 1955368.

Kuo, D. and Fagan, M.J. (1999) Satisfaction with methods of Spanish interpretation in an ambulatory care clinic. *Journal of General Internal Medicine* 14 (9), 547–550. PMCID: 1496734.

Lee, L.J., Batal, H.A., Maselli, J.H. and Kutner, J.S. (2002) Effect of Spanish interpretation method on patient satisfaction in an urban walk-in clinic. *Journal of General Internal Medicine* 17 (8), 641–645. PMCID: 1495083.

Locatis, C., Williamson, D., Gould-Kabler, C., Zone-Smith, L., Detzler, I., Roberson, J. et al. (2010) Comparing in-person, video, and telephonic medical interpretation. *Journal of General Internal Medicine* 25 (4), 345–350. PMCID: 2842540.

Napoles, A.M., Santoyo-Olsson, J., Karliner, L.S., O'Brien, H, Gregorich, S.E. and Perez-Stable, E.J. (2010) Clinician ratings of interpreter mediated visits in underserved primary care settings with ad hoc, in-person professional, and video conferencing modes. *Journal of Health Care of the Poor and Underserved* 21 (1), 301–317.

Ngo-Metzger, Q., Sorkin, D.H., Phillips, R.S., Greenfield, S., Massagli, M.P., Clarridge, B. et al. (2007) Providing high-quality care for limited English proficient patients: The importance of language concordance and interpreter use. *Journal of General Internal Medicine* 22 (Suppl 2), 324–330. PMCID: 2078537.

Parsons, L. and Day, S. (1992) Improving obstetric outcomes in ethnic minorities: An evaluation of health advocacy in Hackney. *Journal of Public Health Medicine* 14 (2), 183–191.

Patil, S. and Davies, P. (2014) Use of Google Translate in medical communication: Evaluation of accuracy. *BMJ* 349:g7392. PMCID: 4266233.

Price, E.L., Perez-Stable, E.J., Nickleach, D., Lopez, M. and Karliner, L.S. (2012) Interpreter perspectives of in-person, telephonic, and videoconferencing medical interpretation in clinical encounters. *Patient Education and Counseling* 87 (2), 226–232. PMCID: 4059012.

Prince, D. and Nelson, M. (1995) Teaching Spanish to emergency medicine residents. *Acadamic Emergency Medicine* 2 (1), 32–36; discussion 6–7.

Ramsey, K.W., Davis, J. and French, G. (2012) Perspectives of Chuukese patients and their health care providers on the use of different sources of interpreters. *Hawaii Journal of Medicine of Public Health* 71 (9), 249–252. PMCID: 3443847.

Wu, A.C., Leventhal, J.M., Ortiz, J., Gonzalez, E.E. and Forsyth, B. (2006) The interpreter as cultural educator of residents: Improving communication for Latino parents. *Archives of Pediatric and Adolescent Medicine* 160 (11), 1145–1150.

Ziguras, S., Klimidis, S., Lewis, J. and Stuart, G. (2003) Ethnic matching of clients and clinicians and use of mental health services by ethnic minority clients. *Psychiatric Services* 54 (4), 535–541.

7 Language Concordance Between Limited English Proficient Patients and Their Clinicians

Dana Canfield and Lisa C. Diamond

Introduction

Patients with language barriers are at risk of impaired communication with their clinicians and thus disparities in care. Professional interpreters and truly bilingual clinicians can reduce disparities owing to language barriers. Despite knowledge that the use of professional interpreters improves patient care for patients who are limited English proficient (LEP), research from the US, Australia and New Zealand has shown that clinicians underuse language services in favor of their own, often limited, non-English skills (Atkin, 2008; Diamond *et al.*, 2009, 2012a, Gadon *et al.*, 2007; Gray *et al.*, 2011). This fact, combined with the rapid growth of the LEP population in English-language dominant countries and the complex discussions that take place in clinical care, highlights a compelling unmet need for standards to guide the use of non-fluent language skills by clinicians with LEP patients. This chapter will review the literature on language concordance and the relationship between clinician language proficiency and quality of care. While other countries have noted low compliance with interpreter use (Atkin, 2008; Gray *et al.*, 2011), this chapter focuses on the US, where more research has been done to evaluate clinician non-English language use with LEP patients.

Effective communication between physicians and patients is essential to the provision of high-quality, patient-centered health care (Institute of Medicine, 2001). Patients with LEP have poorer healthcare processes and outcomes (Wisnivesky *et al.*, 2009; Pippins *et al.*, 2007; Hu & Covell, 1986; Lauderdale *et al.*, 2006; Woloshin *et al.*, 1995; Weinick & Krauss, 2000). Although socioeconomic and insurance status explain some of these associations, disparities in care for people with LEP persist even when these factors are taken into consideration, suggesting that language and culture also play a role (DuBard & Gizlice, 2008). There are policies regarding access to language services that affect the way healthcare organizations provide care to patients with LEP in the US (see Chapter 2). The National Standards on Culturally and Linguistically Appropriate Services (CLAS Standards) in Health Care include four standards that outline adequate provision of linguistic access services and are considered mandates (US Department of Health and Human Services (Office of Minority Health), 2013). First, healthcare organizations should make language assistance services, including bilingual staff and interpreter services, available to patients with LEP free of charge, in a timely manner, during all hours of operation. Second, patients with LEP must be informed in their preferred language of their right to receive language services, both verbally and in writing. Third, family and friends of patients should not be used as interpreters (unless requested by the patient), and healthcare organizations must assure the proficiency of language services being offered by interpreters and bilingual staff. Fourth, healthcare organizations must have signage and written patient information in the languages commonly seen in their service area (US Department of Health and Human Services (Office of Minority Health), 2013). Absent from these regulations is any specific guidance on when clinicians can appropriately use their non-English language skills with LEP patients, particularly when clinicians are not completely fluent. In order to establish standards for clinician non-English language use with LEP patients to promote language concordant care, it is necessary to gain an accurate picture of how language services are currently being used, and more specifically, why clinicians are not using interpreters. To this end, some fundamental questions must be answered:

How Well are Healthcare Organizations Meeting the Needs of Patients with LEP? Are These Needs being Met with Language-concordant Physicians?

US federal regulations require that healthcare organizations make language services available (US Department of Justice, 1964). One of these requires that healthcare organizations assure that those providing language services are competent to do so and notes that using untrained people as interpreters should be avoided (US Department of Health and Human Services (Office of Minority Health), 2013). The Joint Commission's standards require that hospitals define qualifications for interpreters and cite 'trained bilingual staff,' which could include physicians, as one reasonable way to address the language needs of LEP patients (The Joint Commission, 2010).

However, the level of compliance with these regulations is low. Many hospitals are not in compliance with the language-related CLAS standards, despite the fact that they are considered federal mandates. In one national study of hospitals, the majority of hospitals surveyed were not providing language assistance in their less commonly requested languages, only informing patients of their right to request language services in English, relying on family members or untrained staff as interpreters, and providing vital documents, such as consent forms and advance directives, in English only (Diamond et al., 2010).

Questions surrounding how hospitals should fund this mandate and the availability of language-concordant providers underlie this lack of adherence to federal regulations; in many cases, hospitals lack a clear source of funding to provide interpreter services and have a deficit of providers and staff who are trained interpreters. Given that reimbursement for professional interpreters is not covered by private insurance (except in California) or Medicare, and only covered by Medicaid in 15 states, it is not known how healthcare organizations can finance these services (Perkins & Youdelman, 2008). Further, while applicants for medical residency are linguistically diverse, their languages tend not include those spoken by the US LEP population, leading to a mismatch between languages spoken by providers and patients (Diamond et al., 2014a).

It is therefore unsurprising that the use of language services for LEP patients has only minimally improved in recent years. Between 2004 and 2010, there was only a modest increase in pediatricians' use of language services, with only 55.8% of pediatricians using professional interpreters in 2010 compared with 49.7% in 2004 (DeCamp et al., 2013). While it is encouraging that there has been any increase in physician's use of interpreters, it is not commensurate with the increased number of LEP patients and falls drastically short of being adequate.

To address this discrepancy, it is necessary to know the specific language needs and preferences of patients. Similarly, data is needed to identify the mismatch between provider and patient race, ethnicity and language. This also relies on a picture of the demographics of both providers and patients, but the data needed to address these issues is inconsistently collected. The importance of collecting patient race, ethnicity and language data was underscored by the 2009 Institute of Medicine Report 'Race, Ethnicity, and Language Data: Standardization for Health Care Quality Improvement', and indeed, hospitals are collecting these data for patients at increased rates. Health plans and healthcare organizations were more likely in 2010 to collect data on patient race, ethnicity and language preferences than they were in 2006 (Nerenz et al., 2013). More recently, the Institute for Diversity issued a report entitled 'Diversity and Disparities' which showed a continued increase in the collection of patient race, ethnicity and language preference data between 2011 and 2013. This report also showed a slight increase in the utilization of these data to identify disparities in treatment or outcomes in an effort to provide more equitable care, from 20% of hospitals in 2011 to 22% in 2013. However, there has been no increase in the collection of corresponding race, ethnicity and language proficiency data of providers (Nerenz et al., 2013), rendering studies of concordance challenging.

Taken together, these findings highlight potential sources of inequitable care that, while perhaps improving, are nonetheless persistent. Of particular concern are the lack of compliance with the CLAS standards, the continued lack of provider race, ethnicity and language proficiency data, and the failure of the majority of hospitals to use the data they are collecting about patient demographics to identify disparities and design interventions to provide more equitable care.

Is there an Association between Language Concordance and Better Quality of Care and Outcomes for Patients with LEP?

Studies have shown that language concordance between patients and providers results in improved healthcare quality and outcomes. Language concordance between patients and clinicians leads to better patient satisfaction with care. Patients receiving language-concordant care are less likely to have questions about their care (Green et al., 2005), and patients receiving language-discordant care report worse interpersonal care and give lower ratings to their providers (Ngo-Metzger et al., 2007). Medication adherence also declines when patients receive language-discordant care, as shown in a study of asthmatic patients which demonstrated that patients with language-discordant care were slightly more likely to miss an appointment and to go to the emergency room than those with language-concordant care (Manson, 1988). Patient understanding of diagnoses and treatment is also worse with language discordance. In a study of Spanish-speaking patients, patients who reported that no interpreter was necessary for their visit rated their own understanding of their disease to be 'good' to 'excellent' 67% of the time, compared with 57% of patients who used an interpreter and 38% of those who thought an interpreter should have been used (Baker et al., 1996). Another study of Spanish-speaking patients found that patient functioning and well-being for patients with diabetes was greater when language-concordant care was provided (Perez-Stable et al., 1997). Patient perception of patient-centeredness was found to be higher in a study of Spanish-speaking diabetic patients with language-concordant physicians, probably because those physicians were more likely to elicit their patient's problems and concerns (Fernandez et al., 2004). More health education is given to LEP patients with language-concordant providers, with language-concordant physicians more likely to document diet and physical activity counseling compared with language-discordant pairs (Ngo-Metzger et al., 2007; Eamranond et al., 2009). Given all of these findings, it is no surprise that having a language-concordant provider leads to fewer emergency department visits, less likelihood of missing medications and lower costs (Manson, 1988; Jacobs et al., 2007; Carter-Pokras et al., 2004).

In addition to better quality of care and outcomes, the risk of malpractice concerns is lower for LEP patients with language-concordant physicians, leading to healthcare that is more cost-effective. Physicians who have trouble understanding patients as a result of a language barrier are more likely to order extra tests or ask for consultant opinions to avoid malpractice, indicating two sources of inefficient spending (Chen et al., 2011). A study of Latino patients with diabetes revealed that glycemic control in patients with language-concordant physicians was better (Fernandez et al., 2011). Given that improved glycemic control is at the foundation of diabetes management and prevention of complications which would require hospitalization and expensive treatment, this indicates another area where language-concordant care can lead to better outcomes and decreased cost.

Studies evaluating the impact of language concordance on quality of care and outcomes therefore indicate that having a language-concordant physician is of great benefit to LEP patients and to healthcare systems.

How do Clinicians Actually Provide Language Services to LEP Patients in Practice?

A commentary by Schenker et al. (2008) described four factors that should be considered when deciding whether and how an interpreter should be used in clinical settings: the accessibility of interpreter services; patient preferences; the clinical scenario; and the degree of language gap between patient and physician. The availability of interpreter services varies widely among institutions and, even when interpreters are readily accessible, the quality of and the wait time for interpreter services may deter providers from using them, particularly in urgent situations. Patient preference for interpreters can be difficult to assess when a language barrier exists, and many patients are unaware of their legal right to a professional interpreter at no cost. The power imbalance between physicians and patients might discourage patients from requesting that an interpreter be used over the physician's non-fluent language skills, further obscuring the physician's perception of the patient's preference. The clinical scenario can also be an unavoidable deterrent to using language services; in an emergency, care must be provided whether or not language assistance is available. However, in non-urgent situations, clinicians tend to be less likely to request an interpreter for a seemingly straightforward encounter, potentially causing them to miss important information that changes the diagnosis and course of treatment. Finally, partial fluency of either the patient or physician in the other's language can cause a misevaluation of the degree of the language gap, leading the physician to be overly confident in the mutual comprehension of the dialogue (Schenker et al., 2008).

A more recent commentary by Hsieh (2015) drew many of the same conclusions about the factors that commonly influence whether interpreter services are called upon by clinicians. The results of this study echo Schenker's comments about the role of accessibility of interpreter services and the urgency of the clinical scenario, adding to them the common scenario in which a family member acts as the interpreter, and the possible implications this could have on patient privacy and autonomy. Providers seem to be willing to use family members as interpreters in many situations, citing reluctance primarily when there is the perception of a controlling or manipulative dynamic between the family member and patient. Regarding partially fluent physicians using their own language skills to communicate with patients, the commentary emphasized that, while reliance on these skills should not substitute for a trained interpreter, their use should not be entirely discouraged, referring to a 2002 study that demonstrated an increase in patient satisfaction and a reduction in the need for interpreters for pediatric emergency physicians treating uncomplicated conditions (ear pain, sore throat, lacerations, vomiting and diarrhea) using the skills gained from completing a 10-week course in medical Spanish (Mazor et al., 2002). However, it is important to note that the satisfaction gained by the LEP parents of the patients in this study was mainly related to the increase in rapport built between families and physicians, with parents being more likely to agree with statements such as 'the physician was concerned about my child' and 'made me feel comfortable', and that neither clinical outcomes nor communication errors were studied (Mazor et al., 2002). In general, the Hsieh study highlighted the various ways in which providers' use of their language skills and reliance on use of untrained interpreters, such as family members, lead to compromised patient care (Hsieh, 2015).

Previous qualitative research has shown that resident physicians weighed the potential benefits of providing language-concordant care, which included saving time, against the difficulties of obtaining and using an interpreter (Diamond et al., 2009). One study found that physician-centered communication, in which the primary goal is to gather clinical information rather than to address patient concerns, causes resident physicians to be less likely to call an interpreter, which comes at the cost of development of physician–patient rapport (Diamond et al., 2009). Together with a lack of awareness of the many issues associated with using an untrained interpreter out of convenience, these issues form two of the reasons why resident physicians are less likely to call interpreters (Diamond et al., 2009). Another qualitative study from 2014 provided further insight into the reasons why physicians neglect to call interpreters, pointing out that the judgment made to forego an interpreter is highly situational. In the absence of enforced regulations about when to call an interpreter, providers frequently feel conflicted about whether to 'get by' or to 'get help'. Further, this decision is not always made in the patient's best interest, with a provider's own time constraints and the ease of finding an interpreter frequently dictating whether interpreter services are used (Parsons et al., 2014). This theme of providers inappropriately deeming interpreter services unnecessary is echoed by a 2011 study in which physicians with medium- and even low-level Spanish skills reported frequent use of ad-hoc interpreters and of their own skills (Diamond et al., 2012a).

As a result of the inconsistent and situational nature of provider decision-making regarding whether to rely on their own limited language skills or call an interpreter, research into the role of language proficiency testing of physicians has emerged. A 2012 study revealed that simply administering a 20 minute, telephone-based Spanish proficiency test decreased the comfort of non-fluent resident physicians who were using Spanish in straightforward clinical encounters, from 64% of residents reporting comfort prior to testing to 51% afterwards (Lion et al., 2012). As previously discussed, some seemingly straightforward scenarios may have a level of complexity that providers miss altogether when they are only able to communicate with patients in very basic terms, and administering language proficiency tests could improve patient care by preventing such oversights. Another study showed that self-reported Spanish proficiency of providers was not predictive of their performance on a proficiency test and that, regardless of actual proficiency, most who claim any level of skill will communicate with patients without an interpreter (Lion et al., 2013). This finding underscores the need to administer proficiency tests, not to discourage providers from attempting to build rapport with a patient in the patient's language, but to raise clinicians' awareness of their own limitations in communication, which has greater clinical significance – a concept that will be further discussed later in the chapter.

Research is needed to better characterize the factors influencing physicians' use of interpreters so that appropriate interventions to increase interpreter use among non-fluent physicians can be designed. While these studies have uncovered the lack of standardization when it comes to the use of interpreters and demonstrated a role for proficiency testing in solving this problem, they have not addressed the issue of how to go about measuring proficiency.

How Should Clinician Language Proficiency be Measured and/or Regulated?

Evidence suggests that care provided by language-concordant physicians is more patient-centered (Fernandez et al., 2004), associated with greater patient satisfaction (Green et al., 2005; Ngo-Metzger et al., 2007) and results in fewer emergency department visits (Manson, 1988). Research is needed to help establish a standard of fluency reporting for clinicians who intend to provide language-concordant care. Non-medical fields are more advanced in developing standardized descriptions of professional linguistic proficiency. For example, in the 1950s, after determining that 75% of US Foreign Service officers failed to meet a useful proficiency level for their work-related languages, the US Foreign Service Institute began developing and validating fluency testing methods that resulted in a standard scale for language proficiency. The scale has been revised and validated by the Interagency Language Roundtable (ILR), an organization now comprising representatives from academia, government and non-government organizations.

The ILR scale and other related scales could become the basis for establishing a standard of fluency reporting for clinicians (Diamond & Reuland, 2009). In this chapter, we use the ILR scale as an example because it is the only brief, validated tool that has been adapted to capture proficiency in a medical setting (Diamond et al., 2012b). When physicians in a large, multi-specialty group were asked to transition from reporting their own language skills on a non-validated scale to the ILR scale, there was a substantial variation in the self-reported ILR ratings for physicians who had previously reported their skills as 'Medical/Conversational' on the non-validated scale (Diamond et al., 2012b). Given that these self-reported metrics for fluency are published on providers' websites and used by patients who are choosing a provider, they carry a weight that has historically been overlooked. A change as simple as updating a published scale to one that is more accurate and precise could improve the care delivered to LEP patients by guiding them toward providers whose language skills better match their own (Diamond et al., 2012b).

Even for non-fluent speakers, providing language-concordant care may be appropriate and even desirable in some settings and circumstances (Fernandez et al., 2004; Jacobs et al., 2007). However, with interactions that are only partially language concordant, there are obvious concerns for quality of care and patient safety, again emphasizing the need to establish standards of fluency. On the ILR scale, speakers who can give straightforward instructions in a language but may use awkward or incorrect phrasing, together with speakers who can communicate effectively in most social and professional situations but have difficulty communicating some abstract topics, constitute the 'middle of the ILR range' (Diamond & Reuland, 2009). Resources used for fluency testing should therefore be directed primarily toward clinicians in this skill range who intend to provide language-concordant care (Diamond & Reuland, 2009). By identifying and administering proficiency tests to providers who fall into this middle category of fluency, healthcare organizations can ensure that physician fluency is not significantly lower than their self-reported level, and appropriately implement policies on interpreter use and documentation (Diamond & Reuland, 2009). The incidence of partially concordant interactions will thereby be reduced.

In addition to evaluating and ranking a physician's overall proficiency in a language, there must be attention given to the context in which they will be using that language. Different levels of language proficiency may be needed for different clinical circumstances. For example, a physician may be fluent in a non-English language but unable to provide psychiatric care or high-stakes medical/surgical treatment in that language (Regenstein et al., 2013). Examples of high-risk encounters where interpreters should always be used are end-of-life or advanced care planning discussions, high-stakes genetic counseling and trauma, physical or sexual assault (Regenstein et al., 2013). In addition to these context-driven cues as to when an interpreter should be used, there are 'red flags' clinicians should be educated about that indicate when the use of an interpreter has become critical. Among such indications are 'word finding', in which a physician cannot think of a good word to describe a concept, 'rephrasing', in which a patient displays lack of comprehension during teach-back communication with the physician, and 'emotional disconnect', in which a patient displays an emotional response that seems discordant with the conversation (Regenstein et al., 2013). Research is needed to further demarcate scenarios in which clinicians of various fluency levels should seek an interpreter.

In essence, without a clear, standardized measure of a provider's language skills, patients, hospitals and physicians themselves remain ignorant of a piece of information that has the power to shape a patient encounter. It is thus in the best interest of all parties to adopt a standardized scale for describing the language skills of physicians, and for further research to be done to reveal situations where physicians providing language-concordant care should be especially vigilant.

Are Clinicians Aware of Their Own Limitations When Speaking Another Language?

With regard to fluency self-assessment, studies show conflicting evidence about clinicians' awareness of their own linguistic skills. One study showed that physicians' self-reported Spanish fluency was strongly associated with their Spanish-speaking patients' reports of optimal patient-centered communication (Fernandez et al., 2004). Another study showed that medical students accurately assessed their own level of Spanish language proficiency when compared with their performance on a standardized oral fluency test. This finding applied to students who reported their own skills as greater than 'novice' capability and who were interested in medical Spanish coursework, indicating that ability and interest may play a role in determining the accuracy of self-assessment (Reuland et al., 2009).

In contrast, a large study of clinicians who were also functioning as interpreters for LEP patients showed that one in five had language proficiency levels that were inadequate. The study included non-clinician dual-role staff interpreters and found the same rate of inadequate proficiency (Moreno et al., 2007). A later study sought to reveal the factors associated with accuracy of self-assessment compared with an oral language proficiency test for staff functioning in a dual role as interpreters. It found that both higher education and being born outside of the US were indicators of passing the language competency test. It further showed that accurate self-assessment of abilities comes from education in the skill set; dual-role interpreters with prior interpreter training were more accurate in their assessment of their skills (Diamond et al., 2012c). These findings indicate a vital role for interpreter training for all bilingual providers and staff, regardless of education, country of origin or self-reported fluency.

For clinicians and staff members working with LEP populations, training and proficiency assessments have the potential to not only improve outcomes and patient care, but also to improve job satisfaction for physicians. A 2014 study demonstrated that residents rated their own self-efficacy in caring for LEP patients as low, possibly leading to low satisfaction, and concluded that strategies that promote resident self-efficacy and assess non-English language proficiency should be part of training curricula. This study further concluded that exposing trainees to best practices in interpreter-based encounters might lead to improved resident satisfaction (Hernandez et al., 2014). Another approach to improving self-efficacy in residents caring for LEP patients is to improve their fluency in a language spoken by LEP communities earlier on in their training. A 2012 study showed that medical students with intermediate to advanced baseline Spanish fluency who took part in a post-year 1 Spanish language international health immersion rotation were more likely to improve their Spanish fluency than those in US-based coursework alone (Reuland et al., 2012). However, while it is clear that early exposure to a language spoken by the LEP community is a positive part of a medical education, it is important to recognize that not all medical Spanish curricula are created equally, and that they vary widely in their effectiveness (Hardin & Hardin, 2013). A study of emergency department interns demonstrated the possibility that participating in a medical Spanish program could even increase the rate of medical errors by instilling providers with a false sense of fluency, causing them to be unaware of when their communication was discordant. Minor errors were found in more than half of interactions these physicians with patients, and major errors in 14% of interactions (Prince & Nelson, 1995).

Even for providers with skills in a language spoken by LEP patients, knowing one's own limitations and how to best utilize interpreters is essential. One study, mentioned previously, showed that, when physicians reporting fluency in a non-English language self-assessed their skills using an adapted version of the ILR scale, they were likely to reclassify their level of skill afterwards (Diamond et al., 2012b), indicating that more accurate measures of proficiency are needed. Simply administering such an assessment probably leads to better patient care by not only giving providers a more objective measure of their proficiency, but also through their more accurate self-classification, alerting their patients to the degree of language gap between patients and physicians.

Conclusions

It is important that medical trainees and providers are taught that, while attempting to communicate with patients across a language barrier may be done in good faith, it can sometimes perpetuate health disparities faced by patients who do not speak the dominant language of the country they live in (Diamond & Jacobs, 2010). A curriculum geared toward reducing health disparities in the context of language barriers is essential, and should include instruction on red flags that indicate when a physician needs to call an interpreter and how to work with professional interpreters, and should address the use of ad hoc interpreters (Diamond & Jacobs, 2010). Research has shown that curricula in each of these areas do not have to be long or exhaustive (Jacobs et al., 2010). A 1.5 hour curriculum in a large, urban medical school was shown to significantly raise medical student knowledge of language barriers in health care (Jacobs et al., 2010).

As noted earlier, adhering to a standardized scale of proficiency provides patients and physicians with increased transparency with regard to whether language-concordant care can be provided. Although physicians with low or high self-reported fluency are likely to provide an accurate assessment of their skills, providers with some fluency are more prone to inaccuracy and may require further testing (Diamond et al., 2014b). For any curriculum in language barriers and interpreter use to be useful, it is first necessary for physicians to have a basic understanding of their own skills and limitations.

Taking all of the recent findings in this arena into account, it is therefore clear that, through a combination of standardized measurement of language proficiency of clinicians who report some level of fluency in a non-English language and curricula geared toward improving clinician knowledge of the health disparities imposed by language barriers, as well as how to reduce them by proper use of interpreting services, patients will be better cared for by their physicians.

References

Atkin, N. (2008) Getting the message across-professional interpreters in general practice. *Australian Family Physician* 37 (3), 174–176.

Baker, D.W., Parker, R.M., Williams, M.V., Coates, W.C. and Pitkin, K. (1996) Use and effectiveness of interpreters in an emergency department. *JAMA* 275 (10), 783–788.

Carter-Pokras, O., O'Neill, M.J., Cheanvechai, V., Menis, M., Fan, T. and Solera, A. (2004) Providing linguistically appropriate services to persons with limited English proficiency: A needs and resources investigation. *American Journal of Management of Care* 10 (Special issue), Sp29–Sp36.

Chen, J., Fang, H. and Rizzo, J.A. (2011) Physician–patient language concordance and malpractice concerns. *Medical Care* 49 (11), 1040–1044.

Commission, T.J. (2010) *Advancing Effective Communication, Cultural Competence, and Patient- and Family-Centered Care: A Roadmap for Hosptials*. Oakbrook Terrace, IL: The Joint Commission.

DeCamp, L.R., Kuo, D.Z., Flores, G., O'Connor, K. and Minkovitz, C.S. (2013) Changes in language services use by US pediatricians. *Pediatrics* 132 (2), e396–e406.

Diamond, L.C. and Jacobs, E.A. (2010) Let's not contribute to disparities: The best methods for teaching clinicians how to overcome language barriers to health care. *Journal of General Internal Medicine* 25 (Suppl 2), S189–S193.

Diamond, L.C. and Reuland, D.S. (2009) Describing physician language fluency: Deconstructing medical Spanish. *JAMA* 301 (4), 426–428.

Diamond, L.C., Schenker, Y., Curry, L., Bradley, E.H. and Fernandez, A. (2009) Getting by: Underuse of interpreters by resident physicians. *Journal of General Internal Medicine* 24 (2), 256–262.

Diamond, L.C., Wilson-Stronks, A. and Jacobs, E.A. (2010) Do hospitals measure up to the national culturally and linguistically appropriate services standards? *Medical Care* 48 (12), 1080–1087.

Diamond, L.C., Tuot, D.S. and Karliner, L.S. (2012a) The use of Spanish language skills by physicians and nurses: Policy implications for teaching and testing. *Journal of General Internal Medicine* 27 (1), 117–123.

Diamond, L.C., Luft, H.S., Chung, S. and Jacobs, E.A. (2012b) 'Does this doctor speak my language?' Improving the characterization of physician non-English language skills. *Health Service Research* 47 (1 Pt 2), 556–569.

Diamond, L.C., Moreno, M., Soto, C. and Otero-Sabogal, R. (2012c) Bilingual dual-role staff interpreters in the health care setting: Factors associated with passing a language competency test. *International Journal of Interpreter Education* 4 (1), 5–20.

Diamond, L., Grbic, D., Genoff, M., Gonzalez, J., Sharaf, R., Mikesell, C. and Gany, F. (2014a) Non-English-language proficiency of applicants to US residency programs. *JAMA* 312 (22), 2405–2407.

Diamond, L., Chung, S., Ferguson, W., Gonzalez, J., Jacobs, E.A. and Gany, F. (2014b) Relationship between self-assessed and tested non-English-language proficiency among primary care providers. *Medical Care* 52 (5), 435–438.

DuBard, C. and Gizlice, Z. (2008) Access to care, and receipt of preventive services among US Hispanics. *American Journal of Public Health* 98 (11), 2021–2028.

Eamranond, P.P., Davis, R.B., Phillips, R.S. and Wee, C.C. (2009) Patient–physician language concordance and lifestyle counseling among Spanish-speaking patients. *Journal of Immigrant and Minority Health* 11 (6), 494–498.

Fernandez, A., Schillinger, D., Grumbach, K., Rosenthal, A., Stewart, A.L., Wang, F. and Perez-Stable, E.J. (2004) Physician language ability and cultural competence. An exploratory study of communication with Spanish-speaking patients. *Journal of General Internal Medicine* 19 (2), 167–174.

Fernandez, A., Schillinger, D., Warton, E.M., Adler, N., Moffet, H.H., Schenker, Y., Salgado, M.V., Ahmed, A. and Karter, A.J. (2011) Language barriers, physician–patient language concordance, and glycemic control among insured Latinos with diabetes: The Diabetes Study of Northern California (DISTANCE). *Journal of General Internal Medicine* 26 (2), 170–176.

Gadon, M., Balch, G. and Jacobs, E. (2007) Caring for patients with limited English proficiency: The perspectives of small group practitioners. *Journal of General Internal Medicine* 22 (Suppl 2), 341–346.

Gray, B., Stanley, J., Stubbe, M. and Hilder, J. (2011) Communication difficulties with limited English proficiency patients – clinician perceptions of clinical risk and patterns of use of interpreters. *New Zealand Medical Journal* 124 (1342), 23–38.

Green, A.R., Ngo-Metzger, Q., Legedza, A.T., Massagli, M.P., Phillips, R.S. and Iezzoni, L.I. (2005) Interpreter services, language concordance, and health care quality. Experiences of Asian Americans with limited English proficiency. *Journal of General Internal Medicine* 20 (11), 1050–1056.

Hardin, K.J. and Hardin, D.M. (2013) Medical Spanish programs in the United States: A critical review of published studies and a proposal of best practices. *Teaching and Learning Medicine* 25 (4), 306–311.

Hernandez, R.G., Cowden, J.D., Moon, M., Brands, C.K., Sisson, S.D. and Thompson, D.A. (2014) Predictors of resident satisfaction in caring for limited English proficient families: A multisite study. *Academic Pediatrics* 14 (2), 173–180.

Hsieh, E. (2015) Not just 'getting by': Factors influencing providers' choice of interpreters. *Journal of General Internal Medicine* 30 (1), 75–82.

Hu, D.J. and Covell, R.M. (1986) Health care usage by Hispanic outpatients as function of primary language. *Western Journal of Medicine* 144 (4), 490–493.

Institute of Medicine (2001) *Crossing the Quality Chasm: A New Health System for the 21st Century*. Washington, DC: The National Academies Press, Committee on Quality of Health Care in America.

Jacobs, E.A., Sadowski, L.S. and Rathouz, P.J. (2007) The impact of an enhanced interpreter service intervention on hospital costs and patient satisfaction. *Journal of General Internal Medicine* 22 (Suppl 2), 306–311.

Jacobs, E.A., Diamond, L.C. and Stevak, L. (2010) The importance of teaching clinicians when and how to work with interpreters. *Patient Education and Counseling* 78 (2), 149–153.

Lauderdale, D.S. et al. (2006) Immigrant perceptions of discrimination in health care: The California Health Interview Survey 2003. *Medical Care* 44 (10), 914–920.

Lion, K.C. et al. (2012) Impact of language proficiency testing on provider use of Spanish for clinical care. *Pediatrics* 130 (1), e80–e87.

Lion, K.C. et al. (2013) Clinical Spanish use and language proficiency testing among pediatric residents. *Academic Medicine* 88 (10), 1478–1484.

Manson, A. (1988) Language concordance as a determinant of patient compliance and emergency room use in patients with asthma. *Medical Care* 26 (12), 1119–1128.

Mazor, S.S. et al. (2002) Teaching Spanish to pediatric emergency physicians: Effects on patient satisfaction. *Archives of Pediatric and Adolescent Medicine* 156 (7), 693–695.

Moreno, M.R., Otero-Sabogal, R. and Newman, J. (2007) Assessing dual-role staff-interpreter linguistic competency in an integrated healthcare system. *Journal of General Internal Medicine* 22 (Suppl 2), 331–335.

Nerenz, D.R., Veselovskiy, G.M. and Carreon, R. (2013) Collection of data on race/ethnicity and language proficiency of providers. *American Journal of Management of Care* 19 (12), e408–e414.

Ngo-Metzger, Q. et al. (2007) Providing high-quality care for limited English proficient patients: The importance of language concordance and interpreter use. *Journal of General Internal Medicine* 22 (Suppl 2), 324–330.

Parsons, J.A.B., Natalie A., Smith-Gorvie, E. and Hudak, P.L. (2014) To 'Get by' or 'get help'? A qualitative study of physicians' challenges and dilemmas when patients have limited English proficiency. *BMJ Open* 4 (6).

Perez-Stable, E.J., Napoles-Springer, A. and Miramontes, J.M. (1997) The effects of ethnicity and language on medical outcomes of patients with hypertension or diabetes. *Medical Care* 35 (12), 1212–1219.

Perkins, J. and Youdelman, M. (2008) Summary of State Law Requirements: Addressing Language Needs in Health Care. See http://www.healthlaw.org/library/item.174993 (accessed 21 July 2015).

Pippins, J.R. et al. (2007) Association between language proficiency and the quality of primary care among a national sample of insured Latinos.[See comment.] *Medical Care* 45 (11), 1020–1025.

Prince, D. and Nelson, M. (1995) Teaching Spanish to emergency medicine residents. *Academic Emergency Medicine* 2 (1), 32–36; discussion 36–37.

Regenstein, M., Andres, E. and Wynia, M.K. (20013) Appropriate use of non-English-language skills in clinical care. *JAMA* 309 (2), 145–146.

Reuland, D. et al. (2009) Accuracy of Self-assessed Spanish fluency in medical students. *Teaching and Learning in Medicine* 21 (4), 305–309.

Reuland, D.S. et al. (2012) Effect of Spanish language immersion rotations on medical student Spanish fluency. *Family Medicine* 44 (2), 110–116.

Schenker, Y. et al. (2008) Navigating language barriers under difficult circumstances. *Annals of Internal Medicine* 149 (4), 264–269.

The Joint Commission (2010) *Advancing Effective Communication, Cultural Competence, and Patient- and Family-centered Care: A Roadmap for Hosptials*. The Joint Commission: Oakbrook Terrace, IL.

US Department of Health and Human Services (Office of Minority Health) (2013) National Standards for Culturally and Linguistically Appropriate Services (CLAS). See http://minorityhealth.hhs.gov/templates/browse.aspx?lvl=2&lvlID=15 (accessed 3 May 2015).

US Department of Justice (1964) Title VI of the Civil Rights Act.

Weinick, R.M. and Krauss, N.A. (2000) Racial/ethnic differences in children's access to care. *American Journal of Public Health* 90 (11), 1771–1774.

Wisnivesky, J.P. et al. (2009) Assessing the relationship between language proficiency and asthma morbidity among inner-city asthmatics. *Medical Care* 47 (2), 243–249.

Woloshin, S. et al. (1995) Language barriers in medicine in the United States. *JAMA* 273 (9), 724–728.

8 Breaking the Silence: Identifying the Needs of Bilingual Speakers in Health Care

Gwerfyl Roberts

Despite the growing commitment in health care to establish communicative competence with service users, the language needs of bilingual speakers often remain invisible, leading to the marginalization of vulnerable groups and compromising the quality of their care. Nevertheless, with the revitalization of many of the world's indigenous minority languages, healthcare systems must adapt to legislative change and advances in language policy. This chapter reviews the research evidence from bilingual Wales, UK that contributes to our understanding of the dynamics of bilingual healthcare communication and examines the implications for implementing the evidence from an individual and organizational perspective.

Introduction

Engaging patients as partners in health and involving them in decisions about care and treatment options is fundamental to patient-centered care (Légeré et al., 2008). Nevertheless, when language and cultural barriers arise in consultations, shared decision-making is inevitably compromised (Edwards et al., 2009) and people are less likely to receive the care they need, understand its significance, comply with treatment and derive satisfaction from care delivery (Jacobs et al., 2006). While professional interpreters can help bridge the linguistic gap between practitioners and patients (Karliner et al., 2007), clinical outcomes and satisfaction with care are enhanced when both parties speak the same language and understand the cultural context in which communication takes place (Fernandez et al., 2004; Freeman et al., 2002; Jacobs et al., 2007; Ngo-Metzger et al., 2007; Perez-Stable, 1997). This is not surprising since language is more than just a means of communication.

Although it plays a crucial role in transmitting information safely and effectively, language also helps people assert their identity and express their thoughts, feelings and anxieties, especially at times of stress (Grosjean, 2010). Thus, language is a way of establishing common ground for communication and understanding in health care that helps capture the lived experience of service users and foster therapeutic relationships (Gerrish, 2001). Nevertheless, even when practitioners and patients share a common language, communication barriers may persist, especially where patients are bilingual and where they are denied opportunities to use their primary language (Misell, 2000; Office of the French Language Commissioner, 2009).

In countries, such as the US, Canada, Australia, New Zealand and the UK, the majority of the population are monolingual English speakers. Healthcare providers within these countries have thus traditionally adopted the responsibility of offering English as a common language, with the expectation that minority language speakers adapt their language use to align with that of their predominantly English-language healthcare systems. Thus, despite the official status bestowed over the years on minority languages, such as French in Canada, Maori in New Zealand, Irish in Ireland and Welsh in Wales, public expectations for their use in health care remain low (Misell, 2000; Office of the French Language Commissioner, 2009). However, patients are often vulnerable and anxious on accessing health care; and although they may appear bilingual in both official languages, to varying degrees, they will often lose command of their English language in a healthcare context and revert to their primary language to fulfil different cognitive, emotional and social functions (Iaith, 2012; Office of the French Language Commissioner, 2009). Nevertheless, because of the legacy of language deference amongst minority language speakers and the expectation in English-dominant contexts that 'they all speak English anyway' (Office of the French Language Commissioner, 2009; Welsh Government, 2016), they are often hesitant to ask for services in their primary language. Service users with mental health problems or learning disabilities, older people and preschool children raised through a minority language have been shown to be particularly vulnerable in this respect, although they are often the least capable of demanding their language rights (Misell, 2000; Office of the French Language Commissioner, 2009). Other bilinguals who are less vulnerable but who use their minority language on a daily basis will often feel more comfortable expressing themselves and communicating their health needs in their primary language, thus enabling them to become active participants in their care. Thus, despite the expectation that, nowadays, most official minority language speakers in English-dominant settings are bilingual to some degree, their communication with their English-dominant healthcare system may be compromised by a distinct language and cultural barrier. Thus, 'understanding the role language differences play in medical encounters and their impact on clinical outcomes must necessarily include an understanding of the larger context in which language takes place' (Gregg & Saha, 2007: 369). In the context of intercultural communication, this inevitably means taking account of the full language profile of bilingual speakers as well as developing an awareness of the wider sociopolitical factors that influence a language's power, prestige and status.

Research on bilingualism has increased significantly over recent years, demonstrating its psychological, social and emotional components (Bhatia & Ritchie, 2006). However, for minority language speakers in English-dominant contexts, their ability to speak English, and hence their bilingual attainment, means that their specific language and cultural needs are often overlooked. Thus, their needs in health care are often invisible and misunderstood, with grave implications for the quality of care delivery (Office of the French Language Commissioner, 2009; Misell, 2000). With the increasing diversity of populations in developed countries where the majority speak two or more languages, and the enhanced status of indigenous minority groups, language and cultural competence in health care is under mounting scrutiny (Department of Health, 2012; National Health and Medical Research Council, 2005; US Office of Minority Health, US Department of Health and Human Services, 2001). Moreover, in countries such as Wales and Canada, which promote the use of two official languages, there is legislative and policy commitment to embed bilingualism within healthcare organizations and deliver an 'active offer' of language services according to patient needs (Office of the French Language Commissioner, 2009; Welsh Government, 2012a).

Given the dearth of evidence to inform bilingual healthcare communication, this chapter sets out to locate bilingualism within the experiential domain of healthcare users and providers.

Set within the bilingual context of Wales, UK, it reports on a scoping review of the research evidence that captures the perceptions of service users and practitioners about bilingualism in healthcare communication, with a specific focus on Welsh speakers as minority language users of an English-dominant healthcare system. Drawing on recent theoretical perspectives on bilingualism and with reference to the wider global research literature on language barriers in health care, the review sets out to enhance our understanding of the dynamics of bilingual healthcare communication for official language minority speakers in an English-dominant healthcare setting; and consider the implications for implementing the evidence from an individual and organizational perspective.

The Bilingual Context of Wales

In the bilingual context of Wales, where over half a million people (19% of the population) are Welsh-speaking (Office for National Statistics, 2012), the indigenous Welsh language is afforded equal and official status with

English in the conduct of public business (Welsh Language (Wales) Measure, 2011). Moreover, the *National Language Plan* (Welsh Government, 2012b: 42) acknowledges that 'strengthening Welsh-language services in health care is regarded as a priority since, for many, language in this context is more than just a matter of choice – it is a matter of need'.

Historical context of the Welsh language

Despite such rhetoric, the Welsh language has not always been afforded the prestige and status it receives today. Indeed, its history is one of dominance in the face of English oppression since the unification of Wales under English rule during the 16th century. In light of its exclusion from public administration throughout this period, the language was marginalized and its status eroded. This led to a state of diglossia (in the sense of Fishman, 1967) in Wales whereby Welsh was confined to the personal domains of everyday life. This shift had a detrimental impact on people's attitudes toward Welsh and the confidence of its speakers who inherited a legacy of inferiority about their language which contributed toward its rapid decline (Davies, 2007). Whilst, over the years, the changing political landscape of Wales has played a significant part in the revival of the Welsh language, as minority language speakers (May, 2012), Welsh-speakers still experience discriminatory attitudes, language oppression and language assimilation, all of which have a detrimental effect on their opportunities to engage effectively with healthcare services (Welsh Government, 2012a; Welsh Language Commissioner, 2014).

Legislative and policy drive for the Welsh language in health care

In spite of its troubled history, the devolution of Wales in 1999 proved a significant turning point for the Welsh language, which is now at the core of its national identity (Welsh Government, 2012b), legislative frameworks (Council of Europe, 1992; Welsh Language (Wales) Measure, 2011) and health and social care strategic intent (Welsh Government, 2012a; 2016).

The equality principle embedded in the Welsh Language Act (1993) was strengthened in the Welsh Language (Wales) Measure 2011, which provided the Welsh language official status in Wales alongside English, made provision for promoting and facilitating the use of the language and established the role of the Welsh Language Commissioner. Meanwhile, amidst growing concerns regarding the impact of failures to deliver Welsh language services in the health sector, particularly to vulnerable groups (Misell, 2000), the Welsh Government published its *Strategic Framework for Welsh Language Services in Health, Social Services and Social Care* (Welsh Government, 2012a) and follow-on framework (Welsh Government, 2016), aptly named *More Than Just Words*. This confirmed the way in which meeting the linguistic needs of service users is inextricably linked to providing good quality, safe and compassionate care. Adopting the 'active offer' approach embedded in Canadian legislation (Official Languages Act, 1985), the framework represents a significant shift in moving the responsibility from the user to ask for services through the medium of Welsh to the service which must ensure it provides them. The principle was later endorsed by the Welsh Language Commissioner in the report of her first statutory Inquiry which focused exclusively on the Welsh language in primary healthcare services (Welsh Language Commissioner, 2014).

Thus, reflecting on the legislative and policy context in Wales, the principles of language equality are clearly embedded in current healthcare strategies where bilingual services are deemed fundamental for the provision of quality care. Understanding the nature of bilingual communication is fundamental to the effective delivery of these services.

Bilingualism

Bilingualism is generally regarded as the term for speaking one or more languages or as a cover term for multilingualism (Myers-Scotton, 2006). Yet Baker and Jones (1998) argue that, given its elusive nature, bilingualism defies a simple definition. Whilst there is a need to differentiate between bilingualism as an attribute of the individual, and bilingualism as a societal characteristic, they are intrinsically linked. In order to appreciate the distinctive elements of bilingualism, Baker (2011) reminds us of some of its important dimensions which demonstrate that individual bilingualism is far more complex than simply having access to two languages (see Table 8.1).

Table 8.1 Key dimensions of bilingualism (after Baker, 2011)

Language dimension	Feature
Ability	Productive and receptive abilities may be varied. Ability is thus on a continuum that varies among speakers
Use	Domains of acquisition and use are varied. Different languages are used for different purposes
Balance of two languages	One language is usually more dominant than the other. Equal ability or use of both languages is rare
Choice	When bilinguals are in contact, their language choice depends on their individual attitudes, identity and preferences
Switch	When bilinguals are in contact, a speaker may switch languages deliberately or subconsciously to accommodate the perceived preference of the listener

Given the significance of person-centered communication in health care (Legaré et al., 2008), an understanding of bilingualism is crucial for quality care. For example, practitioners should be aware of the important distinction between language ability and use when assessing bilingual clients, and thus tailor their communication accordingly. Moreover, insight is also required into the unique and varied language proficiencies of individuals across their language domains, their confidence and readiness to use their languages in different contexts and the internal and external factors that facilitate or impede this choice.

Bhatia and Ritchie (2006) claim that bilingualism is a widespread global phenomenon with over two-thirds of the world's children growing up in a bilingual environment. On this basis, it is somewhat surprising that, as a concept, it receives so little attention in the growing body of research literature on language barriers in health care. While there is a wealth of research reporting the challenges faced by service users with 'limited English proficiency' and 'non-English speakers', bilingualism does not feature to any great extent in this discourse; the focus is largely on the mismatch imposed by predominantly monolingual English provider organizations, such as those in the US, Australia and parts of the UK. Nevertheless, this does not deny the fact that many of these client groups are bilingual, speaking their own minority languages and English to varying degrees. Neither does it deny the efforts of provider organizations in other nation states, such as Canada, or devolved countries, such as Wales (where two official languages reside), to provide an 'active offer' of bilingual services (Office of the French Language Commissioner, 2009; Welsh Government, 2012a, 2016).

However, the argument here is that, more often than not, the literature on language barriers in health care depicts monolingualism (in English) as its frame of reference and it is this which is perceived as the norm, with bilingualism viewed as the problematic exception. Auer and Wei (2007) labor the point that, despite significant progress in research on multilingualism over the years, the monolingual ideology remains dominant and many people and organizations still have misconceived ideas about multilingualism. Thus, language barriers in health care may not be inherent to bilingualism per se but arise out of a certain historical and attitudinal context in which it is perceived as a problem, or creates problems. This scoping review sets out examine the perceptions of service users and practitioners, as reported in research studies from Wales, about the use and role of language in a bilingual health care context.

Methodology

In line with the methodological framework outlined by Arksey and O'Malley (2005), later refined by Levac et al. (2010), the aim of the scoping review was to 'clarify a complex concept and refine subsequent research inquiries' (Levac et al., 2010: 1). The concept under scrutiny was bilingualism in healthcare communication, as featured in the research literature emerging from Wales. The review set out to examine the research evidence exclusive to Wales that captured the perceptions of service users and practitioners about bilingualism in healthcare communication. The decision to limit the search to studies published after 2000 coincided with the development of the US CLAS standards (Office of Minority Health, US Department of Health and Human Services, 2001) and the first desk-top review of Welsh language services in the National Health Service in Wales (Misell, 2000). Although there was no intention to appraise the quality of the research, one of the key strengths of a scoping review is its potential to provide a rigorous and transparent method for mapping the area under focus in a relatively short period of time (Arksey & O'Malley, 2005). The search strategy was developed from the research question and included the following search terms in combination: Welsh; Wales; bilingual; language; culture; awareness; attitudes; sensitivity; service users; practitioners; health care. A range of different sources were accessed, including:

- electronic databases, such as ASSIA, LLBA, MEDLINE, SSA and Google Scholar;
- reference lists;
- hand searching of key journals, such as *International Journal of Bilingualism* and *Journal of Transcultural Nursing*; and
- existing networks and relevant organizations, such as LLAIS, NHS Wales Welsh Language Unit, Care Council for Wales and the Welsh Language Commissioner.

Findings and Discussion

On the basis of the strategy outlined above, five relevant research studies were identified, the details of which are outlined in Table 8.2. Of these five studies, the first was commissioned by the Welsh Government, adopting a mixed-methods approach, to focus exclusively on the perceptions of healthcare professionals about language awareness in practice (Roberts et al., 2004). Further analysis of the data may be found in Irvine et al. (2006) and Roberts et al. (2007). The following two small-scale studies adopted a qualitative approach to focus on the perceptions of Welsh-speaking service users and providers about Welsh language provision in the context of mental health (Madoc-Jones, 2004) and third sector services (Prys, 2010). The two remaining studies represented larger commissioned works, adopting qualitative methods, to focus on the experiences of a broader cohort of Welsh-speaking service users and their perceptions of health and social care (Iaith, 2012;

Table 8.2 Research studies included in scoping review

Author(s) and year of publication	Design	Sample	Methods	Findings
Madoc-Jones (2004)	Qualitative survey	Purposive sample of Welsh-speaking mental health service users (n = 5)	Face-to-face semi-structured interviews	Being bilingual shapes individual experiences of mental health services amongst Welsh-speakers. Current service provision is inadequate in meeting their linguistic needs
Roberts et al. (2004)	Two-phased mixed-methods survey Phase 1: Postal questionnaire survey Phase 2: Qualitative survey	Phase 1: Random stratified sample of healthcare professionals across Wales (n = 1968) Phase 2: Purposive stratified sample of survey respondents (n = 83)	Phase 1: Postal survey using structured questionnaires Phase 2: Face-to-face semi-structured interviews	Organizational as well as individual factors are important in responding to language needs in health care
Prys (2010)	Qualitative survey	Purposive sample of Welsh-speaking service users (n = 25) and service providers (n = 23) from third sector organizations	Telephone and face-to-face semi-structured interviews	Despite identifying a preference for Welsh language services from third sector providers, Welsh speakers are rarely offered language choice, and they are unlikely to make demands because of their vulnerability
Iaith (2012)	Qualitative survey	Purposive sample of Welsh-speaking health and social care service users and their carers (n = 51) from four priority groups: children; older people; mental health service users; and people with learning disabilities	Telephone and face-to-face semi-structured interviews	Welsh-speakers report deficits in Welsh language provision in health and social care which compromise the quality of care. As minority language speakers, their low expectations and disempowerment militate against their ability to challenge the delivery of services
Beaufort Research (2014)	Two-phased mixed-methods surve Phase 1: Telephone questionnaire survey Phase 2: Qualitative survey	Phase 1: Representative quota sample of Welsh speakers across Wales (n = 1010) Phase 2: Purposive sample of survey respondents (n = 120)	Phase 1: Telephone survey using structured questionnaires Phase 2: Face-to-face semi-structured interviews	Welsh-medium services are provided on the basis of demand rather than need

Welsh Language Commissioner, 2014). All in all, this provided a wealth of rich data for analysis, reported in Welsh and English, according to the language preference of the research respondents.

In line with the Framework Analysis approach (Ritchie & Lewis, 2003), respondents' perceptions were examined for content, and coded and categorised accordingly. Five broad themes emerged, as follows, and these will be discussed in turn:

- acknowledgment of the significance of bilingualism;
- perceived models of bilingualism;
- bilingualism and expression;
- bilingualism and emotion;
- bilingualism and cultural identity.

Acknowledging the significance of bilingualism

The first theme to emerge from the scoping review is the extent to which practitioners acknowledge or fail to acknowledge the significance of bilingualism for service users (see Box 8.1). It appears that, where this is denied, there is a risk of relinquishing the power and rights of clients to speak for themselves, thereby driving their bilingualism into the shadows. Some of the negative perceptions illustrated here are of grave concern since, in the absence of bilingual practitioners, facilitating language choice for service users often hinges on the language attitudes and sensitivity of those from the dominant language group (Cioffi, 2003; Misell, 2000; Timmins, 2002; Vezina et al., 2014). Nevertheless, speakers inevitably make subjective evaluations about the value of their own language variety and those within their wider community and, because different varieties are valued differently, a person's linguistic repertoire can prove to be a significant source of symbolic power (Myers-Scotton, 2006).

As a theoretical model derived from sociolinguistics and first introduced by Giles et al. (1977), the model of ethnolinguistic vitality seeks to identify and explain language attitudes in society whereby the vitality of a language is influenced by its status, demography and institutional support. Since bilingual communication generally involves members of different ethnolinguistic groups of unequal power and status, speakers are more likely to converge to the language of the group which is deemed to have the highest vitality (e.g. English) than to the language of lower prestige (e.g. Welsh; Sachdev & Giles, 2006). Thus, 'the low expectations of the majority of Welsh speakers, as speakers of a traditionally marginalized, minority language, as well as an underpinning reluctance or inability on the part of often disempowered individuals to complain about healthcare services, both militate against the ability to effectively challenge the services being delivered' (Iaith, 2012: 6).

Nevertheless, as we can see from the last respondent (see Box 8.1), a shift toward person-centered communication enables the practitioner to actively engage in a systematic evaluation of the patient's language profile in an attempt to realign power differentials through language. Clearly, there is a risk that patients may feel patronized by the attempts of practitioners to accommodate their language use. Thus, language often has to be negotiated, whether explicitly or implicitly, and those negotiations can be quite complicated (Myers-Scotton, 1993). Nevertheless, there is evidence to suggest that, on the whole, 'Welsh-speaking patients appreciate any efforts, however small, to acknowledge their language and culture and to communicate with them at least partially in Welsh' (Misell, 2000: 75).

Box 8.1: Acknowledging the Significance of Bilingualism

'Gofynodd neb i mi pa iaith oeddwn i am ddefnyddio. Doeddwn i ddim am wneud fuss. Y perygl oedd y byddan yn fy ngweld fel rhyw fath o Welsh nash.' (No one asked me what language I wanted to use. I wasn't going to make a fuss. The danger was that they'd see me as some sort of Welsh nationalist.) (Service user, Madoc-Jones, 2004: 221)

'Er mwyn hwyluso mynediad at y gwasanaeth on i angen ar frys, ac on i mewn galar, nes i just neud o'n Saesneg a nes i'm gofyn an wasanaeth yn y Gymraeg ... achos oni'n meddwl ... os mae rhywun yn gofyn am wasanaeth Cymraeg, mae'n hirach.' (In order to facilitate access to the service that I urgently needed, and I was grief stricken, I just did it in English and I didn't ask for a Welsh service ... because I thought, ... if someone asks for a Welsh language service, it takes longer ...) (Service user, Prys, 2010: 193)

'Ond mae rhywun yn mynd i weld ymgynghorydd a'r 'consultant' – naturiol wedyn yn Saesneg 'de, dw i ddim yn disgwyl dim arall 'lly i ddweud y gwir.' (But when one goes to see the consultant and the advisor ... it's natural then that it's in English, I don't expect anything else to tell you the truth.) (Service user, Beaufort Research, 2014: 34)

'I've been working with a man regularly, weekly for about six months, before I realised that Welsh was his first language.' (Practitioner, Roberts et al., 2004: 37)

'I think, for the patient, the priority is their health, it's not the language.' (Practitioner, Roberts et al., 2004: 29)

> 'Fe'i gorchmynnwyd gan fwy nag un nyrs i siarad Saesneg ... 'You should speak English so that I can understand', meddai'r nyrs wrthi. Doedd gan amryw o'r staff ddim amgyffred o'r angen i ddeall anghenion emosiynol claf Cymraeg ei hiaith a dryslyd ei meddwl.' (She was instructed by more than one nurse to speak English .... 'You should speak English so that I can understand you', the nurse said to her. Many of the staff had no idea about the need to understand the emotional needs of a Welsh-speaking patient who was confused.) (Relative, Iaith, 2012: 17)
>
> 'I can normally gauge who speaks Welsh and who can't ... Firstly, I look at their name. If they've got a Welsh name ... also if their cards are written in Welsh – their get well cards – I'll have a quick peek at them, and, if they're written in Welsh, again, I know they speak Welsh, and sometimes you can just overhear them, one word might be a Welsh word because they just tend to mix English and Welsh don't they? So, if they do that, that's when I'll know they speak Welsh.' (Practitioner, Roberts *et al.*, 2004: 37)

Perceived models of bilingualism

The second theme derived from the review illustrates the theory proposed by Grosjean (1985, 2008) that there are two contrasting views of bilingualism. Both are illustrated in the voices of the practitioners and service users captured in Box 8.2. The first practitioner adopts a monolingual or fractional view whereby she evaluates bilingual clients as 'two monolinguals in one person' (Grosjean, 2008: 10), each client perceived to be equally and fully fluent in both English and Welsh. Arguably, this viewpoint is unfair since bilinguals tend to use their two languages in different situations and with different people. Hence, their languages will be stronger in different domains (Baker, 2011; Grosjean, 2008; Myers-Scotton, 2006). Nevertheless, the fractional model suggests that bilinguals should demonstrate proficiency comparable to that of monolinguals in both languages. Given that this is rarely the case, bilinguals may be denigrated; this can alter their self-image and undermine their confidence to use their language (Johnstone & Kanitsaki, 2008, 2009). This can have a marked effect in health care and prevent bilingual clients from speaking their chosen language or being assessed effectively. It may also impact on the readiness of practitioners to use their minority language in the healthcare context (Drolet *et al.*, 2014; Garrett *et al.*, 2008; Roberts & Paden, 2000; Vezina *et al.*, 2014).

An alternative, holistic view of bilingualism offered by Grosjean (2008) takes account of the fact that bilinguals are not the sum of two complete or incomplete monolinguals but that they have a unique linguistic profile where both languages are constantly interacting and their use of language is context-bound. Grosjean (1997) termed this phenomenon the 'complementarity principle' whereby 'bilinguals usually acquire and use their languages for different purposes, in different domains of life, with different people. Different aspects of life often require different languages' (Grosjean, 2008: 23). This helps shed light on the true configuration of the bilingual's repertoire; the way in which language skills may change over time; the need for clinical assessments that are appropriate to the domains of language use; and the reasons why regular bilinguals are not usually very effective translators or interpreters.

Thus, the complementarity principle (Grosjean, 1997) dispels some of the deep-rooted myths about bilingualism in health care, as identified by Misell (2000) and the Office of the French Language Commissioner (2009), such as:

- health service users who speak two languages are completely bilingual;
- language is not all that important in health care;
- there is no need for bilingual services.

By and large, the practitioners cited within this theme recognize the importance of language in different domains of their clients' lives and switch purposively and sensitively from one language to another to meet their needs. This notion of switching is discussed in more detail in the next theme that explores bilingualism and expression.

Box 8.2: Perceived Models of Bilingualism

'All Welsh speakers speak very good English and are very capable of taking home the message we want in English.' (Practitioner, Roberts *et al.*, 2004: 25).

'(Roedd) defnyddio'r dwy iaith yn confuso'r un bach, a just defnyddio un iaith – a'r Saesneg fysa hwnna, oedd y recommendation.' (Using two languages was confusing the child, and just using one language – and that was English – was the recommendation.) (Relative, Beaufort Research, 2014: 33)

'Byddan nhw'n trio dweud rhywbeth ac ych chi'n trio'u helpu nhw ac mae hynny'n helpu da'r berthynas.' (They try saying something (in Welsh) and you try helping them and that helps the relationship.) (Service user, Iaith, 2012: 16)

'(Byddwn i'n) gofyn i rywun pa iaith mae nhw eisiau siarad – os ydy nhw'n gyfforddus yn y Saesneg neu fod eisiau newid i'r Gymraeg.'

> ((I would) ask someone which language they want to speak – if they're comfortable in English or they want to switch to Welsh.) (Practitioner, Roberts *et al.*, 2004: 103)
>
> 'I would use my minimal Welsh, e.g. 'diolch' (thank you) with patients – words I am comfortable with – to make patients feel comfortable.' (Practitioner, Roberts *et al.*, 2004: 104)
>
> 'Mae siarad Cymraeg yn teimlo'n fwy cartrefol er mod i'n siarad Saesneg yn dda.' (Though I speak English well, I feel more homely speaking Welsh.) (Service user, Madoc-Jones, 2004: 218)
>
> 'For dying patients, providing opportunities to talk about the affairs of the heart and sympathise in their preferred language is very important indeed.' (Practitioner, Roberts *et al.*, 2004: 105)

Bilingualism and expression

Grosjean (1985, 1997, 2008) depicts a bilingual person as a unique speaker and an integrated whole, where one language should not be examined without considering the other. This is a key factor in exploring the way in which bilingualism affects language functioning, such as expression, which is the focus of this next theme. Although most of the service users represented in Box 8.3 are bilingual, they explain that switching to Welsh makes it easier for them to express themselves and explain their symptoms. This, they suggest, enhances the flow and depth of the conversation whereby they feel more able and ready to disclose personal matters and concerns, particularly at times of stress.

Grosjean (2008) claims that, in conversations, bilinguals are continually making decisions (albeit largely unconsciously) about which language to use and to what extent they will draw on their other language (if at all). He proposed that, in their everyday lives, bilingual speakers find themselves in various language modes that correspond to positions on a monolingual–bilingual continuum. When communicating with other bilinguals who share their two languages, bilinguals find themselves in a bilingual mode where language mixing is likely to occur through code-switching or borrowing, that is, the use of two language varieties in the same conversation (Myers-Scotton, 2006) or, more precisely, the insertion of words or phrases from one language into sentences from another language. Rather than view this as interference, it is now well established that code-switching is a valuable linguistic strategy that helps bilinguals clarify meaning, ease tension and communicate friendship, all of which are key to effective communication in a healthcare context (Baker & Jones, 1998).

Nevertheless, it is important to note that language choice in a bilingual context is seldom neutral since there are processes at work that motivate speakers to modify their speech in response to the listener. This phenomenon is explained by Sachdev and Giles (2006) in their Communication Accommodation Theory (CAT) where they suggest that people emphasize or minimize social differences between themselves and their listeners through altering their speech styles. There are, inevitably, a number of reasons why bilinguals switch from one language to another, the most obvious example being when they are unable to find the right words. Nevertheless, there are also social and psychological factors at work that influence speakers to lay down markers of social integration, solidarity and differentiation. Given that the perceived status and power of languages in a bilingual context are rarely equal and while acknowledging the wider power disparities inherent in healthcare encounters, the scope for accommodation is thus significant. This ability to adapt language thus offers a strategy that promotes harmony between individuals which can facilitate and support the all-important relationship between the client and practitioner. In contrast, language choices that appear patronizing (hyperaccommodation) encourage divergence which can lead to anger and dissatisfaction amongst listeners and considerable embarrassment for the speakers as well.

According to CAT (Sachdev & Giles, 2006), individuals use communication to an extent to signal their attitudes toward each other, and in gauging the response, they can evaluate the social distance between them. Adapting their communication style, either through, for example, changing the register of the language in a monolingual setting or by switching language in a bilingual context, is called 'speech accommodation', and it is based on the social psychological models of similarity-attraction and intergroup distinctiveness. Convergence takes place when a person, in conversation, tries to imitate the other person's speech patterns in order to be friendly, denote closeness or identify with the other person. This behavior may be exhibited through a wide range of linguistic and non-verbal features, including code-switching, where converging to a common linguistic style has been shown to reduce uncertainty and interpersonal anxiety whilst enhancing mutual understanding (Gudykunst, 1995).

CAT is well illustrated in a classic study reported by Bourhis et al. (1989), who adopted a survey approach to examine the perceptions of physicians, student nurses and patients about their use of 'medical' and 'everyday' language in their interactions in a hospital setting. While the doctors reported converging to the 'everyday' language of their patients, the patients and student nurses did not perceive their speech as converging. Similarly, patients reported attempting to converge to the 'medical language' of health professionals but this was not corroborated by the physicians. The student nurses were perceived by all groups to be converging to the 'everyday language' of patients and were thus identified as important 'communication brokers' in health care. 'Medical language' was seen as problematic for patients whilst 'everyday language' was deemed to improve their understanding.

A systematic review of healthcare literature published between 1990 and 2001 (Brown & Draper, 2003) set out to explore the use of patronizing patterns of speech and modified forms of address in conversations between nurses and other health workers, and older people. The findings confirmed that over-accommodation with older people was rife, fostering dependence and lowered self-esteem.

Turning our attention to bilingual accommodation, Roberts (1994), in an ethnographic study of the use of the Welsh language in an acute bilingual healthcare setting in West Wales, demonstrated how bilingual nurses converged to using Welsh with Welsh-speaking patients to provide comfort and reassurance. This strategy was well received by patients and shown to be a powerful tool for establishing caring relationships which patients perceived as therapeutic. These effects are corroborated in the themes emerging from our literature synthesis where efforts to converge to Welsh with Welsh-speaking clients appear to instil feelings of satisfaction and fulfilment (see Box 8.3).

In stark contrast to convergence, divergence occurs when a person accentuates speech differences in order to ensure distance, consolidate power and authority and denote separateness. While consumerism, partnership, advocacy and power sharing are all part of the current rhetoric in health care (Murphy, 2011), the evidence from the language barriers in the healthcare literature suggests that language barriers continue to adversely affect patients in terms of their access to health services, comprehension and adherence, quality of care, and patient and provider satisfaction (Schwei *et al.*, 2016). This raises fundamental questions about the relative power of clients and the way in which the practitioner–client relationship reflects an imbalance of power around issues of control and compliance which are often mediated through language.

Despite the increasing emphasis on the importance of therapeutic interactions as the key to caring relationships, historically, healthcare professionals have exerted power and control over clients through their use of language, through a variety of approaches such as: control of information (Macleod Clarke, 1982); the use of persuasion (Hewison, 1995); control of the agenda (Macleod Clarke, 1982; Hewison, 1995); the pluralization of the client (Lanceley, 1985); the use of softeners (Lanceley, 1985); inappropriate terms of endearment (Hewison, 1995; Bowie, 1996); over-familiarity (Wyn Siencyn, 1995; Bowie, 1996); and over-accommodation (Brown & Draper, 2003). Accentuating language and cultural differences through divergence can add to this power disparity (see Box 8.1). Moreover, monolinguals may not view bilingual code-switching in a positive light, misinterpreting its attributes as poor mastery of language, with derogatory connotations. For example, in a qualitative survey of healthcare staff and service user participants in Australia ($n = 145$), Johnstone and Kanitsaki (2008) demonstrated that language prejudice operated directly and indirectly at all levels whereby 'limited English proficiency' speakers or those who spoke English proficiently as a second language but with a 'heavy accent' were at risk of being evaluated negatively as communicatively and rationally incompetent (Johnstone & Kanitsaki, 2008: 28). While this is how speakers are generally perceived by members of the dominant culture, its impact can have far-reaching effects in health care.

Box 8.3: Bilingualism and Expression

'Mae e lot yn rhwyddach i ni. Wy'n fwy rhugl yn Gymraeg. Mae e'n teimlo'n fwy personol. Ych chi'n gallu sôn am eich gofidiau.' (It's a lot easier for us. I'm more fluent in Welsh. It feels more personal. You can talk about your worries.) (Service user, Iaith, 2012: 43)

'Weithiau mae'n anodd i mi ddweud be dwi am ddweud yn Saesneg.' (Sometimes I can't say what I want to say in English.) (Service user, Madoc-Jones, 2004: 219)

'Dywedwch chi'n awr bod ni hefo rhywun Saesneg smo i'n gallu explainio 'run peth yn Saesneg ac ni'n gallu gneud yn Gymraeg. Ni'n gallu deud yn rhwyddach yn Gymraeg nag yn Saesneg. Alle ni ddeud e'n Saesneg ond so fo ddim mor rhwydd ag yn y Gymraeg. Cymraeg yw'n iaith gyntaf.' (Say now that we are with someone who's English speaking, we can't explain in the same way in English as we can in Welsh. We can say it easier in Welsh than in English. We could say it in English but it's not as easy as in Welsh, Welsh is our first language.) (Service user, Prys, 2010: 192)

'Yn Gymraeg, dwi'n gallu siarad am brofiadau a phetha personol iawn. Mae'n haws gwneud hynny yn Gymraeg. Dyw'r llif ddim yna yn Saesneg. Dach chi'n gorfod cyfieithu, yn arbennig pan dach chi'n sôn am rywbeth sydd mor bwysig i ni fel teulu.' (In Welsh, I can talk about experiences and really personal things. It's easier to do that in Welsh. The flow isn't the same in English. You have to translate, especially when you're talking about something which is so important to us as a family.) (Service user, Iaith, 2012: 50)

'Os nad oes modd i'r claf esbonio'n glir yn Saesneg, mae'n gallu cael effaith mawr ar y diagnosis a fel 'yn ni'n trin nhw.' (If the patient can't explain clearly, in English, this can have a huge effect on the diagnosis and how we treat them.) (Practitioner, Roberts et al., 2004: 26)

> 'Sa'r prawf yn decach ... ella sa'n 'neud gwahaniaeth i'r canlyniad meddygol, os dach chi'n cael siarad eich iaith eich hun dach chi'n gallu mynegi eich hun yn well o ran be dach chi'n 'i deimlo a'i gofio'. (If the test was fairer ... maybe it would have made a difference to the medical results, if you can speak your own language you're able to express yourself better, about what you feel and remember.) (Service user, Beaufort Research, 2014: 31)
>
> 'Mae o wedi bod yn deall Saesneg cystal â chi a fi ond tostrwydd wedi neud o'n awr yn tefe. Roedd ei Saesneg yn alright chi'n gwybod, mae e wedi cael ei godi'n Gymraeg ond oedd e yn deall Saesneg ond yn awr Cymraeg yw ei iaith e, dyw o ddim yn deud gair o Saesneg.' (He used to understand English as well as you and me, but the illness has taken him now. His English was alright you know, he was raised in Welsh but he understood English, but now Welsh is his language, he doesn't say a word of English.) (Practitioner, Prys, 2010: 192)

Thus, there are a host of conditions which enable bilingual speakers to express themselves more effectively in their chosen language. Practitioners need to be aware of the external forces at play that influence patients' use of language and adopt appropriate strategies for accommodating their speech styles to meet individual needs.

Bilingualism and emotion

Language is our main vehicle for classifying and expressing emotions, and it is widely accepted that these are often shaped by the social and cultural context in which they are experienced (Altarriba & Morier, 2006). Inevitably, being bilingual raises questions about how speakers use their different languages to express feelings and emotions. This is particularly important in the context of mental health where language is crucial in helping to construct meaning; and communication is an essential component of therapeutic interventions. Within the broader context, Jacobs et al. (2006: 111) claim that 'the conversation between physician and patient has long been recognized to be of diagnostic importance and therapeutic benefit'.

The next theme to emerge from the scoping review focuses on bilingualism and emotion where respondents offer vivid accounts of the way in which language colors their emotions and helps them identify with their inner feelings or self and relay experiences as they happened. The voices captured in Box 8.4 on the one hand make reference to the barriers associated with attempting to relay emotions in a second language, whilst, on the other hand, alluding to the fact that switching languages can also guard against sharing uncomfortable or painful thoughts. Reviewing the research in this emerging field helps make sense of these experiences and validate perceptions.

Cognitive psychologists have long been interested in the way in which emotion is represented and expressed since this is key to enhancing our understanding of the mental processes that influence health and well-being (Altarriba, 2006). More recently, in response to increasing diversity in health care, their attention is drawn to the dynamics of language use in the assessment and treatment of bilingual patients and the way in which emotion is encoded. This interest is based on the understanding that the role of language in therapy is central to effective treatment and that bilingualism should be perceived as a strength rather than a deficit (Santiago-Rivera & Altarriba, 2002).

Reviewing the body of research emerging from North America, Altarriba and Morier (2006: 252) conclude that, 'in cases of psychological assessment and diagnosis, a bilingual may appear to present him- or herself in different ways depending on the language used'. This finding is substantiated by our Welsh respondents who, when speaking Welsh with staff, felt more comfortable and more able to express their feelings freely. Switching to English was either impossible under the circumstances or marked a distinct change in their persona. Similar reports emerge from a research study of the experiences of Francophones in Ontario living with HIV or AIDS, where a respondent explains, 'It is much more comfortable to speak about my emotions in French. It is much more natural to share my emotions in French instead of English' (Samson & Spector, 2012: 664).

Bilinguals usually report their first or primary language to be their most emotional language, carrying with it more associations and connotations. Having access to two languages, they are thus offered the option of choosing one system or the other (or both simultaneously) in an effort to express whatever they are feeling (Grosjean, 2008; Altarriba & Morier, 2006). Non-equivalence between language concepts may partly account for this choice but code-switching may also occur as a protective measure where words themselves may elicit different emotions in the bilingual's first and second language. For example, Bond and Lai (1986) demonstrated that bilingual students from the University of Hong Kong found it easier to discuss more embarrassing topics in their second rather than primary language. Altarriba and Morier (2006: 258) conclude that findings such as these seem to suggest a 'distancing function inherent in a bilingual's second language'. Thus, in order to avoid describing unpleasant or even painful emotions, bilinguals may switch from one language to another as a coping strategy (Santiago-Rivera & Altarriba, 2002). These findings are substantiated by Pavlenko's (2012) comprehensive review of the empirical research in the field that demonstrates how bilinguals process verbal stimuli differently in their respective languages, leading her to coin the term, 'disembodied cognition'.

Another phenomenon that has come to light in recent years is the way in which memory retrieval for bilinguals is enhanced when events are recounted in the language in which the event occurred. Reviewing a body of evidence derived from studies of autobiographical memory, Schrauf and Durazo-Arvizu (2006) conclude that there is empirical evidence to suggest that, when bilinguals recall first language memories from childhood in a second language, there is a loss of emotional intensity. Moreover, when the language of retrieval reflects the language of encoding, there is more intensity to the emotion that is remembered. This phenomenon is clearly illustrated by the last respondent (see Box 8.4), where the highly charged event occurred in Welsh, evoking with it strong feelings and emotions. Recounting the event in English proved particularly challenging for this client.

Many of the respondents represented in this theme alluded to the fact that speaking Welsh made them feel more themselves and that speaking English felt unreal or unnatural. This is a familiar perception amongst bilinguals since it is argued that 'language is one of the main organizing principles which gives a form and meaning to our experience' (Davies, 2002: 28). Nevertheless, such claims have fueled fierce debate over the years about the way in which speakers conceptualize and understand the world, and the extent to which this is influenced by the structure of their language. Whilst the notion that language categorically determines thought is now heavily contested, it is more widely accepted that the distinctiveness of language can influence thought in more subtle ways that are evident in the testimonies of bilingual speakers (de Groot, 2010).

Adopting a lengthy online questionnaire maintained on the Birbeck College and administered between 2001 and 2003, Dewaele and Pavlenko set out to explore this phenomenon among bilinguals and consider to what extent they felt like different people when speaking different languages, whether they were perceived as different by listeners and whether they behaved differently. The survey was completed by 1039 bilingual and multilingual speakers and the findings summarized by Pavlenko (2008). While the survey was subject to the customary limitations of an online survey, the questions about different selves elicited many emotional responses and these were captured within four main sources of perceptions of different selves, namely, linguistic and cultural differences; distinct learning contexts; different levels of language emotionality; and different levels of language proficiency. Pavlenko (2006: 26–27) concluded that 'Reflections of bilingual writers and explorations by linguists and psychoanalysts show that languages may create different, and sometimes incommensurable, worlds for their speakers who feel that their selves change with the shift in language'. This phenomenon is clearly borne out among our Welsh-speaking respondents who feel more themselves speaking Welsh.

Box 8.4: Bilingualism and Emotion

'Roedd hi'n lyfli ond o'n i'n teimlo'n afreal iawn yn siarad Saesneg ... Tase hi'n siarad Cymraeg, fydden ni wedi cyrraedd rhywle arall.' (She was lovely, but I felt unreal talking in English ... If she spoke Welsh, we would have reached somewhere else.) (Service user, Iaith, 2012: 24)

'Dywedais fy mod i'n hapus i siarad yn Saesneg ond yna gofynodd i mi drafod fy mywyd a fy nheimladau. Doedd gen i ddim y geiriau.' (I said I was OK speaking English to him, but then he wanted to talk about my life and feelings. I didn't have the words.) (Service user, Madoc-Jones, 2004: 219)

'Dydyn nhw ddim yn cael gwir farn rhywun. Fedra i'm dweud sut dwi'n teimlo. Fedra i'm ei roi o mewn geiriau ... Dwi di dweud mwy wrthoch chi na dwi'n dweud wrthyn nhw. Mae'n saffach dweud dim byd.' (They don't really have somebody's true opinion. I can't say how I feel. I can't put it into words ... I've said more to you than I tell them. It's safer not to say anything.) (Service user, Iaith, 2012: 25)

'(Mae'r Gymraeg) yn bwysig iawn i mi, dwi'n teimlo mwy fel fy hun yn Gymraeg, mwy cyffyrddus – Cymro ydw i.' ((The Welsh language) is very important to me. I feel more myself in Welsh, more comfortable – I'm Welsh.) (Service user, Madoc-Jones, 2004: 218)

'Gyda'r henoed, dwi'n credu fod o'n eitha' pwysig bod nhw'n – oes oes rhywun i gael, fyddai lot well 'da nhw i siarad 'da rhywun yn Gymraeg – just i wneud nhw deimlo'n fwy cyfforddus dwi'n credu i ddechrau efo fo – yn enwedig os ma' fe ambiti rhywbeth fel iechyd.' (With the elderly, I believe that it is quite important that they – if there is someone available, they would much prefer to speak to someone in Welsh – just to make them more comfortable to start with – especially if it's about something like health.) (Practitioner, Roberts et al., 2004: 25)

'Oedd o 'just' yn gwneud pethe'n haws bod ni'n siarad Cymraeg, trafod yn Gymraeg unrhyw broblema oedd gynnon ni, ac oedd o fwy agos atoch chi mewn ffordd mwy cartrefol.' (It just made things easier that we spoke Welsh, could discuss any problems that we had in Welsh, and it made it feel closer and more comfortable.) (Service user, Beaufort Research, 2014: 16)

'Oedd y pethe o'n ni'n trio eu trafod yn y cyfarfodydd wedi digwydd yn Gymraeg – y teimladau, popeth i gyd yn Gymraeg. Oedd y sefyllfa yr un

> mwyaf anodd i fi yn fy mywyd. Mae Saesneg fi'n iawn ond pan ych chi'n gyfarwydd â sefyllfa yn Gymraeg – y teimladau, y dadleuon i gyd yn Gymraeg, ac ych chi'n gorfod neud hynny dan bwysau mawr, mae e'n anodd ofnadwy yn Saesneg.' (The things we were trying to discuss in the meetings had happened in Welsh – the feelings, everything in Welsh. The situation was the most difficult one for me ever. My English is OK but when something has happened to you in Welsh – the feelings, the arguments all in Welsh, and you have to do it all under a lot of pressure, it's terribly difficult in English.) (Service user, Iaith, 2012: 46)

Bilingualism and cultural identity

Language is not simply about communication since it also provides a means of establishing and asserting identity. For the bilingual speakers represented in this next theme (see Box 8.5), speaking Welsh communicates a special sense of connect and belonging which helps build trusting relationships.

As explained by Aitchison and Carter (1994: 57),

> Not only does (language) carry a view of the environment, using the word in its proper inclusive sense, but through its vocabulary and its structure, through the associations generated by its literature, through the symbol which it is and the symbols which it transmits, it creates a distinctive identity which is at once a derivative of tradition and an expression of the past.

O'Hagan (2001) affirms this important link between language, ethnicity and cultural identity from the Irish perspective by drawing on the work of Ó Riagáin, who states:

> Language is in the first instance a means of communication. But it is a lot more than that. It is a communal tool, developed and refined by its users, to express their ideas, their beliefs, their feelings. It reflects a people's development, their shared historical experience and their sense of community. It is a receptacle where a people's most intimate and finest thoughts can be recorded, stored and transmitted, not only to other contemporary members of the community, but even from one generation to the other. It is the mainspring of culture. (Ó Riagáin 1998: 154).

Clearly, for bilingual speakers, a key aspect of their self is embodied in their language and its sociocultural associations. Their language thus carries meaning beyond words, and this helps them identify with speakers of the same language. In the bilingual healthcare context, this leads to a greater rapport and solidarity among minority language speakers, which has been shown to enhance satisfaction with care provision, as evidenced in studies from Wales (Misell, 2000), Northern Ireland (O'Hagan, 2001), Sweden (Heikkila & Elman, 2000; Heikkila *et al.*, 2007) and Canada (Samson & Spector, 2012).

Nevertheless, it is evident that the effective delivery of bilingual healthcare services cannot rely solely on the language proficiency of practitioners since it also demands a heightened awareness of language across the workforce and an appreciation of its inherent cultural dimensions. With its roots in educational linguistics, particularly second language acquisition, language awareness is defined as:

> an understanding of the human faculty of language and its role in thinking, learning and social life. It includes awareness of power and control through language, and the intricate relationships between language and culture. (Van Lier, 1995: xi)

In other words, language awareness requires not only knowledge about language but also a critical awareness that considers 'how languages or styles of language reflect and sustain differences in power and status' (Baker & Jones, 1998: 633). Indeed, sociolinguists, such as Gumperz (1972), suggest that 'communicative competence' can only be achieved through a heightened awareness and understanding of the broader context in which language takes place. The final respondent in this theme (see Box 8.5) offers a sobering example of the way in which a stark lack of cultural and language awareness on the part of a practitioner can strip an individual of his dignity and self-worth.

In an attempt to provide equity of service and overcome health disparities, there is evidence of growing commitment in the UK (Department of Health, 2012; Welsh Government, 2012a, 2016), US (Office of Minority Health, US Department of Health and Human Services, 2001), Canada (Office of the French Language Commissioner, 2009), Australia (National Health and Medical Research Council, 2005) and New Zealand (New Zealand Ministry of Health, 2006) toward tailoring services that are sensitive to a wide range of cultural and communication needs.

Heavily embedded in Leininger's (1988) trans-cultural nursing theory from the US, early interpretations of cultural competence in health care were aligned with

> a formal area of study and practice focussed on comparative holistic cultural care, health, and illness patterns of people with respect to differences and similarities in their cultural values, beliefs, and lifeways with

the goal to provide culturally congruent, competent, and compassionate care. (Leininger 1997: 342)

Since Leininger's (1988) early work, a number of conceptual frameworks have been established to guide cultural competence in health care. Many of these frameworks identify common constructs and depict cultural competence on a continuum from critical awareness and cultural knowledge through to skills development, practice and application (Balcazar et al., 2009). More importantly, a few extend the scope of cultural competence beyond the level of the individual practitioner to include an organization's capacity to integrate the principles and values of cultural competence into its policies and structures. This comprehensive approach is reflected in the CLAS Standards (Office of Minority Health, US Department of Health and Human Services, 2001), which are based on the Cross et al. (1989: iv–v) conceptual definition of cultural competence:

> Cultural and linguistic competence is a set of congruent behaviours, attitudes and policies that come together in a system, agency or among professionals that enables effective work in cross-cultural situations. 'Culture' refers to integrated patterns of human behaviour that include the language, thoughts, communications, actions, customs, beliefs, values and institutions of racial, ethnic, religious or social groups. 'Competence' implies having the capacity to function effectively as an individual and an organization within the context of the cultural beliefs, behaviours and needs presented by consumers and their communities.

Thus, while still endorsed by her followers and refined over the years, Leininger's (1997) static and uniform view of culture that focuses exclusively on the cognitive domain has been heavily criticized (Campesino, 2006; Johnson & Munch, 2009; Williamson & Harrison, 2010). It is argued that her approach obscures the broader sociopolitical context of colonized and marginalized people and the power differences inherent in health care (Culley, 2000; Gustafson, 2005). Moreover, even in her recent work, Leininger (2007) overlooks the significance of language in the construction of cultural identity and the power dimensions that influence language use among minority language speakers.

In response to increasing health inequalities among the indigenous Maori population of New Zealand and with its roots embedded in post-colonial theory (Anderson et al., 2003), a new concept of cultural safety in health care began to emerge (Ramsden, 2002). This, argues Wepa (2003), moves beyond the concept of cultural competence to analyzing power imbalances, institutional discrimination and colonization, as they apply to health care. It considers the impact of colonial processes on the ongoing relationship between indigenous and non-indigenous people and how this affects health and the dynamics of health care. Embracing the concept within the Canadian healthcare system, Smye and Browne (2002: 47) propose that:

> ### Box 8.5: Bilingualism and Cultural Identity
>
> 'Mi gliciais i hefo hi yn syth. Mae ei gwreiddiau a'i magwraeth lai na 10 milltir o lle 'magwyd i. Roedd hi felly yn gwybod o ble roeddwn i yn dod, nid yn unig yn ddaearyddol, ond yn ieithyddol a diwylliannol. Fedra i ddim dechra disgrifio pa mor allweddol oedd hi i roi'r hyder imi y bydden i'n gallu gofalu am X. Roeddwn i yn ei thrystio hi yn llwyr ac yn gwybod ei bod hi'n siarad hefo fi mewn ffordd lle roeddwn i'n gwybod ei bod hi yn fy neall i.' (I clicked with her immediately. Her roots and upbringing were within 10 miles of where I'd been brought up. So she knew where I came from, not just in terms of geography but linguistically and culturally. I can't begin to describe how vital she was in giving me the confidence to believe that I could care for X. I trusted her implicitly and I knew she was talking to me in a way that showed me she understood.) (Service user, Iaith, 2012: 51)
>
> 'Mae hwn yn mynd i swnio'n od ond ar ôl tua tair wythnos, daeth gweithiwr cymdeithasol i'm gweld a oedd yn gallu siarad Cymraeg. Roedd y profiad yn debyg i atgyfodiad oherwydd roedd yn gallu gwneud y pethau bach fel siarad am *Pobl y Cwm* ac roedd beth oedd yn digwydd yn y rhaglen yn fy ngwneud i mi deimlo'n normal eto.' (After about three weeks, a social worker who could speak Welsh came to see me and it was like coming alive again – it seems silly but being able to talk about *Pobl y Cwm* (Welsh-language soap opera) and what was happening made me feel normal again.) (Service user, Madoc-Jones, 2004: 219)
>
> 'Odd hi'n siarad Cymraeg ac yn dod o'r un math o gefndir. Odd mam yn gallu ei thrystio hi i fynd â nhad mas. Oedd dad yn dwlu arni hefyd.' (She spoke Welsh and came from the same background. My mother could trust her to take my father out. My father doted on her too.) (Relative, Iaith, 2012: 50)
>
> 'Recognising a patient through their own language means that you recognise them as a whole person.' (Practitioner, Roberts *et al.*, 2004: 108)
>
> 'Dylent wneud 'effort' i ddysgu ar y lleiaf, dylent ein cyfarch yn Gymraeg ... Byddai yn gwneud gwahaniaeth. Byddai yn dangos parch i'r iaith ac i siaradwyr Cymraeg. Byddai yn codi ysbryd.' (They should make an effort to learn at least, they should greet us in Welsh ... It would make a difference. It would show respect towards the language and towards

> Welsh speakers. It would raise our spirits.) (Service user, Beaufort Research, 2014: 52)
>
> 'Doeddwn i ddim yn teimlo bod croeso i mi ar y ward, doedd dim deunydd Cymraeg a doedd y staff ddim yn barod i gydnabod fy Nghymreictod ac felly ro'n i'n gyndyn i siarad gyda nhw, ond anfonwyd ... o'r nefoedd.' (I didn't feel welcomed on the ward, there were no Welsh materials and the staff didn't seem prepared to recognise my Welshness, this made me reluctant to speak with them, but (name of Welsh-speaking psychiatrist) was a god send.) (Service user, Madoc-Jones, 2004, pg 221)
>
> 'Wedyn mi ffoniais i (gwasanaeth) – a'r ymateb ges i wedyn oedd o'n ffiaidd, gofyn am enw'r claf, ac mi ddywedais i (enw), a dyma nhw'n dweud sut wyt ti'n sillafu hwn, ac mi sillafais fy enw tair gwaith, a wedyn ges i 'that's not a name it's a meaningless jumble of letters' (Then I rang the (service) – and the response I had was vile, they asked for the name of the patient, and I said (my name) and they said 'how do you spell that?' And I spelled my name out three times, and the response was 'that's not a name, it's a meaningless jumble of letters'.) (Service user, Beaufort Research, 2014: 45)

> Cultural safety is concerned with fostering an understanding of the relationship between minority status and health status as a way of changing nurses' attitudes from those which continue to support current dominant practices and systems of health care to those which are more supportive of the health of minority groups.

The Welsh speakers represented in this review demonstrate how language is a key aspect of their cultural identity. The anti-oppressive approach embedded within the concept of cultural safety reminds us of the importance of historical, cultural, social and political processes in our engagement with them as bilingual speakers, and informs our thinking about tackling language discrimination and oppression.

Study Limitations

Scoping studies are gaining popularity as a methodology for reviewing health research evidence but the approach continues to attract debate and discussion in the literature, particularly around methodological rigor (Levac et al., 2010). For complex interventions, such as bilingual healthcare communication, this scoping study has enabled the mapping of the evidence from the perspectives of service users and providers in the bilingual context of Wales. Nevertheless, a wider review of the policy literature may have identified further issues that have a bearing on the nature of practice in a bilingual context. Decisions around which studies to include in this scoping study were made by a single author. Despite her expertise in the field, an iterative team approach to selecting studies may have enhanced the rigor of the research (Levac et al., 2010).

Conclusions and Recommendations

This scoping review set out to examine the research evidence from the bilingual context of Wales that captures the perceptions of service users and practitioners about bilingualism in healthcare communication, with a specific focus on Welsh speakers as minority language users of an English-dominant healthcare system. The varied and vivid accounts offer a wealth of data that shed light on our understanding of the dynamics of bilingual healthcare communication in this context and offer scope for enhancement at an individual and organizational level. Whilst the findings relate specifically to the Welsh context, they are substantiated in parts by the global evidence, thus indicating the scope for transferability and the potential for wider research. In drawing on the theoretical and empirical evidence, the voices of those who are generally silenced are heard and the perceptions of bilingual service users are validated.

The findings confirm that language is more than just words. It offers scope for individuals to express their social and cultural identity and provides an important vehicle for conveying thoughts and emotions. Nevertheless, for bilingual speakers, language choice in health care is rarely a balanced choice since it is strongly influenced by the context in which communication takes place and its inherent power dimensions. Moreover, bilingual speakers process language in a dynamic, complex and purposeful way which takes account of their full linguistic repertoire in both languages. All of these findings offer a very clear message to healthcare services to adapt their practice and policies to meet the dynamic needs of bilingual speakers as part of their commitment toward person-centered, therapeutic communication as well as equitable care.

At an *individual level*, the review demonstrates a need to integrate language awareness and theories of bilingualism into core curricula around healthcare communication, whilst supporting language learning that is fit for purpose and reflects the local demographic profiles of client groups.

At an *organizational level*, the review gives strength to the 'active offer' principle where the responsibility for language choice sits with the provider rather than the service user, reflecting Betancourt et al.'s (2003) framework of cultural competence and Wynia and Matiasek's (2006) 'promising practices' for strong leadership, designated champions and systematic language planning that adopts a whole-system approach.

Finally, with a view to directing *further research*, the review gives strength to the proposal by Segalowitz and Kehayia (2011) for building an interdisciplinary research agenda that is theory driven and problem solving, to build the evidence for bilingual healthcare communication.

Nevertheless, implementation of the evidence base is challenging in the face of such complex interventions as bilingual communication in health care, particularly where the empirical evidence is limited and so too is the scope of systematic reviews (Pawson, 2006). In this case, adopting methodologies derived from implementation science (Damschroder *et al.*, 2009: 5) offers access to a wider breadth of evidence from different perspectives to establish an alternative approach to evidence synthesis which emphasizes 'the dynamic interplay between individuals and the organisation in which they work, and how that interplay influences individuals and organisational behaviour change'.

The evidence suggests that such interplay is a critical factor in the delivery of language-appropriate services in health care where language use in a bilingual context is reliant not only on the knowledge, skills and attitudes of healthcare providers but also on the readiness of organizations to embed language awareness into their organizational strategies and operational systems. Implementing the 'active offer' principle thus requires a commitment by practitioners and provider organizations to adopt new ways of working, yet little is known about the mechanisms that influence their interactions in this respect and impact on transforming care experiences.

This scoping review offers a resounding call for action at a strategic, operational and individual level to enhance language-appropriate practice for bilingual speakers and redress the balance of power. Arguably, the evidence to inform the organizational cultural shift required of the 'active offer' principle is complex and contextual and beyond the scope of systematic reviews. Nevertheless, the realist approach (Pawson, 2006) offers an alternative means of evidence synthesis that has been shown to enhance our understanding of such complex social interactions. Broadening the scope for collating evidence from a range of individual and organizational perspectives while adopting novel approaches for synthesis and evaluation offers far-reaching opportunities to shed light on the complexities of language use within a bilingual context, and the mechanisms that drive or counter the 'active offer' principle.

A realist approach is thus proposed that acknowledges that the world is an open system, with structures and layers that interact to form mechanisms and contexts. Rather than identifying simple cause-and-effect relationships, realistic evaluation activity is concerned with finding out about 'what mechanisms work, in what conditions, why, and to produce which outcomes?' As Pawson (2006: 74) explains, 'A realist approach means synthesizing complexity to go beyond reportage and summary of existing states of affairs. The point after all is to support fresh thinking to revise

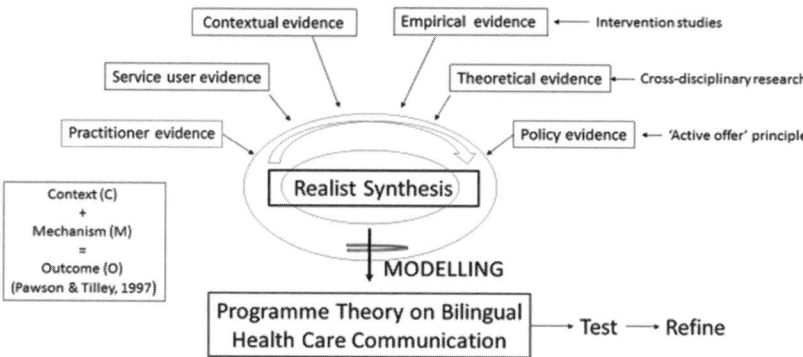

Figure 8.1 Realist synthesis framework

policy and launch it in new circumstances.' Thus, on this basis, a realist synthesis is recommended, bringing together all the evidence, from a practitioner, service user, contextual, empirical, theoretical and policy base to develop a program theory on bilingual healthcare communication for testing and refining (see Figure 8.1). In this way, there is scope to bring bilingual speakers out of the shadows to receive safe, dignified communication and quality care.

References

Aitchison, J. and Carter, H. (1994) *A Geography of the Welsh Language*. Cardiff: University of Wales Press.

Altarriba, J. (2006) When is a first language more emotional? In A. Pavlenko (ed.) *Bilingual Minds: Emotional Experience, Expression and Representation* (pp. 232–256). Clevedon: Multilingual Matters.

Altarriba, J. and Morier, R. (2006) Bilingualism: Language, emotion and mental health. In T. Bhatia and W. Ritchie (eds) *The Handbook of Bilingualism* (pp. 250–280). Oxford: Blackwell Publishing.

Anderson, J., Perry, J., Blue, C., Browne, A., Henderson, A., Khan, K., Reimer-Kirkham, S., Lynam, J., Semeniuk, P. and Smye, V. (2003) Rewriting cultural safety within the postcolonial and postnational feminist project: Toward new epistemologies of healing. *Advances in Nursing Science* 26 (3), 196–214.

Arksey, H. and O'Malley, L. (2005) Scoping studies: Towards a methodological framework. *International Journal of Research Methodology* 8, 19–32.

Auer, P. and Wei, L. (2007) Introduction: Multilingualism as a problem? Monolingualism as a problem? In P. Auer and L. Wei (eds) *Handbook of Multilingualism and Multilingual Communication* (pp. 1–14). Berlin: Mouton de Gruyter.

Baker, C. (2011) *Foundations of Bilingual Education and Bilingualism* (5th edn). Bristol: Multilingual Matters.

Baker, C. and Jones, S. (1998) *Encyclopaedia of Bilingualism and Bilingual Education*. Clevedon: Multilingual Matters.

Balcazar, F., Suarez-Balcazar, Y. and Taylor, T. (2009) Cultural competence: Development of a conceptual framework. *Disability and Rehabilitation* 31 (14), 1153–1160.

Beaufort Research (2014) *Research Report: Welsh-medium Primary Care Services Research*. Cardiff: Beaufort Research. See http://www.comisiynyddygymraeg.org/English/Publications%20List/Health%20Inquiry%20-%20Beaufort%20Research%20Report.pdf

Betancourt, J., Green, A. and Carrilo, J. (2003) Defining cultural competence: A practical framework for addressing racial/ethnic disparities in health and health care. *Public Health Reports* 118, 293–302.

Bhatia, T. and Ritchie, W. (eds) (2006) *The Handbook of Bilingualism*. Oxford: Blackwell Publishing.

Bond, M. and Lai, T. (1986) Embarrassment and code-switching into a second language. *Journal of Social Psychology* 126, 179–186.

Bourhis, R., Roth, S. and MacQueen, G. (1989) Communication in the hospital setting: A survey of medical and everyday language use amongst patients, nurses and doctors. *Social Science and Medicine* 28 (4), 339–346.

Bowie, I. (1996) Terms of address: Implications for nursing. *Journal of Advanced Nursing* 23, 113–119.

Brown, A. and Draper, P. (2003) Accommodative speech and terms of endearment: Elements of a language mode often experienced by older adults. *Journal of Advanced Nursing* 4 (1), 15–21.

Campesino, M. (2006) Beyond transculturalism: Critiques of cultural education in nursing. *Journal of Nursing Education* 47 (7), 298–304.

Cioffi, R. (2003) Communicating with culturally and linguistically diverse patients in an acute care setting: Nurses' experiences. *International Journal of Nursing Studies*, 40 (3), 299–306.

Council of Europe (1992) *European Charter for Regional or Minority Languages*. Brussels: Council of Europe. See http://www.coe.int/t/dg4/education/minlang/textcharter/default_en.asp

Cross, T., Bazron, B., Dennis, K. and Isaacs, M. (1989) *Towards a Culturally Competent System of Care Volume I*. Washington, DC: Georgetown University Child Development Center, CASSP Technical Assistance Center.

Culley, L. (2000) Working with diversity: Beyond the factfile. In L. Finlay and A. Bullman (eds) *Changing Practice in Health and Social Care*. London: Sage.

Damschroder, L., Aron, D., Keith, R., Kirsh, S., Alexander, J. and Lowery, J. (2009) Fostering implementation of health services research findings into practice: A consolidated framework for advancing implementation science. *Implementation Science* 4, 50; doi: 10.1186/1748-5908-4-50.

Davies, D. (2002) The significance of the Welsh language and culture in the health care services. In The All Wales Network Committee for Arts, *Speaking the Invisible: Culture, Identity and Psychiatry* (pp. 23–45). Cardiff: NHS Wales.

Davies, J. (2007) *A History of Wales*. London: Penguin.

De Groot, A. (2010) *Language and Cognition in Bilinguals and Multilinguals: An Introduction*. Hoboken, NJ: Taylor and Francis.

Department of Health (2012) *Department of Health Equality Objectives Action Plan 2012–2016*. London: Department of Health.

Drolet, M., Savard, J., Benoît, J., Arcand, I., Savard, S., Lagacé, J., Lauzon, S. and Dubouloz, C. (2014) Health service for linguistic minorities in a bilingual setting: Challenges for bilingual professionals. *Qualitative Health Research* 24 (3), 295–305.

Edwards, M., Davies, M. and Edwards, A. (2009) What are the external influences on information exchange and shared decision-making in healthcare consultations: A meta-synthesis of the literature. *Patient Education and Counselling* 75, 37–52.

Fernandez, A., Schillinger, K., Grumbach, A., Stewart, F., Wang, F. and Perez-Stable, E. (2004) Physician language ability and cultural competence: An exploratory study of communication with Spanish-speaking patients. *Journal of General Internal Medicine* 19 (2), 167–174.

Fishman, J. (1967) Bilingualism with and without diglossia; diglossia with and without bilingualism. *Journal of Social Issues* 23 (2), 29–38.
Freeman, G., Rai, H., Walker, J., Howie, D., Heaney, D. and Maxwell, M. (2002) Non-English speakers consulting with the GP in their own language: A cross-sectional survey. *British Journal of General Practice* 52, 36–38.
Garrett, P.W., Dickson, H.G., Lis-Young, Whelan, A.K. and Roberto-Forero, R. (2008) What do non-English-speaking patients value in acute care? Cultural competency from the patient's perspective: A qualitative study. *Ethnicity and Health* 13 (5), 479–496.
Gerrish, K. (2001) The nature and effect of communication difficulties arising from interactions between district nurses and South Asian patients and their carers. *Journal of Advanced Nursing* 33 (5), 566–574.
Giles, H., Bourhis, R. and Taylor, D. (1977) Towards a theory of language in ethnic group relations. In H. Giles (ed.) *Language, Ethnicity, and Intergroup Relations* (pp. 307–348). New York: Academic Press.
Gregg, J. and Saha, S. (2007) Communicative competence: A framework for understanding language barriers in health care. *Journal of General Internal Medicine* 22 (S2), 368–370.
Grosjean, F. (1985) The bilingual as a competent but specific speaker–hearer. *Journal of Multilingual and Multicultural Development* 6, 467–477.
Grosjean, F. (1997) Processing mixed language: Issues, findings and models. In A. Groot and J. Kroll (eds) *Tutorials in Bilingualism: Psycholinguistic Perspectives* (pp. 225–254). Mahwah, NJ: Lawrence Elbaum Associates.
Grosjean, F. (2008) *Studying Bilinguals*. Oxford: Oxford University Press.
Grosjean, F. (2010) *Bilingual: Life and Reality*. Cambridge, MA: Harvard University Press.
Gudykunst, W. (1995) Anxiety/uncertainty management (AUM) theory: Current status. In R. Wiseman (ed.) *Intercultural Communication Theory* (pp. 5–58). Thousand Oaks, CA: Sage.
Gumperz, J. (1972) Sociolinguistics and communication in small groups. In: J. Pride and J. Holmes (eds) *Sociolinguistics* (pp. 203–224). Harmondsworth: Penguin.
Gustafson, D. (2005) Transcultural nursing theory from a critical perspective. *Advances in Nursing Science* 28 (1), 2–16.
Heikkila, K. and Elman, S. (2000) Health care experiences and beliefs of elderly Finnish Immigrants in Sweden. *Journal of Transcultural Nursing* 11 (4), 281–289.
Heikkila, K., Sarvimaki, A. and Ekman S. (2007) Culturally congruent care for older people: Finnish care in Sweden. *Scandinavian Journal of Caring Sciences* 21, 354–361.
Hewison, A. (1995) Nurses' power in interactions with patients. *Journal of Advanced Nursing* 21, 75–82.
Iaith (2012) *Welsh Speakers' Experiences of Health and Social Care Services*. Newcastle Emlyn: Iaith. See http://www.wales.nhs.uk/sites3/Documents/415/120208welshresearchreporten%5B1%5D.pdf
Irvine, F., Roberts, G., Jones, P., Spencer, L., Baker, C. and Williams, C. (2006) Communicative sensitivity in the bilingual healthcare setting: A qualitative study of language awareness. *Journal of Advanced Nursing* 53 (4), 1–13.
Jacobs, E., Chen, A., Karliner, L., Agger-Gupta, N. and Mutha, S. (2006) The need for more research on language barriers in health care: A proposed agenda. *The Millbank Quarterly* 84 (1), 111–113.
Jacobs, E., Sadowski, L. and Rathous, P. (2007) The impact of an enhanced interpreter service intervention on hospital costs and patient satisfaction. *Journal of General Internal Medicine* 22 (Suppl 2), 306–311.
Johnson, Y. and Munch, S. (2009) Fundamental contradictions in cultural competence. *Social Work* 54 (3), 220–231.

Johnstone, M. and Kanitsaki, O. (2008) Cultural racism, language prejudice and discrimination in hospital contexts: An Australian study. *Diversity in Health and Social Care* 5, 19–30.

Johnstone, M. and Kanitsaki, O. (2009) Engaging patients as safety partners: Some considerations for ensuring a culturally and linguistically appropriate approach. *Health Policy* 90, 1–7.

Karliner, L., Jacobs, E., Chen, A. and Mutha, S. (2007) Do professional interpreters improve clinical care for patients with limited English proficiency? A systematic review of the literature. *Health Services Research* 42 (2), 727–754.

Lanceley, A. (1985) Use of controlling language in the rehabilitation of the elderly. *Journal of Advanced Nursing* 10, 125–135.

Légaré, F., Ratté, S., Gravel, K. and Graham, I.D. (2008) Barriers and facilitators to implementing shared decision-making in clinical practice: Update of a systematic review of health professionals' perceptions. *Patient Education and Counselling* 73 (3), 526–535.

Leininger, M. (1988) Leininger's theory of nursing: Culture, care, diversity and universality: A theory of nursing. *Nursing Science Quarterly* 2 (4), 152–160.

Leininger, M. (1997) Transcultural nursing research to transform nursing education and practice: 40 years. *Image: The Journal of Nursing Scholarship* 29 (4), 341–347.

Leininger, M. (2007) Theoretical questions and concerns: Response from the Theory of Culture Care Diversity and Universality Perspective. *Nursing Science Quarterly* 20, 9–13.

Levac, D., Colquhon, H. and O'Brien, K. (2010) Scoping studies: Advancing methodology. *Implementation Science* 5, 69.

Madoc-Jones, I. (2004) Linguistic sensitivity, indigenous peoples and the mental health system in Wales. *International Journal of Mental Health Nursing* 13, 216–224.

May, S. (2012) *Language and Minority Rights: Ethnicity, Nationalism and the Politics of Language.* Oxford: Routledge.

Mcleod Clarke, J. (1982) Nurse–patient communication: An analysis of conversation from surgical wards. In J. Wilson-Barnett (ed.) *Nursing Research: 10 Studies in Patient Care* (pp. 25–56). Chichester: John Wiley.

Misell, A. (2000) *Welsh in the Health Service: The Scope, Nature and Adequacy of Welsh Language Provision in the National Health Service in Wales.* Cardiff: Welsh Consumer Council.

Murphy, J. (2011) Engaging patients and families in e-health. *Nurse Economist* 29 (6), 339–41.

Myers-Scotton, C. (1993) *Social Motivations for Code-switching: Evidence from Africa.* Oxford: Clarendon Press.

Myers-Scotton, C. (2006) *Multiple Voices: An Introduction to Bilingualism.* Oxford: Blackwell.

National Health and Medical Research Council (2005) *Cultural Competency in Health: A Guide for Policy, Partnerships and Participation.* Canberra: National Health and Medical Research Council.

New Brunswick Official Languages Act (2002) See http://laws.gnb.ca/en/ShowPdf/cs/O-0.5.pdf

New Zealand Ministry of Health (2006) *Maori Health Action Plan 2006–2011.* Wellington: Ministry of Health. See http://www.health.govt.nz/system/files/documents/publications/whakatataka-tuarua-action-plan.pdf

Ngo-Metzger, Q., Sorkin, D., Phillips, R., Gereenfield, S., Massagli, M., Clarridge, B. and Kaplan, S. (2007) Providing high quality care for limited English proficient patients: The importance of language concordance and interpreter use. *Journal of General Internal Medicine* 22 (Suppl 2), 324–330.

Office for National Statistics (2012) *Census 2011.* See http://www.ons.gov.uk/ons/rel/census/2011-census/key-statistics-for-local-authorities-in-englandand-wales/rft-table-data-cube-pivot-table.xls (accessed 24 April 2015).

Office of the French Language Commissioner (2009) *Special Report on French Language Health Services Planning in Ontario 2009*. Toronto: Office of the French Language Commissioner. See http://csfontario.ca/wpcontent/uploads/2009/05/FLSC_report_french_health_planning_2009.pdf

Official Languages Act (1985) Canada. See http://laws-lois.justice.gc.ca/eng/acts/o-3.01/

O'Hagan, K. (2001) *Cultural Competence in the Caring Profession*. London: Jessica Kingsley.

Ó Riagáin, D. (1998) A European overview, with some examples: A lecture in the Ulster Tongue series of events. Linen Hall Library, Belfast. In K. O'Hagan, *Cultural Competence in the Caring Profession*. London: Jessica Kingsley.

Pavlenko, A. (2006) Bilingual selves. In A. Pavlenko (ed.) *Bilingual Minds: Emotional Experience, Expression and Representation* (pp. 1–33). Clevedon: Multilingual Matters.

Pavlenko, A. (2008) Emotion and emotion-laden words in the bilingual lexicon. Keynote article. *Bilingual Language Cognition* 11 (2), 147–164.

Pavlenko, A. (2012) Affective processing in bilingual speakers: Disembodied cognition? *International Journal of Psychology* 47 (6), 405–428.

Pawson, R. (2006) *Evidence-based Policy: A Realist Perspective*. London: Sage.

Pawson, R. and Tilley, N. (1997) *Realistic Evaluation*. London: Sage.

Perez-Stable, E., Napoles-Springer, A. and Miramontes, J. (1997) The effects of ethnicity and language on medical outcomes of patients with hypertension or diabetes. *Medical Care* 35 (12), 1212–1219.

Prys, C. (2010) Use of Welsh in the third sector in Wales. *Contemporary Wales*. 23 (1), 184–200.

Ramsden, I. (2002). Cultural safety and nursing education in Aotearoa and Te Wapiounamu. Unpublished PhD, University of Victoria, Wellington.

Ritchie, J. and Lewis, J. (2003) *Qualitative Research Practice: A Guide for Social Science Students and Researchers*. London: Sage.

Roberts, G. (1994) Nurse patient communication within a bilingual healthcare setting. *British Journal of Nursing* 3 (2), 60–67.

Roberts, G. and Paden, L. (2000) Identifying the factors influencing minority language use in healthcare education: A European perspective. *Journal of Advanced Nursing* 32 (1), 75–83.

Roberts, G., Irvine, F., Jones, P., Spencer, L., Baker, C. and Williams, C. (2004) *Report of a Study of Welsh Language Awareness in Healthcare Provision in Wales*. Cardiff: Welsh Assembly Government. See http://www.wales.nhs.uk/sites3/documents/415/ACF3394.pdf

Roberts, G., Irvine, F., Jones, P., Spencer, L., Baker, C. and Williams, C. (2007) Language awareness in the bilingual healthcare setting: A national survey. *International Journal of Nursing Studies* 44, 1177–1186.

Sachdev, I. and Giles, H. (2006) Bilingual accommodation. In T. Bhatia and W. Ritchie (eds) *The Handbook of Bilingualism* (pp. 353–378). Oxford: Blackwell.

Samson, A. and Spector, N. (2012) Francophones living with HIV/AIDS in Ontario: The unknown reality of an invisible cultural minority. *AIDS Care* 24 (5), 658–664.

Santiago-Rivera, A. and Altarriba, J. (2002) The role of language in therapy with the Spanish–English bilingual client. *Professional Psychology: Research and Practice* 33 (1), 30–38.

Schwei, R., Del Pozo, S., Agger-Gupta, N., Alvarado-Little, W., Bagchi, A., Chen, A., Diamond, L. and Jacobs, E. (2016) Changes in research on language barrier in health care since 2003: A cross-sectional review study. *International Journal of Nursing Studies* 54, 36–44.

Schrauf, R. and Durazo-Arvizu, R. (2006) Bilingual autobiographical memory and emotion: Theory and methods. In A. Pavlenko (ed.) *Bilingual Minds: Emotional Experience, Expression and Representation* (pp. 284–311). Clevedon: Multilingual Matters.

Segalowitz, N. and Kehayia, E. (2011) Exploring the determinants of language barriers in health care (LHBC): Towards a research agenda for the language sciences. *The Canadian Modern Language Review* 67 (4), 48–507.

Smye, V. and Browne, A. (2002) 'Cultural safety' and the analysis of health policy affecting aboriginal people. *Nurse Researcher* 9 (3), 42–56.

Timmins, C. (2002) The impact of language barriers on the health care of Latinos in the United States: A review of the literature and guidelines for practice. *Journal of Midwifery and Women's Health* 47 (20), 80–96.

US Office of Minority Health, US Department of Health and Human Services (2001) The National Culturally and Linguistically Appropriate Services (CLAS) Standards in Health and Health Care. Washington, DC: Office of Minority Health, US Department of Health and Human Services. See http://minorityhealth.hhs.gov/assets/pdf/checked/finalreport.pdf

Van Lier, L. (1995) *Introducing Language Awareness*. London: Penguin.

Vezina, S., Morneault, A., Frigault-Bezeau, B., Gallant, C., Gaumont, F., Checheu, J., Haché, J. and Gautreau, S. (2014) *The Active Offer of Health Services in Both Official Languages in New Brunswick*. Edmunston: University of Moncton.

Welsh Government (2012a) *More than just Words: Strategic Framework for Welsh Language Services in Health, Social Services and Social Care*. Cardiff: Welsh Government.

Welsh Government (2012b) *A Living Language a Language for Living: Welsh Language Strategy 2012–2017*. Cardiff: Welsh Assembly Government.

Welsh Government (2016) *More than just Words: Follow-on Strategic Framework for Welsh Language Services in Health, Social Services and Social care*. Cardiff: Welsh Government.

Welsh Language Act (1993) London: HMSO. See http://www.legislation.gov.uk/ukpga/1993/38/contents

Welsh Language Commissioner (2014) *My Language, My Health: The Welsh Language Commissioner's Inquiry into the Welsh Language in Primary Care*. Cardiff: Welsh Language commissioner's Office.

Welsh Language (Wales) Measure (2011) London: HMSO. See http://www.legislation.gov.uk/mwa/2011/1/contents/enacted

Wepa, D. (2003) An exploration of the experiences of cultural safety educators in New Zealand: An action research approach. *Journal of Transcultural Nursing* 14 (4), 339–348.

Williamson, M. and Harrison, L. (2010). Providing culturally appropriate care: A review. *International Journal of Nursing Studies* 47 (6), 761–769.

Wyn Siencyn, S. (1995) *A Sound Understanding*. Cardiff: CCETSW Cymru.

Wynia, M. and Matiasek, J. (2006) *Promising Practices for Patient-centered Communication with Vulnerable Populations: Examples from Eight Hospitals*. New York: The Commonwealth Fund. See http://www.commonwealthfund.org/~/media/files/publications/fund-report/2006/aug/promising-practices-for-patient-centered-communication-with-vulnerable-populations—examples-from-ei/wynia_promisingpracticespatientcentered_947-pdf.pdf

9 Engaging the Community to Develop Solutions for Languages of Lesser Diffusion

Francesca Gany, C. Javier González, E. Zoe Schutzman and Debra J. Pelto

Introduction

The parents, who were from Mexico, took their infant, who was very ill, to a Fresno clinic, where they were given instructions in Spanish. The parents did not understand the instructions and continued with their same practice, which was to breastfeed the baby. When the baby's vomiting and diarrhea continued, the family returned to the clinic. The clinic staff called Child Protective Services, which charged the parents with negligence for not following the instructions to not breastfeed the baby, who was allergic to lactose. The parents were initially given a Spanish interpreter in court before it was eventually recognized that they did not understand Spanish and had not understood the initial instructions. We were able to provide them with a Mixtec-speaking interpreter. (Leoncio Vásquez Santos, Director, Centro Binacional para el Desarrollo Indígena Oaxaqueño (Binational Center for the Development of Oaxacan Indigenous Communities))

Around the world, an estimated 7102 languages are spoken, not including regional variants and dialects (Lewis *et al.*, 2015). Languages of lesser diffusion, also known as languages of limited diffusion or minority languages, are languages that are spoken by relatively small numbers of people and in limited geographic areas (Mikkelson, 1999). A language of lesser diffusion (LLD) may be the national language of a small country from which a local population has emigrated, may be spoken by a small ethnic minority, such as a refugee population, or may be spoken by an indigenous group. In this chapter we will focus on LLDs found in the US as representative examples of how to address the needs of populations of LLD speakers found throughout the world.

Table 9.1 Estimates of numbers of most commonly spoken languages and aggregated languages of lesser diffusion in the US in 2011

Language	Number of speakers
20 most common responses to the question, 'What language do you speak at home?'	
Only spoke English at home	230,947,071
Spoke another language at home	60,577,020
Most common non-English languages	
Spanish	37,579,787
Chinese (Mandarin and Cantonese)	2,882,497
Tagalog	1,594,413
Vietnamese	1,419,539
French	1,301,443
Korean	1,141,277
German	1,083,637
Arabic	951,699
Russian	905,843
French Creole	753,990
Italian	723,632
Portuguese	673,566
Hindi	648,983
Polish	607,531
Japanese	436,110
Persian	407,586
Urdu	373,851
Gujarati	358,422
Greek	304,928
Total number of speakers of 20 most common languages including English	285,095,805
Speakers of Languages of Lesser Diffusion (all other spoken languages)	6,428,286
Estimated users of American Sign Language (ASL)[a]	Estimate 100,000–1,000,000
Total US Population age 5 and over	291,524,091

Calculations except where noted are based on estimated data from the American Community Survey 2011 (Ryan, 2013).

[a]The Census Bureau does not collect data on sign language use and presumes that users of ASL know English (U.S. Census Bureau, 2013). Those who use ASL are coded as English speakers. ASL users are estimated at 100,000–1,000,000 (Barnett et al., 2011).

There is no universally accepted listing of what languages comprise the LLDs. Languages of lesser diffusion are defined in the local context. The National Council on Interpreting in Health Care (NCIHC), which has an LLD Work Group, does not specify a national list for the US because even a widely known language, if spoken by few people within a particular geographic area, can be seen as an LLD for that geographic region (R. Balistreri, personal communication, D. Pelto, NCIHC LLD Work Group, 2015). The Northern Virginia Area Health Education Center considers any language other than the five most frequently spoken in their region to be LLDs (NVAHEC, 2013). The International Medical Interpreters Association provides two lists of non-LLDs. These are the 10 most frequently spoken languages in the US and the 20 most frequently spoken languages in the US. All others are considered minority languages (IMIA, 2015). In a large metropolitan area, it may be useful to consider LLDs as those other than the 20 most frequently spoken languages, while in a less diverse area, it may be useful to think of those other than the five to 10 most frequently spoken languages. These number over 300 in the US and include Indo-European languages such as Albanian, Romanian, Panjabi and Ukrainian; Asian and Pacific Island languages such as Burmese and Hmong, and minority Chinese languages such as Formosan and Wu; Native North American languages such as Choctaw, Dakota, Ojibwa and Navajo; Hebrew; African languages such as Amharic, Bantu, Cushite and Swahili; and other languages native to Mesoamerica and South America such as the Mayan languages, the Oto-Manguen languages, the Uto-Aztecan languages and Quechua (Table 9.1; US Census Bureau, 2010). About 6.4 million people in the US reported speaking a language at home other than the top 20 most commonly spoken, and about 11.7 million reported that they speak a language other than the top 10 most commonly spoken. About 2 million of these stated that they spoke English 'less than very well', i.e. are limited English proficient (LEP) (US Census Bureau, 2010). These individuals require an interpreter in a healthcare encounter if their providers are not fluent in their languages (The Joint Commission, 2014; USDOJ, 2015a, 2015b). Trained LLD interpreters may not be readily available (R. Balistreri, personal communication, D. Pelto, NCIHC LLD Work Group, 2015), especially in languages that have recently moved into an area. This chapter will address how to predict the need for interpreters of LLD, and potential avenues of LLD interpreter workforce development.

Predicting and Assessing Language Access Needs

It may be challenging to identify those who speak an LLD and need interpretation. If the speakers of an LLD feel stigmatized, in some cases following histories of oppression against their ethnic group, group members could be hesitant to profess their identity and language needs (N. Adelson, personal communication regarding Asociación Mayab, D. Pelto, 2015). Speaking up to say that one does not fluently speak or understand an official or dominant language can be imagined to be a weakness or something shameful. In this situation, as illustrated in the anecdote that opens this chapter, a patient who is an indigenous person from Latin America who migrates to the US may be assumed to be fluent in Spanish, and a Spanish/English interpreter may be mistakenly assigned (Mikkelson, 1999; L. Vásquez Santos, personal communication regarding Centro Binacional para el Desarrollo Indígena Oaxaqueño, D. Pelto, 2015). Alternatively, the patient may say he/she speaks a locally dominant language, and might not even think to ask to speak in his/her preferred language.

The question, 'In what language do you feel most comfortable speaking with your doctor or nurse?' (Hasnain-Wynia *et al.*, 2007) or 'In what language do you prefer to receive your medical care?' (Karliner *et al.*, 2008) should be accompanied by a question asking from which country and region or town the patient has emigrated. 'I Speak' language identification cards, which are often available in the US in a limited number of languages and could be tailored for an institution's languages, may also be useful, especially for languages which are commonly written (American Institutes for Research, 2005). If the patient does not identify a language from an 'I Speak' card, and the provider does not speak a language the patient understands, there are two potentially expedient ways to identify the patient's preferred language: either through the institution's language services office or through a remote telephone interpretation contractor (V. Sosa, personal communication, D. Pelto, 2015). If the institution has an onsite language service, their staff should be experts in assessing the patient's preferred language and locating an interpreter. They can suggest possible countries of origin to the patient. Once the patient has identified his/her country of origin, and if possible, a region, the country listing of languages from the free web edition of 'Ethnologue: Languages of the World' should be read to the patient (Lewis *et al.*, 2015). The Ethnologue site is searchable by country, and provides listings of both immigrant and native languages. One can also examine an area map, available from Ethnologue, with the patient (L.L. Ford, A. Isidro & J. Williams, personal communication regarding IndigenousInterpreting + , a service of Natividad Medical Foundation, D. Pelto, 2015). Reviewing country language lists and a map may be particularly useful to identify the languages of patients from Mexico, for example, as Mexico has 68 languages and 364 variants (Lewis *et al.*, 2015). Once a likely language is identified, it should be confirmed by locating someone (who either speaks that language or one that is very close to it that is mutually intelligible) to speak with the patient to make a final determination of what language should be used for interpretation. The remote interpretation contractor may be aware of a recently arriving language group in the region because of an increase in requests for a particular language. The contractor can be contacted to assess the patient over the phone. In sum, it is important to ask the patient's preferred language as recommended above, to use language mapping or, alternatively, to contact the language services contractor to identify patients' preferred languages.

The magnitude of institutional language access need should be determined by assessing both the need among patients currently seen in the healthcare institution and the unmet need throughout the institution's catchment area.

Within the institution, periodic Language Needs Assessments should be conducted. The data could be obtained from data that are already available in an electronic medical record or from separate patient surveys. In addition to asking, 'What language do you feel most comfortable speaking with your doctor or nurse?' (Hasnain-Wynia et al., 2007), electronic medical record and survey questions may include other questions that can help inform care, such as: 'How well do you speak English (very well, well, not well, or not at all)?' (Institute of Medicine, 2009). While Shin and Bruno (2003) suggest asking the question, 'What language do you speak at home?', we would instead ask, 'What languages do you speak at home?' as more than one language may be spoken, including more than one language of lesser diffusion (i.e. Mixtec and Nahuatl). As patient literacy is important for understanding written information and instructions, we would suggest adapting Hasnain-Wynia et al.'s (2007) question, 'In which language would you feel most comfortable reading medical or healthcare instructions?' to read 'The doctor and/or nurse will speak with you about your medical condition and your healthcare instructions. We would also like to provide you with written information to take home with you. In what language(s) would you like to receive written information about your condition and medical care? Do you have family members or friends whom you would like to read this information? If yes, what language should it be in?' A regular data query or survey administration schedule should be determined (e.g. on the same schedule as a Community Health Needs Assessment).

At the community level, data on shifting language trends may be collected through consultation with community advisory boards and other agencies and organizations in the institution's catchment area (such as schools, health departments, community groups, faith based organizations, and local and regional refugee and immigrant-serving organizations), and through state and local Census data. The methods for data collection could include surveys, focus groups and key informant interviews with agency and community leaders. Researchers in schools of public health and anthropology programs may be able to contribute to updating needs assessments. The US Department of State and resettlement agencies participating in the Reception and Placement Program are good sources of information about anticipated settlement patterns of new residents (Bureau of Population, Refugees and Migration, 2014; Vega, 2014). Section 501(r) of the Affordable

Care Act requires that tax-exempt hospital facilities conduct a Community Health Needs Assessment and adopt an implementation strategy at least once every three years (Patient Protection and Affordable Care Act, 2010). The language access data and the plan for meeting the community's needs should form an important component of an institution's Community Health Needs Assessment.

Modalities of Interpretation of Languages of Lesser Diffusion

As with the more commonly spoken languages, the interpretation for LLDs may be provided in-person, or remotely via telephone or video. Remote services offer the potential convenience of being able to access an interpreter in a comparatively short time, eliminating the delays of transportation or rescheduled appointments (Masland et al., 2010), and of pooling resources for less commonly spoken languages. Some patients may prefer the anonymity of a remote telephone interpreter, while others might prefer an in-person interpreter. Remote interpretation by video offers the same potentially rapid access as telephone interpreting, and enables the interpreter, patient and provider to see an image, albeit limited, of each other. Interpretation of LLDs may take place using any of these modalities.

Because it is uncommon to study an LLD as a second language (Goldberg et al., 2015), the most likely interlocutors for those who speak an LLD are native speakers who also speak a more commonly spoken language such as English or Spanish. If the interpreter speaks the LLD and another language such as Spanish, but not English, the method of relay interpreting – interpreting from the source language (the preferred language of the patient) to an intermediate language by one interpreter, and then from the intermediate language to the dominant language by a second interpreter – can be used (Mikkelson, 1999). For example, it may be difficult to find a K'iche/English interpreter for a Guatemalan immigrant who speaks K'iche Maya and does not speak Spanish or English. However, there may be a K'iche/Spanish interpreter who can interpret from K'iche to Spanish, and a second, Spanish/English interpreter available who can interpret from Spanish into English. This may be cumbersome, and more expensive, because of the need to locate and pay two qualified people, and because of the extra time needed to translate all the discourse from one language to two others. However, relay interpreting may be the only possibility for some LLDs. In time, as the children of the immigrant generation are educated and grow to adulthood in the US, they have the potential to be trained as professional interpreters, in order to interpret from the original language directly into English (L. Vásquez Santos, personal communication regarding Centro Binacional para el Desarrollo Indígena Oaxaqueño, D. Pelto, 2015).

Identifying and Developing Interpretation Services Resources for LLDs

Once an interpreting need has been identified for a particular LLD, a healthcare institution should work to ensure that a trained professional interpreter is available as needed. Untrained persons, minors and family members should not be used as interpreters (US Department of the Treasury, 2001; Smedley et al., 2003; Wilson-Stronks & Galvez, 2007; Federal Interagency Working Group on Limited English Proficiency (LEP), 2014). Untrained interpreters will not have learned the code of ethics and standards of practice. Family members may bias an interpretation, and there is no possibility of maintaining confidentiality. Patients may not wish to fully disclose their medical history or issues of concern when someone close to them is present. Asking a child to interpret for an adult is problematic for several reasons, including that it imposes role-reversal, in which the child becomes the support for and the authority over the parent/adult (Gilbert, 2005). LLD interpreters can potentially be identified through the pool of current staff interpreters. The institution can check with any remote or face-to-face interpretation agencies under contract to see what access they have to interpreters of a specific LLD and, if appropriate, inform the agencies that the institution anticipates a growing need for a particular language. The institution can also reach out to local agencies that may already be employing trained LLD interpreters, such as schools, immigrant-serving organizations and the social service and court systems. In an acute emergency, an institution may need to ask if there are other employees who speak the LLD. However, many immigrant communities are small or close-knit, therefore, the patient may be reluctant to speak openly in front of another community member, and an untrained interpreter has not absorbed the ethics, standards and methods of interpretation (see below). The need to maintain confidentiality, protect patient privacy and translate directly without revising content should be impressed upon an employee asked to interpret in an emergency situation, and alternative resources should be identified or developed as soon as possible.

If there is no source of trained interpreters, and it appears that there is an emerging population whose language access needs are going unmet, efforts should be made to collaborate with the local community to develop interpreting resources. Organizations such as immigrant service and legal service organizations with similar interpreting needs, cultural centers and places of worship are potential sources to either identify, or collaborate in developing, interpreting resources and services.

The ability to speak both the LLD and a dominant language does not by itself qualify a person as an interpreter. Training in the ethics (National Council on Interpreting in Health Care, 2004), standards of practice (National Council on Interpreting in Health Care, 2005) and methods of interpretation, along with key vocabulary, are necessary to effectively interpret in the medical setting. Because some LLD-speaking communities are small or exist in isolated pockets in the US, or in their countries of origin, where everyone knows each other or each other's family, it is especially important for interpreters to be trained to maintain confidentiality, both during the medical encounter and afterwards when interacting with the patient in the community, or with other community members who could know the patient. These ethical standards should also be explained to the patient with the goal of diminishing the fear of a potential loss of confidentiality. However, because such fear may linger and detract from a patient's ability to communicate openly, a patient may prefer to communicate via an anonymous interpreter over the telephone to avoid subsequent contact with a local interpreter. National certification through the National Board of Certification for Medical Interpreters is only offered in six languages, none of which are LLDs (NBCMI, 2012). Therefore, there is no interpreter certification for LLDs.

Programs that provide LLD interpreters have often been developed as collaborative efforts between healthcare providers, LLD-speaking communities and interpretation educators. Each brings a special perspective to the effort. Communities of LLD speakers know when and how their community is challenged in accessing and receiving medical services. They are likely to have observed similar problems in accessing social and educational services, communicating with law enforcement or interacting with the legal system. Key opinion leaders and gatekeepers will have access to the community for purposes of formally surveying needs and identifying potential interpreters. Interpreting training programs can be accessed to collaborate in the design and delivery of the interpreter training. To train a small number of students, collaborating with an experienced certified interpreter may be sufficient. Identifying an instructor who speaks the language of the trainees can facilitate the LLD-specific learning activities. Securing collaboration in competency testing and periodic refresher training is also helpful.

There are many interpreter training programs around the country through which training can be obtained for groups and individuals. If a healthcare institution plans to train several interpreters, it may be possible to obtain onsite tailored training and periodic refresher training. Ideally this should be led by at least one instructor who speaks the LLD(s) of interest, to clarify medical vocabulary in the LLD, to ensure comprehension of concepts and to facilitate and evaluate role playing.

Overview of LLD Medical Interpreting Training Programs and Initiatives

Below we describe our own training program, The Medical Interpreting Training Program, and five others that have developed services in response to the need for LLD language access. The Medical Interpreting Training Program, a program of the Immigrant Health and Cancer Disparities Service of Memorial Sloan Kettering Cancer Center, was developed to eliminate language and cultural barriers to health care. The Medical Interpreting Training Program provides interpreter language screening, bilingual assessment and training, and provider training to deliver services in collaboration with interpreters. Interpreter training includes instruction for interpreters of dominant languages (such as Spanish, Chinese, Russian or Arabic) and for speakers of LLDs. Below we describe our approaches to common challenges in training interpreters of LLDs. We employ as a case example training which was tailored for interpreters of Burmese, Nepalese, Somali and Karen, which we provided for a client who had recently started a health program for refugees. The Navajo Nation Community Health Representatives Program, housed within the Navajo Nation Department of Health, employs paraprofessionals who provide language services for Navajo speakers within the context of their health screening, promotion and education duties. Navajo Nation Community Health Representatives (CHRs) interpret for patients and providers during medical encounters and speak in Navajo during their health promotion visits with their patients. Below we describe this program's efforts to link their patients, many of whom are elderly, isolated, dispersed over a vast geographic area and diagnosed with a chronic illness, to medical care and services, information and education through the work of Navajo-speaking CHRs. As in general it is the older generation who exclusively or primarily speak Navajo, the younger CHRs polish their language and interpreting skills along with their health promotion skills. Centro Binacional para el Desarrollo Indígena Oaxaqueño, a community-based organization with headquarters in Fresno, California, was created to serve the indigenous immigrant communities who had relocated from Oaxaca, Mexico. Centro Binacional para el Desarrollo Indígena Oaxaqueño provides training to interpreters of Mexican indigenous languages and interpretation services for the medical, justice and social service sectors, within the context of their other civic and community development and cultural programs. Below we describe their history and their efforts to sustainably provide interpretation training and services. Organization Maya K'iche was formed as a cultural organization to promote Mayan language and culture among K'iché Mayan immigrants in the New Bedford, Massachusetts area. They perform interpreting services in area legal and clinical settings. Their interpreters have received training organized by the State of Massachusetts. Organization Maya K'iche does not currently have a contractual agreement with the local hospital, and payment arrangements are not regularized, potentially limiting the future sustainability of their medical interpreting services. Asociación Mayab was formed as a civic and cultural organization to serve immigrants from the Yucatan Peninsula who relocated to the San Francisco Bay area. In addition to their community cultural and educational programs, they provide training for indigenous interpreters, and act as a not-for-profit employment agency for interpreters and agencies needing interpreters for clinical and legal settings. Indigenous Interpreting +, a service of Natividad Medical Foundation, was started to respond to the language needs within Natividad Medical Center of Monterey County, California. They have designed training and an optional six-month practicum for their indigenous interpreters, and provide both training and interpretation services to other organizations. Below we describe each of the five programs in greater detail, including their formation, training program, modalities of providing services and the challenges they face.

The Medical Interpreting Training Program, Immigrant Health and Cancer Disparities Service

The Medical Interpreting Training Program, now housed at Memorial Sloan Kettering Cancer Center's Immigrant Health and Cancer Disparities Service, was created during our tenure at New York University in 1989. The program is a founding member of the NCIHC and is an adviser to the Certification Commission for Health Care Interpreters. The program incorporates the following key components: (a) screening for bilingual skill; (b) screening for and evaluation of interpreter skill and performance; (c) training in medical interpreting, including role and ethics, cultural and linguistic competency, interpreter techniques, consecutive and simultaneous interpreting (proximate and remote) and sight translation; (d) training for providers on how to work effectively with medical interpreters; and (e) training for national certification (in cases in which the language is certifiable). A cadre of qualified medical interpreters act as language coaches who instruct, supervise and evaluate medical interpreters. The medical interpreting training model utilizes a multilingual approach whereby the didactic instruction is delivered in English and the practicum is language specific, to address the subtleties of every language pair (including colloquial and medical terminology). The Medical Interpreter Training Program also includes: (a) a virtual language laboratory where students practice interpreting and receive feedback from their language coaches and/or peers (González & Gany, 2010); (b) the Program for Medical Interpreting Services and Education (PROMISE), which trains interpreters and assists them in finding jobs; (c) the Remote Simultaneous Medical Interpreting system, which utilizes remote interpreters to interpret in the simultaneous model (Gany et al., 2007a, 2007b); and (d) the Virtual Interpreting Training and Learning (VITAL) Program, a distance learning program for medical interpretation (González & Gany, 2010).

The Medical Interpreting Training Program has conducted LLD language-specific training in Burmese, Nepalese, Somali and Karen for an organization which operates a clinic serving refugee populations. The 10 day (80 hour) intensive medical interpreting training program consisted of a morning multilingual large-group didactic session and an afternoon language-specific small-group practicum, which included extensive role-play exercises. The lead instructor was responsible for the general management of the classes and for supervising the other instructors. LLD instructors conducted screening evaluations for bilingual skill and translated didactic materials and evaluation instruments that had not been developed in the LLD languages. The ideal criteria for the LLD instructors include being a trained medical interpreter (preferably certified nationally) with at least five years of experience interpreting in healthcare settings and at least three years of instruction experience; having sufficient linguistic knowledge to allow the ability to discern, process and convert language nuances to encourage concept-based interpretation and avoid literalism; and completion of a 20 hour workshop on the program's student-centered methodology.

The following challenges common to training LLD interpreters were addressed:

(1) The difficulty in recruiting bilingual instructors: In some cases we could not identify local instructors, making it necessary to incur additional fees for travel and training for instructors, and in some cases to train by telephone and video. For one language (Karen), we were not able to identify an instructor for our first training. To address this deficit, an especially strong student was assigned to help teach, and additional study groups were organized. For a later training in Karen, we were able to identify an instructor whose skills were still developing. Trainees in the class were asked to support the instructor in teaching the material. Because of the difficulty finding strong instructors who were bilingual in Karen–English, it was especially difficult to evaluate potential interpreters and to perform the final assessment in Karen.

(2) The difficulty in recruiting strong interpreter student candidates – because the communities from which the potential trainees were recruited were relatively new to the area, it was challenging to find as many trainees with strong bilingual skills as originally planned. To cope with this deficit, we included more peer exchanges than usual during the language-specific portion of the training so that the trainees could also learn from each other. In the end, the students developed strong self-awareness techniques to self-evaluate and learned to disclaim their limitations during real interpreted encounters.

(3) The limited pre-existing didactic materials and testing instruments – all materials had to be adapted and translated into all four languages. We recommended that the Karen interpreters collaborate to improve the materials as a continuing education strategy.

(4) The lack of linguistic and cultural equivalencies between English and the LLDs – this resulted in the need for greater use of explanations of the

concept or word to be interpreted when it cannot be translated by a single word. For example, in Somali, 'colonoscopy' is 'baaris lagu sameeyo mindhicirka weyn gudihiisa' ('screening done inside the big colon') and lesion is 'is-beddel lagu arko xubin ama oogada markuu xanuun ku dhaco' ('a change seen on a tissue or on the skin when it is inflamed/infected'). We emphasized communicative techniques such as requesting clarification to help to fully grasp a concept and provide an accurate interpretation through an adequate explanation of the concept.

The Community Health Representatives Program of the Navajo Nation

The Community Health Representatives Program of the Navajo Nation was created through a Navajo Nation public health advocacy process during the 1950s–1960s (M.-G. Begay, personal communication regarding Navajo Nation Community Health Representatives Program, D. Pelto, 2015). The program was initially funded by the Indian Health Service. It transferred to the Navajo Nation in 1968 and is now operated by the Navajo Nation Department of Health. Initially, speaking Navajo was not an official requirement for the CHRs as in the 1960s most Navajo, including the CHRs, spoke Navajo. Since that time, there has been a language shift toward English among younger people, but most elders still speak Navajo and many do not speak English well. Because CHRs primarily work with elderly non-English speaking Navajo, they speak Navajo with their patients and interpret between patients and healthcare providers. The Navajo Nation CHRs are paraprofessionals who care for individual patients and perform health assessments and community needs assessments. All of the patient education and health screening is performed using the Navajo language, and CHRs interpret between patients and non-Navajo-speaking providers.

As part of their required public health training, many Navajo Nation CHRs take a Navajo medical terminology course as an elective at Diné College. The CHRs receive informal training in interpreting and translation (e.g. of letters from insurers) from senior staff and peers on an ongoing basis during occasional trainings and staff meetings, when they also discuss issues of dialect and generational differences in language use. Newly hired CHRs shadow experienced CHRs to gain more exposure to medical terminology and methods of interpretation.

Like many of those who interpret LLDs, the Navajo Nation CHRs find the issue of linguistic and cultural equivalency to be challenging. Many Navajo elders are not familiar with electronic and biomedical technology, making discussion of medical problems and procedures very difficult. There are generational differences in Navajo speech such that elders use different terms than younger people. Only some of the CHRs read and write in Navajo.

Centro Binacional para el Desarrollo Indígena Oaxaqueño

Centro Binacional para el Desarrollo Indígena Oaxaqueño (Binational Center for the Development of Oaxacan Indigenous Communities, or CBDIO) was started in 1993 by the Frente Indígena Oaxaqueña Binacional (Binational Indigenous Oaxacan Front, or FIOB), an affiliation of organizations, communities and individuals who work on issues facing Mexican indigenous communities in Mexico and those who have migrated to the US (CBDIO, n.d.). FIOB began CBDIO to respond to the needs of the immigrant indigenous community of the Fresno, California area. At that time, local service providers assumed that all Mexican immigrants spoke Spanish, thus, language was a barrier for indigenous immigrants from the state of Oaxaca (L. Vásquez Santos, personal communication regarding Centro Binacional para el Desarrollo Indígena Oaxaqueño, D. Pelto, 2015). CBDIO began the Indigenous Interpreter Project in 1996 to train their own community members as interpreters in medical, legal, school and social service settings. The first training of 12 interpreters took place in 1996, facilitated by professional interpreters from the International Language Institute of Monterrey. The curriculum focused on techniques, legal terminology and professional ethics. In 1999, in response to a growing demand for medical services among indigenous people living in California, in collaboration with Healthy House of Merced, CBDIO held a series of intensive trainings, totaling 80 hours, focusing on professional interpretation in health settings, medical terminology, confidentiality and anatomy. The trainees spoke Mixtec, Zapotec, Triqui and Chatino, as well as Spanish and in some cases, English.

CBDIO's interpreter training includes medical terminology, techniques for interpreting including using first person instead of third person, ethics, confidentiality, standard of practice, role playing and vocabulary development to cope with the lack of direct indigenous translations for many English and Spanish words. In addition to Healthy House of Merced, CBDIO has collaborated with other agencies including the Natividad Medical Center and Monterey Institute. Past trainees who have gained experience are invited to return and take part in subsequent training, and are encouraged to continue their education and exposure to the field and to network with each other to continue developing their skills. As of 2015, the Oaxacan community has been present for over 20 years in the Fresno and Los Angeles areas, and more people speak English, enabling CBDIO to shift from relay interpreting to bilingual interpreting directly into English. CBDIO itself provides interpreting services through the assignment of program staff and the agency director on an ad hoc basis. CBDIO asks the client agencies to pay for their services but finds that there is resistance on the part of some hospitals and clinics, who know that CBDIO is dedicated to the well-being of the community and will probably provide interpreting free of charge if needed (L. Vásquez Santos, personal communication regarding Centro Binacional para el Desarrollo Indígena Oaxaqueño, D. Pelto, 2015).

Organization Maya K'iche

Organization Maya K'iche began as a grassroots culture and education group in New Bedford, Massachusetts in 1995 (Capetillo-Ponce & Abreu-Rodriguez, 2010), registering as a 501(c)3 organization in 1998 (Ortega et al., 2015). Their mission is to support both the Mayan and non-Mayan Central American communities of the New Bedford area, which began to emerge in the early 1980s during a period of civil wars across Guatemala and other Central American countries (Knauer, 2011). The organization's early work focused on education in the K'iche language for children, later shifting to advocacy efforts after a raid on a local factory in 2007 (Vasquez Toness, 2010).

Organization Maya K'iche does not provide training in interpretation. Several individuals associated with Organization Maya K'iche, though, have received training from the state of Massachusetts (Health Imperatives, 2011; M. Fallon, 2015, personal communication, D. Pelto). Others who did not complete the formal training were trained more informally, one-on-one by other trained interpreters. Three interpreters associated with Organization Maya K'iche respond to requests from the local hospital, from individual patients and from the legal system (E. Yac, personal communication regarding Organzation Maya K'iche, D. Pelto, 2015.). Organization Maya K'iche does not have a formal contract with the local hospital. According to a representative of the local hospital's language access office, the hospital contracts with a telephone interpreting service which does not provide K'iche services (Anonymous personal communication with representative of Southcoast Health System Inc., D. Pelto, 2015).

Asociación Mayab

Asociación Mayab (previously Asociación Maya Yucateca del Area Bahia (Yucatec Maya Association of the Bay Area)) originated among the Yucatec Maya community in San Francisco in 2004 to provide aid for victims of Hurricane Isidoro. The group evolved into a cultural preservation association, providing lessons in Mayan languages, dance classes and other cultural, health promotion and emergency support programs. Among the founders were individuals with training in medicine and public health, and a certified English–Spanish interpreter. In response to an increasing number of requests for interpretation of Mayan languages, the agency designed a structured comprehensive training. Asociación Mayab began to provide trainings, facilitated by certified interpreters, through a series of weekly 3 hour sessions, beginning with a 6 week program, and later expanding to 8 weeks and then to 12 weeks to more fully address the learning objectives and provide time to practice.

The topics covered in the Asociación Mayab training include the code of ethics; standard of practice; skills and methods needed for both consecutive and simultaneous interpreting; the US legal system and key terminology; and medical terminology. Asociación Mayab serves as an employment referral agency for legal and medical interpreters they have trained. Interpreters provide medical interpreting both in person and remotely. For the most part, they are interpreting into Spanish. However, like CBDIO, Asociación Mayab is finding that the immigrant community they serve has now been in the US long enough that there are individuals with sufficiently strong skills in both indigenous languages and English, so that some interpreters are able to interpret directly from their indigenous language into English, without the need for a second relay interpreter.

Asociación Mayab's interpretation services are supported by fee-for-service arrangements and the training is grant funded. The administrative tasks are substantial. The organization must seek and report on grant funds, receive requests for and assign interpreters, bill medical providers and legal systems, and pay the interpreters. Asociación Mayab representatives describe interpretation as often 'forgotten' in other agencies' budgets and grant applications (N. Adelson, personal communication regarding Asociación Mayab, D. Pelto, 2015; A. Pérez, personal communication regarding Asociación Mayab, D. Pelto, 2015). While they do have some ongoing contracts, including with a local university, they find that some agencies prefer to contract with a remote interpretation agency, which then subcontracts the work to Asociación Mayab. Because Asociación Mayab prioritizes the needs of the local indigenous population, their policy is to provide services under these circumstances even if they have to agree to accept a lower fee, although they still pay the interpreter at the standard professional rate. Although the work pays well, because assignments are part-time and temporary, interpreters are often forced to decline work because taking it would jeopardize their full-time positions, most of which are in the construction or food service industries. Additionally, some interpreters are temporary migrants, returning to their home country after a few years, and re-entry is complicated for many im/migrants. For these reasons, as well as because several Mayan languages are spoken in the San Francisco Bay Area, it is necessary to continually train new interpreters.

Indigenous Interpreting + , a service of Natividad Medical Foundation

Indigenous Interpreting + , a service of Natividad Medical Foundation (NMF), was launched in 2014 after repeated requests for indigenous language interpreting from around the country (L.L. Ford, A. Isidro & J. Williams, personal communication regarding IndigenousInterpreting + , a service of NMF, D. Pelto, 2015). NMF is a not-for-profit organization that raises funds to support Natividad Medical Center (NMC), a safety net hospital owned and operated by Monterey County, California. Salinas, where NMC is located, is home to nearly 28,000 agricultural workers who speak languages indigenous to Mexico and Central America. An effort to build trusting relationships with indigenous communities began with NMF reaching out to local indigenous leaders to ask them about their experience of care at NMC and their health-related needs. The community responded that the most pressing issue was the language barrier between patients and providers. At least 64 languages are spoken by patients at NMC and four of the top 10 languages spoken are indigenous languages (Mixteco, Zapoteco, Triqui & Chatino). Upon realizing that they could not identify interpreters who spoke the indigenous languages common at NMC, NMF asked local indigenous community members to be trained as interpreters. They quickly found that standard training for interpreters, which emphasized formal lectures and used an advanced vocabulary, was not appropriate for the indigenous population, many of whom had limited English proficiency, limited formal education and widely varying cultural values and beliefs.

Indigenous Interpreting+ is creating what they describe as 'the first indigenous interpreting training manual in the United States' (L.L. Ford, A. Isidro & J. Williams, personal communication regarding Indigenous Interpreting+, a service of NMF, D. Pelto, 2015), based on the adaptation of dominant language interpreter training to reflect a culture broker role for their LLD interpreter trainees. The first seven formal modules have been completed, with topics including an introduction to healthcare interpreting, reflective practice, consecutive interpreting, glossary-building, sight translation, note-taking, introduction to simultaneous interpreting, interpreter protocols and introduction to mediation skills. These have been created by national experts in interpreting and interpreter curriculum development, working alongside local speakers of indigenous languages. The development team pilot tests each module with the interpreters and revises the curriculum based on their detailed feedback. The modules are hands-on and activity-based, rather than lecture-based, and integrate frequent interaction and role-playing. Fourteen more modules are planned for a total of 21 modules. After completion of a 40 hour basic training, the interpreters may participate in traineeships within the hospital, requiring 24 hours weekly for a period of six months, for which trainees are paid at the rate of $15 per hour. The trainees and graduates further contribute to the development of the program by building glossaries of medical terms. Indigenous Interpreting+ provides interpreting within NMC, and upon request to outside agencies.

The Indigenous Interpreting+ leadership describes two main challenges (L.L. Ford, A. Isidro & J. Williams, personal communication regarding IndigenousInterpreting+, a service of Natividad Medical Foundation, D. Pelto, 2015). First, they were not initially aware of the 68 languages indigenous to Mexico (Instituto Nacional de Lenguas Indígenas, 2010), that these have 364 variants, and that a speaker of one variant usually does not understand a speaker of another variant. To address this issue, Indigenous

Interpreting+ has instituted a practice of asking indigenous clients to identify where they are from (the closest town or municipality) and, if possible, to point to the location on a map. This is checked against a map of local language use in order to help pinpoint which language and variant the person speaks, after which an indigenous speaker of that language or a nearby language speaks with them to find out if they are mutually intelligible. Still, because there are so many indigenous languages, they cannot always find an interpreter. Second, they have found that cultural issues must be addressed along with language issues. To illustrate, they have found that there is great diversity in indigenous beliefs and practices around various medical issues. For example, a Mixteco focus group participant stated that some indigenous communities believe that having a 'chaplain' come into a room and say prayers near a dying person can actually make the person die, leading the hospital to understand that their offers of a 'chaplain' visit were actually disturbing to some patients' family members. The word 'chaplain' cannot be translated, and the concept does not exist in Mixteco. Another illustration is found in some indigenous ideologies around numbering systems, which are different from what is understood within Western biomedicine, to the effect, e.g. that a pain scale of 1–10 does not have the same meaning.

Discussion

There are several effective methods of providing language services for patients who speak an LLD. First, the institution should include comprehensive measures of current language access needs both within the current patient population and as a component of Community Health Needs Assessments. Data should be collected through interviews with community members, as well as individuals from schools, community boards, immigrant-serving organizations, and cultural and faith-based organizations. Local and state Census data should be monitored for population and language shifts. These data should be complemented by information from the US Department of State and data indicating that new arrivals to the area are anticipated, which can help to predict future needs.

Healthcare institutions should proactively prepare to care for emerging populations of LLD speakers by checking whether any current employees speak the LLD and are willing to be trained and take on an interpreting role. Additionally, institutions should contact remote interpretation agencies currently under contact to see whether they can meet the anticipated needs. If neither current employees nor remote interpretation agencies can meet the required service need, institutions should reach out to community organizations to identify individuals who may already be trained interpreters of the needed LLD(s), or community members who may be interested in being trained in interpreting.

All interpreters should be trained and assessed. The non-profit groups we describe have responded to their community's needs for medical and other interpreting and translating services by working with strong collaborators, including accomplished and nationally known interpreters and educators, to design and providing interpretation training to community members. In some cases, their efforts have been supported by faith-based organizations as well as, in one case, an association of an industry employing immigrant workers which has generously funded research on language needs and training for the local medical setting. These organizations provide language services to agencies that serve LLD-speaking communities, in some cases on a contractual basis. However, it can be challenging for services provided by non-profits to remain sustainable. Possible approaches to these problems include negotiating contracts with healthcare providers, or developing collaborations between non-profit ethnic-specific and/or immigrant-serving groups and agencies to be able to submit joint bids or proposals that address multiple language needs.

Currently the interpreting profession is experiencing increasing demands for professionalization, including increasing hours of formal training, practicum hours and certification. Such demands may be difficult to meet for small organizations and for languages in which there is limited written material on interpretation. Certification is not available in LLDs. A concern that interpreters of some LLDs will find these requirements so burdensome that they will withdraw from interpreting has led to the beginnings of a plan to create an internationally accessible, interactive website for learning interpreting and competency testing, with materials in multiple languages (L. Golley, personal communication, D. Pelto, 2015), in line with the VITAL program described above (González & Gany, 2010).

Acknowledgments

We thank the individuals who agreed to be interviewed about their work, including: Naomi Adelson and Alberto Pérez, Asociación Mayab; Mark Fallon, The Central American Immigrant Worker Community Development Program, Catholic Social Services; Leoncio Vásquez Santos, Centro Binacional para el Desarrollo Indígena Oaxaqueño; Linda L. Ford, Angélica Isidro, Victor Sosa and Jennifer Williams, Indigenous Interpreting + , a service of Natividad Medical Foundation; Mae-Gilene Begay, Navajo Nation; and Edgar Yac, Organization Maya K'iche. This work was supported by NIH P30CA008748. Debra Pelto's work was supported by NIH T32CA009461.

References

American Institutes for Research (2005) A patient-centered guide to implementing language access services in healthcare organizations. Bethesda, MD: Office of Minority Health. Retrieved from http://minorityhealth.hhs.gov/Assets/pdf/Checked/HC-LSIG.pdf (last accessed 3 July 2015).

Barnett, S., McKee, M., Smith, S.R. and Pearson, T.A. (2011) Deaf sign language users, health inequities, and public health: Opportunity for social justice. *Preventing Chronic Disease* 8(2), A45.

Bureau of Population, Refugees, and Migration. (2014) Refugee admissions reception and placement program. Fact Sheet. Retrieved from http://www.state.gov/j/prm/releases/onepagers/228696.htm (last accessed 23 May 2014)

Capetillo-Ponce, J. and Abreu-Rodriguez, G. (2010) Immigration, ethnicity, and marginalization: The Maya K'iche of New Bedford. *Trotter Review* 19 (1), 59–80.

Centro Binacional para el Desarrollo Indígena Oaxaqueño. (n.d.). "Who we are: Background." Retrieved from http://centrobinacional.org/en/about-us/antecedente/ (last accessed 18 May 2015).

Federal Interagency Working Group on Limited English Proficiency (LEP) (2014) Limited English Proficiency (LEP): A federal interagency website. Frequently asked questions. See http://www.lep.gov/faqs/faqs.html#One_LEP_FAQ (accessed 9 July 2015).

Gany, F., Kapelusznik, L., Prakash, K., Gonzalez, J., Orta, L.Y., Tseng, C.-H. and Changrani, J. (2007a) The impact of medical interpretation method on time and errors. *Journal of General Internal Medicine* 22 (Suppl 2), 319–323.

Gany, F., Leng, J., Shapiro, E., Abramson, D., Motola, I., Shield, D.C. and Changrani, J. (2007b) Patient satisfaction with different interpreting methods: A randomized controlled trial. *Journal of General Internal Medicine* 22 (Suppl 2), 312–318.

Gilbert, M.J. (2005) The case against using family, friends, and minors as interpreters in health and mental health care settings. Process of inquiry – communicating in a multicultural environment. From the Curricula Enhancement Module Series. Washington, DC, National Center for Cultural Competence, Georgetown University Center for Child and Human Development.

Goldberg, D., Looney, D. and Lusin, N. (2015) Table 6: Percentage of total language course enrollments for the fourteen most commonly taught languages in 2013. In *Enrollments in Languages Other Than English in United States Institutions of Higher Education, Fall 2013*. New York: Modern Language Association of America. Retrieved from http://www.mla.org/pdf/2013_enrollment_survey.pdf (last accessed 20 January 2017).

González, J. and Gany, F. (2010) VITAL: Virtual interpreting training and learning. *International Journal of Interpreter Education* 2, 148–157.

Hasnain-Wynia, R., Pierce, D., Haque, A., Hedges Greising, C., Prince, V. and Reiter, J. (2007) Health research and educational trust disparities toolkit. See hretdisparities.org (accessed 10 July 2015).

Health Imperatives (2011) Fundamentals of medical interpreting. Retrieved from http://hcsm.org/ahec/fundamentals-medical-interpreting (last accessed 19 May 2015).

Institute of Medicine (2009) *Race, Ethnicity, and Language Data: Standardization for Health Care Quality Improvement*. Washington, DC: The National Academies Press.

Instituto Nacional de Lenguas Indígenas (2010) Catálogo de las lenguas indígenas nacionales: Variantes lingüísticas de México con sus autodenominaciones y referencias geoestadísticas. Retrieved from http://www.cdi.gob.mx/lenguamaterna/catalogo_lenguas_indigenas_mexico_2008.pdf (last accessed 1 May 2015).

International Medical Interpreters Association (2015) Minority language division. See http://www.imiaweb.org/divisions/minority_languages.asp (accessed 15 May 2015).

Karliner, L., Napoles-Springer, A., Schillinger, D., Bibbins-Domingo K. and Pérez-Stable E. (2008) Identification of Limited English Proficient Patients in Clinical Care. *Journal of General Internal Medicine* 23 (10), 1555–1560.

Knauer, L.M. (2011) The Maya of New Bedford: Genesis and evolution of a community, 1980–2010. *Historical Journal of Massachusetts* 39 (1–2), 170–206.

Lewis, M.P., Simons, G.F. and Fennig, C.D. (eds) (2015) *Ethnologue: Languages of the World*, 18th edn. Dallas, TX: SIL International.

Masland, M.C., Lou, C. and Snowden, L. (2010) Use of communication technologies to cost-effectively increase the availability of interpretation services in healthcare settings. *Telemedicine Journal and e-Health* 16 (6), 739–745.

Mikkelson, H. (1999) Course profile: Relay interpreting: A solution for languages of limited diffusion? *The Translator* 5 (2), 361–380.

National Board of Certification for Medical Interpreters (2012) Multiple languages available! See http://www.certifiedmedicalinterpreters.org/multiple-languages-a (accessed 3 July 2015).

National Council on Interpreting in Health Care (2004) *A National Code of Ethics for Interpreters in Health Care*. Washington, DC: The National Council on Interpreting in Health Care. Retrieved from http://www.ncihc.org/assets/documents/publications/NCIHC%20National%20Code%20of%20Ethics.pdf (last accessed 13 May 2015).

National Council on Interpreting in Health Care (2005) *National Standards of Practice for Interpreters in Health Care*. Washington, DC: National Council on Interpreting in Health Care. Retrieved from http://www.ncihc.org/assets/media/ncihc%20national%20standards%20of%20practice.pdf (last accessed 13 May 2015).

Northern Virginia Area Health Education Center (2013) Definition of language of 'lesser diffusion'. See http://www.nvahec.org/lesser_diffusion (accessed 15 April 2015).

Ortega, A.N., Rodriguez, H. P. and Bustamante, A. V. (2015) Policy Dilemmas in Latino Health Care and Implementation of the Affordable Care Act. *Annual Review of Public Health* 36, 525–544.

Patient Protection and Affordable Care Act (2010) 42 U.S.C. § 18001.

Ryan, C. (2013) Language use in the United States: 2011. American Community Survey Reports.

Shin, H.B. and Bruno, R. (2003) *Language Use and English-speaking Ability: 2000*. Washington, DC, US Census Bureau. Retrieved from http://www.census.gov/prod/2003pubs/c2kbr-29.pdf (last accessed 20 January 2017).

Smedley, B.D., Stith, A.Y., Nelon, A.R., Committee on Understanding and Eliminating Racial and Ethnic Disparities in Health Care, Board on Health Sciences Policy and Institute of Medicine (eds) (2003) *Unequal Treatment: Confronting Racial and Ethnic Disparities in Health Care*. Washington, DC, National Academies Press. Retrieved from http://www.nap.edu/catalog/10260.html (last accessed 13 June 2014).

The Joint Commission (2014) A crosswalk of the National Standards for Culturally and Linguistically Appropriate Services (CLAS) in health and health care to The Joint Commission Hospital Accreditation Standards. Oak Brook, IL: The Joint Commission. Retrieved from https://www.jointcommission.org/assets/1/6/Crosswalk-_CLAS_-20140718.pdf (last accessed 27 May 2015).

US Census Bureau (2010) Table 1. Detailed languages spoken at home and ability to speak English for the population 5 years and over for the United States: 2006–2008. Suitland, MD: 2006–2008 American Community Survey. Retrieved from http://www.census.gov/data/tables/2008/demo/2006-2008-lang-tables.html (last accessed 29 April 2015).

US Census Bureau (2013) Language use. Frequently asked questions. See https://www.census.gov/hhes/socdemo/language/about/faqs.html#Q8 (accessed 9 July 2015).

US Department of Justice (2015a) Title VI of the Civil Rights Act of 1964. Federal Coordination and Compliance. Retrieved from https://www.gpo.gov/fdsys/pkg/USCODE-2010-title42/pdf/USCODE-2010-title42-chap21-subchapV.pdf (accessed 26 May 2015).

US Department of Justice (2015b) Executive Order 13166. Limited English proficiency (LEP: A federal interagency website). Retrieved from https://www.lep.gov/13166/eo13166.html (accessed 26 May 2015).

US Department of the Treasury (2001) Guidance to Federal Financial Assistance recipients on the Title VI Prohibition Against National Origin Discrimination Affecting Limited English Proficient Persons. See http://www.justice.gov/crt/about/cor/lep/treaslep.php (accessed 9 July 2015).

Vasquez Toness, B. (2010) *Forced Out, Guatemalans Learn the Power of Invisibility. Invisible Communities*. Boston, MA: WBUR. Retrieved from http://www.wbur.org/2010/05/10/invisible-communities-i (last accessed 24 May 2015).

Vega, G. (2014) Recruitment of interpreter candidates for languages of limited diffusion. LLD Training Tips. Retrieved from www.ncihc.org/lld-training-tips (last accessed 17 May 2016).

Wilson-Stronks, A. and Galvez, E. (2007) Hospitals, language, and culture: A snapshot of the nation. Exploring cultural and linguistic services in the nation's hospitals. A Report of Findings. Retrieved from http://www.jointcommission.org/assets/1/6/hlc_paper.pdf (last accessed 14 August 2016).

10 Chinese Voices: Improving Access to Health Care

Fiona Irvine, Martin Partridge and Echo Yeung

Introduction

The provision of culturally and linguistically sensitive services for black and minority ethnic communities is a constant challenge to the UK health service, especially when the diversity of a particular ethnic group is not fully acknowledged. One such diverse group is the Chinese population of the UK that originates from a number of countries and uses several languages (and dialects) including Mandarin, Cantonese and Hakka. Drawing on three recent research studies undertaken by the authors, this chapter will consider some of the challenges faced by various Chinese people in understanding, accessing and using health services, and will consider examples of good practice that can be implemented within the current confines of limited financial resource.

Background

The Chinese began to settle in the UK in the 19th century when most of them were seafarers, cooks and laundry workers and could be found in the main seaports of Liverpool, London, Bristol and Cardiff (Jones, 1979; Wong & Richman, 2000; Wong, 1989). Since then the Chinese population has continued to grow, and according to the most recent national Census, it has increased significantly by 69% in the last decade from 247,403 in 2001 to 393,141 in 2011; Chinese people now comprise 0.7% of the total population of the UK (Office for National Statistics, 2012). It is estimated that only 29% of the Chinese population were born in the UK; the lowest proportion from all main ethnic minority groups in the country. The remainder of the UK Chinese population are immigrants, nearly 27% of whom originate from mainland China, 23% from Hong Kong, 13% from Malaysia, 10% from Singapore and 7% from Vietnam (Office for National Statistics, 2012).

The Chinese population is now widely geographically dispersed across the UK. Statistical information in 2011 showed that there are high-density Chinese populations in the major UK cities; about a third of the Chinese population lives in London with small clusters in cities such as Birmingham, Manchester, Liverpool and Glasgow. The rest of the Chinese population is widely distributed in urban and rural areas throughout the country (Dobbs et al., 2006; Office for National Statistics, 2012). This pattern of dispersal has emerged mainly because the nature of the catering industry, in which a significant proportion of people from Chinese backgrounds are employed, discourages concentration of the population in one geographical area in order to reduce competition (Chiu & Yu, 2001).

The growth in the population of people from Chinese backgrounds is not exclusive to the UK; there has also been a marked increase in the Chinese population in the US. According to mid-2013 estimates by the United Nations Population Division US, visas issued to Chinese nationals increased by 859% from 22,000 in 2000 to 189,000 in 2013. Clearly, given this sharp rise, the US is an attractive destination for people from Chinese backgrounds and nearly one-quarter of Chinese emigrants chose to settle in the US. Other popular destinations include Canada, South Korea, Japan, Australia, Singapore and the Middle East (Hooper & Batalova, 2015).

The new pace of immigration of people from Chinese backgrounds to English-speaking countries such as the US, Canada, Australia and the UK may explain why Chinese immigrants have limited English language proficiency, with suggestions that 60% of the Chinese population of the UK (Tran, 2009) and 62% of the US cannot speak English fluently (Hooper & Batalova, 2015).

The relatively poor English language proficiency amongst the Chinese population together with the large percentage of the Chinese population who are recent immigrants, their wide geographical distribution and the diversity of countries of origin amongst people from Chinese backgrounds suggest that, in the UK, many Chinese people may have difficulty accessing appropriate support networks in times of need (Rochelle & Shardlow, 2012; Liu et al., 2015; Yeung et al., 2015).

These issues are significant because of the evident underutilization of health and social care services among people from Chinese backgrounds. In the UK, there is over-representation of compulsory admission for serious mental illness and higher referral rates from emergency departments to mental health services among people from Chinese backgrounds. Thus they often come into contact with mental health services only when a crisis arises, which frequently warrants compulsory admission (Care Quality Commission, 2010). Furthermore, low rates of service use at community level and high level of illness severity for those who eventually enter the mental health system (Care Quality Commission, 2010) indicate that there is an underutilization of mental health services.

There is a similar underutilization of social care services in the UK. Only 0.1% (205 out of 156,555) of adults with physical disability in England received services provided or commissioned by local authority adult social care between 2012 and 2013, were from Chinese backgrounds. This compares with 0.7% of the total adult population in England who received social services in the same period (Health and Social Care Information Centre (2013). Underutilization of disability support service is commonplace amongst Chinese people in the UK (Bignall & Butt, 2000; Chahal, 2004) and other Western societies such as the US (Fisher & Glanfield, 2009; Miltiades & Wu, 2008).

The Census data does not record information about the number of people who may have learning disabilities in the UK. However, research has shown that between 2001 and 2021 people with learning disabilities will make up approximately 2% of the general population in the UK (Emerson & Hatton, 2004). These figures were based on the demography of the population and the decrease in mortality of people with learning disabilities in recent years (Emerson & Hatton, 2004). From these figures it can be extrapolated that there will be approximately 7862 people with learning disabilities from Chinese backgrounds within the current population in the UK. However, individuals with learning disabilities from minority ethnic communities are underrepresented as users of specialist learning disability services (Faculty of the Psychiatry of Learning Disability of the Royal College of Psychiatrists, 2011) and this is apparent among people from a Chinese background, where there is low uptake of services for people with learning disabilities in the UK (Poxton et al., 2012), leading to isolation and social exclusion (Mir et al., 2001).

Such underutilization is worrying because the fundamental principle of the NHS is to be open to all based on need. This principle is founded on reducing inequalities in health care and is upheld by the Health and Social Care Act (Department of Health, 2012), which legislates for the duty to reduce inequalities in health and social care across the system. Given the limited English language proficiency of many Chinese immigrants, the provision of interpretation services is one way of helping to address the inequalities they face. Although some health and social care services use professional interpreters, there is no legislation for the provision of such services and no official inspection process for professional interpreting services and agencies tend to vary in quality of provision (Costa, 2013).

In addition, people from Chinese backgrounds face challenges in using and accessing health and social care services. One reason for this is that differences in health beliefs and conceptualization of care needs create barriers to the utilization of services (Green et al., 2006; Liu et al., 2015). This helps to explain why late presentation and underutilization of mainstream services are common among people from Chinese backgrounds in the UK (Liu et al., 2015; Yeung et al., 2015). Similarly, in the US, whilst health insurance levels for this population are higher than in the overall immigrant population, they are lower than that of the native-born population, and this serves to limit access to health services (Hooper & Batalova, 2015).

These challenges of understanding, accessing and using services led to three separate research studies being undertaken by the authors that focused on mental health services (Yeung et al., 2012), social care services (Irvine et al., 2014; Yeung et al., 2015) and learning disability services (Partridge, 2013) for people from a Chinese background in the UK.

Methodology

The first study (Yeung et al., 2012) used a phenomenological approach to understand the experiences of pathways to care of Chinese people living with a diagnosis of severe mental illness (Pathways to Mental Health Care Study). Semi-structured interviews were conducted to elicit the subjective views of their pathway experiences. All of the interviews were undertaken by a bilingual Cantonese and English researcher. A convenience sampling approach was used to recruit participants who were from Chinese backgrounds, were aged between 18 and 65 and had a diagnosis of severe mental illness. Individuals who formed their social networks and became involved in the pathway to care journey were also interviewed. Participants were recruited through a number of Chinese community projects that provided services for Chinese people affected by mental health problems. In total, 51 interviews concerning 16 Chinese people with severe mental illness were undertaken. This included 13 interviews with people living with severe mental illness, 17 interviews with their relatives or friends and 21 interviews with Chinese-speaking community workers. Most interviews with participants and their families (35) were conducted in Cantonese, and 12 interviews with community workers and four with people with mental illness were undertaken in English.

The second study (Irvine et al., 2015; Yeung et al., 2015) adopted a qualitative methodology to explore the experiences of social care of Chinese people with physical disabilities (Chinese Voices of Social Care (CVSC) Study). The early stages of the study took a descriptive approach, using face-to-face semi-structured interviews to capture the experiences of participants; the later stages followed an interpretive approach, using focus groups to facilitate interpretation. Purposive sampling was used to recruit people from a Chinese background, who were aged between 18 and 70, had a physical impairment and were in receipt of social care services within 6 months prior to the time of the interview. Focus groups were then used to open up new perspectives and give deeper understandings on themes which emerged from the interviews (Bradbury-Jones et al., 2009). Individual interviews were conducted by two bilingual researchers and one English-speaking researcher.

Twenty-six interviews were carried out in the preferred language of participants; 18 interviews were conducted in a Chinese dialect, including 16 in Cantonese and two in Mandarin, and eight interviews in English. Fourteen participants who had taken part in the interviews agreed to attend the focus groups; two focus groups were conducted in Cantonese and one in English.

The third study (Partridge, 2013) used a qualitative ethnographic methodology that involved participant observations, semi-structured interviews and thematic analysis to explore the ways in which residential and day care, Chinese-specific services and mainstream organizations included adults with learning disabilities from Chinese backgrounds (Including People with Learning Disabilities Study). A strong reflexive approach was adopted in which the researcher's experiences and responses to the research settings formed part of the research material (Etherington, 2004). Key informants provided specific cultural knowledge that added to the researcher's observations and the understanding of participants' experiences of the service they used. In total, participants included eight people with learning disabilities who were from Chinese backgrounds, five family/carers, five service managers, 10 staff and two sessional workers who were all aged 18 and over. They were observed in the residential and/or day service setting and took part in interviews. In some cases a Mandarin, Cantonese or Hakka speaking interpreter was used. Participants originated from Hong Kong, Mainland China, Vietnam, Malaysia and the UK. Participants lived in and around a city in the West Midlands, England. The researcher spent three months respectively in two Chinese-specific services and one mainstream social care service in the West Midlands city.

Challenges and Solutions

From each of the studies there was clear evidence that people from Chinese backgrounds faced linguistic and cultural challenges that impacted on the way that they understood, accessed and used health and social care services; and that in some situations pragmatic solutions had been identified to help overcomes such challenges. We will draw on the findings of the three studies to explore these issues through the chapter. Throughout, pseudonyms have been used to protect the identity of the participants.

Understanding services

Being able to understand the nature and extent of available services was a challenge for the participants in our studies, and we heard stark accounts from people who, owing to limited understanding, failed to access appropriate and available services and instead relied on personal resources or services from their home countries to address their needs. For example, two participants in the Pathways to Mental Health Care Study had a history of mental illness before they came to the UK. However, they did not know how to access mental health services because information about the services was produced only in English, which they were not able to understand.

In one case, Mei had a long history of mental illness prior to her move to the UK, but she had no contact with mental health services for the first seven years that she resided there. It was not until she reached a crisis point, when the police were called, that she finally accessed mental health services.

Mandy had a diagnosis of severe mental illness, and she realized she had to take medication to keep her well. She was very concerned about the lack of prescription after she came to the UK. She explained:

> We tried to buy the medication from the chemist but people there said that they could not sell the medication to me. I didn't know I had to see that kind of doctor (psychiatrist) until my daughter was born. (Interview conducted in Cantonese)

Similar accounts emerged from the CVSC, whereby service users' failure to understand social care services was given as a reason for failing to obtain support early, as illustrated in the following accounts:

> I didn't know what service was available, I just knew that I could try but I didn't know what exactly I should be asking for. (Mr Lau, interview conducted in Cantonese)

> I didn't get in touch with anyone because I didn't know where to go or how to get help ... I didn't know what I was entitled to. (Angela, interview conducted in English)

Not knowing where and how to access social care was one of the reasons for not getting support early and, in this study, focus group members confirmed that they had to wait for a crisis before support was forthcoming from social care. In many cases this occurred only when their health deteriorated to the extent that they required hospital treatment.

Participants in the Including People with Learning Disabilities Study had little or no voice, and their family/carers or those working in the services tended to make decisions for them. For most, their independence and the choices they made seemed conditional on their families, who were seen as key people in their lives. This was because they had remained dependent through staying within the family, who saw it as their duty to speak for them, thus the voices of people with learning disabilities were silenced. The ethnographic nature of this study, amongst people with an intellectual disability who were already embedded in services, meant it was not possible to tease out whether their personal understanding of the services had proved to be a challenge to accessing and using appropriate services.

Accessing services

Accessing appropriate services in the UK proved to be one of the foremost challenges for people from Chinese backgrounds who were in need of assistance from health and social care services. In the Pathways to Mental Health Care Study it was because of language difference that many people experienced difficulties accessing mental health services when they first became unwell. Many did not know where and how to contact services and had to involve relatives for help. However, even when their help was secured, relatives still struggled with access to services and 'I didn't know what to do' was frequently mentioned in the interviews with relatives when their family members became mentally unwell. For example, Lai's mother explained:

> It was very difficult, now at my age (70's), I can't read, don't know any English. I don't know how to sort out the problems ... It is very troublesome. (Interview conducted in Cantonese)

Susan's father in law said:

> We didn't know what to do. At that time, we had nowhere to go for help ... Every time when it happened, we were at a loss. (Interview conducted in Cantonese)

And Fai's wife related the following account:

> At that time (of husband's relapse), I couldn't speak any English; I couldn't put a sentence in English together. I had to drag the doctor, pulled his arms. I asked him to go to my house to see my husband. (Interview conducted in Cantonese)

In the CVSC study it was similar issues with language difference that created barriers to accessing social care services:

> I don't know how to access services because I don't know English, I don't know how to ask for the information I need. (Focus Group 2, conducted in Cantonese)

Moreover, several participants in the CVSC study encountered difficulties understanding social care because literature about services was only available in the English language. Unable to comprehend disability literature compounded the problems with language difference and created a barrier to negotiating access to social care. This partly explains why many participants reached social care only at a crisis point.

Participants were further confused and felt unable to take part fully during the assessment process because they were not able to communicate effectively with the English-speaking social workers who undertook individual assessments to establish the need for services, as illustrated in Ann's account:

> You know when you cannot speak the language, you cannot communicate with others. It's very troublesome ... even if the social worker comes to see us; it's no good if we cannot communicate with them. (Interview conducted in Cantonese).

Failure to engage fully in the assessment process thus created the potential for people either to be denied services or to receive insufficient or inappropriate services.

Participants in the Including People with Learning Disabilities study accessed the Chinese-specific (rather than mainstream) services that were the subject of the study through family connections. Since no one in the study had gained access to this service through conventional means, the suggestion is that, without personal networks, the availability of such services may not be broadcast or, alternatively, access would be denied.

Indeed this suggestion is confirmed by Amanda, the manager of a Chinese Service Centre, who stated:

> As the only Chinese [service in this area] – we never promote any direct services for people with learning disability – never – that's never been one of our – services ... I think the only – what we can provide is – activities – but they need to have support there to take responsibility. (Interview conducted in English)

In all cases the research revealed that the support that Amanda referred to was provided by family/carers.

Conversely, gaining access into a mainstream (rather than Chinese) organization for people with learning disabilities was through the conventional route whereby social workers conducted assessments to establish needs and recommend access to the service. Although this process of access appears to be more readily navigable, it was not without its problems. Unlike the Chinese services where the family was seen as an important link between the family member with a learning difficulty and the service, in the mainstream service, family contact was minimal. This was despite *Valuing People* (Department of Health, 2001), a UK Government White Paper that focuses on learning disabilities and sets out an agenda for action in developing social care services with an emphasis on inclusion for people with learning disabilities, and which recommends that supporters of people with learning disabilities should be included in decision making through person-centered planning. For some service users, this process of accessing services appeared to be an isolating experience. It was especially poignant for Tang-Wei, a 42-year-old man with autism and a learning disability who was living in a mainstream residential unit for people with learning disabilities. Tang-Wei was subject to an incorrect outcome from an initial speech and language assessment, through which he was labeled as having no language skills. His family was not consulted on this matter. However, it was later acknowledged that he spoke some Cantonese but this was not identified on his entry to the mainstream residential service. The erroneous assessment meant that the likelihood of Tang-Wei communicating in his own language was further reduced and was thus a disabling barrier to his inclusion within the residential facility:

> Obviously there is a language barrier which is a problem but with a lot of these guys because of the autism there is always going to be a kind of communication barrier there ... like I said before ... I didn't really take in a lot of things that I notice about [Tang-Wei] which I presumed was his autism, is actually as you said, is his culture, that's quite – you know – surprising, and it's helped me to understand him a bit more I think.
> (Kate, Residential Support Worker, interview conducted in English)

This study suggested that, for people with learning disabilities, having family connections raised a number of issues in terms of accessing services. For some, family acted as an agent to facilitate entry, while for others family were not so involved. It seemed that knowing someone from the 'in group' enabled easier access to services and seemed more effective than being an 'outsider'. This was a common issue in the Chinese-specific services in this study since access to such services was conditional on their behavior and their family links. The findings suggest that people with learning disabilities in the Chinese-specific and mainstream services in this study were 'disabled' either by the role which family took in acting for their relatives with learning disabilities or by the exclusion of family views in favor of professional perspectives. Thus family connections can be an enabling factor, but can also constrain or limit the participation of a person with learning disabilities, both by being overly controlling and by being absent.

Using services

As Tang-Wei's experience suggests, having gained access to health and social care services, the challenges faced by people from Chinese backgrounds did not diminish. For example, the issue of English language proficiency was a continuing challenge for people as they navigated through their health and social care journeys.

When people with mental illness in the Pathways to Mental Health Care Study encountered language barriers, they could become unstuck, as Mei's Chinese-speaking worker pointed out:

> Because she cannot speak English, she cannot make appointments to see her doctor. If it is simple conversation, she can manage it. However, the appointment system is very complicated. When she rang the number, there is the message to tell her to press this button then another. She cannot do it; she is unable to follow it. (Interview conducted in English)

Other respondents struggled with similar difficulties:

> I can't even pick up the phone and talk to my social worker, the receptionist of my social worker ... doctor surgery ... they speak English, I don't understand them. ... Language difference is a big problem. I don't understand what people are saying. I am not able to communicate what I want to say. (Mandy, interview conducted in Cantonese)

Family members also encountered such problems and had to use different strategies to communicate with mental health professionals. For example, Carman's father said:

> When the psychiatrist tried to explain to me about her problems, I did not understand what that meant, schizophrenia? I had to ask him to write it down. When I got home, I had to look up in the dictionary. (Interview conducted in Cantonese)

Ideally, interpretation services would be in place for consultations with health and social care professionals. However, this need was often overlooked, with taxing consequences for service users and family members, as illustrated in the account of Elaine's father and Tina's mother:

> At the beginning, I couldn't understand what the doctor was talking about, I couldn't understand ... there was no interpreter ... After a while, the doctor explained to me about her illness, he said it was schizophrenia. It was after a while, some people explained to me. It was only later on there was an interpreter. (Elaine's father, interview conducted in Cantonese)

> The Chinese community worker from (name of another city) came to visit us with a support worker when Tina first became unwell. I contacted him recently when Tina had a relapse; he told me that because of the funding issue, he could not provide the services for people living in another city. I think the services provided by Chinese speaking workers

are very important. It really helps as they can share your worries, someone to talk to you to ... as we live in a small town, we are neglected by the local authority. (Tina's mother, interview conducted in Cantonese)

Similar accounts arose for the CVSC study, where participants and their families talked of struggling to negotiate encounters with social workers and formal care workers and in these discussions the need for, and the limited provision of, interpreters was a prominent theme:

> At the beginning, the social worker asked an interpreter for help. Now, if they need to speak to me, they will telephone my daughter and ask her to interpret. (Mr Tse, interview conducted in Cantonese)

> When the social worker cannot find an interpreter, she will ask my daughter to help. But you know my daughter lives in another city. It causes her troubles to travel here. (Focus group 1 conducted in Cantonese)

In the Including People with Learning Disabilities, Tang-Wei's experience of communication is a case in point. The mainstream service where he resided was unable to meet his language needs and had little knowledge of his history as an individual or by what cultural norms, values and beliefs he lived. Although there was recognition that he could communicate in Cantonese, with the exception of a limited period when a temporary worker who was a Cantonese speaker from a Chinese background was employed as an interpreter during their summer break from university, limited effort had been made to facilitate communication in Cantonese. Thus Tang-Wei was reduced to making gestures and using single words such as 'wash', 'eat', 'drink', 'sleep', 'go' and 'sit' to make his needs known.

Where Chinese-specific services were in place for people with learning disabilities, their encounters with health and social care professionals was facilitated through the use of Chinese care workers:

> We need to step in and help them, say my client even though he need a sick note from the GP, if he go on his own to ask for note from the GP he can't do that, he can't, he went to GP twice and he forget the sick note, so I need to go with him to get sick note. (Chinese community support worker, interview conducted in English)

Although interpretation or its absence was a particular challenge for people with learning disabilities, it was not the only communication challenge. It seemed that those who used the culturally specific services found it difficult to connect in terms of communication with others in the services even when they spoke the same language. This seemed to reflect other people's attitudes toward them. People with learning disabilities were 'disabled' by the services they used and by their family because they were not included or consulted about their needs; nor were they actively encouraged to exercise choice or control in relationships or activities. For example, during observation in the ethnographic study, staff at the Centre that Lin-Feng attended would only say hello to him if they knew his parents, but there was no conversation or any indication of the staff engaging with him in any other way.

> They just say hello, hello and that's it, no conversation cos [they] doesn't know him very well – and if Amanda is working, yes – but just hello this sort of thing, not deep conversation no. (Lin-Feng's mother, interview conducted in Mandarin)

This lack of inclusion is problematic because it does not take account of the cultural values of family responsibility or the norms associated with such support. The findings suggest that people with learning disabilities in both culturally specific and mainstream services in this study were 'disabled' by being silenced. They were not encouraged to be heard, nor were they consulted on daily issues and/or service development, which had implications for their inclusion and independence.

People using health and social care services did not just face communication challenges and, in our studies, we uncovered examples of people struggling with the attitudes that care providers displayed toward them, which could have a negative impact on their health and quality of life. This applied in relation to people with mental illness:

> The major difficulty was ... I guess the long waiting time, between ... actually seeing a doctor and looking for help ... Sometimes the receptionists aren't very understanding. (Tina, interview conducted in Cantonese)

> The system is not flexible enough, very strict ... You have to give her the medication anyway, one day earlier, it doesn't matter! Getting the prescription really causes a lot of anxiety for her, if there is no medication, it is very difficult for her; she really suffers. (Mandy's husband, interview conducted in Cantonese)

It was also applicable to people in receipt of social care services, where some respondents felt that service providers displayed a lack of compassion:

> It is just like, they (domiciliary workers) do the job and can't really be bothered (to do) more. (Mei Ling's husband, interview conducted in Cantonese)

> I just feel the social worker is treating me like you're just another hopeless case ... And there is a different care worker every time so I never get any sense of continuity. They don't seem very caring. They just come to do the job, and it isn't a very human experience. (Ah Fong, interview conducted in Cantonese)

The situation also resonated for people with learning disabilities, as uncovered in the ethnographic study where some of the staff members' assumptions and attitudes toward people from Chinese backgrounds were observed to be disturbing. For example, on occasions staff would make derogatory remarks such as 'they'll eat anything in China'.

At best these attitudes could be classed as cultural incapacity, where the system or agencies do not intentionally seek to be culturally destructive but rather lack the capacity to help minority clients or communities (Cross, 2001), but at worst, they suggested cultural destructiveness, where according to Cross (2001) attitudes, policies and practices are destructive to cultures and consequently to the individuals within the culture. This was classed by participants in the Pathways to Mental Health Care Study as racial discrimination, as represented in the following data extracts:

> When I was looking for help, I don't know why, I couldn't find the people to help me. I think, somehow, there was racial discrimination here. (Derek, interview conducted in Cantonese)

> Living here (England), is it because we are Chinese? Sometimes they discriminate against us? ... Do you find them discriminating against Chinese people? I really don't know, living in a western society. (Mandy, interview conducted in Cantonese)

Solutions

The challenges that people from Chinese backgrounds with mental illness, physical disabilities and learning disabilities face while trying to understand, access and use health and social care services are glaring. However, the picture is not entirely negative, and our three research studies highlighted instances where individuals, their families, service providers and organizations had identified solutions to avoid or overcome problems.

Participants in the Pathways to Mental Health Care and CVSC studies talked of their steps to draw on personal and family resources to meet their different needs. As there was no mental health literature written in Chinese in the UK, both Margaret and Mandy mobilized their overseas resources and asked friends and family to send them books from Hong Kong and mainland China, respectively. Ann and Carman made more friends by taking part in different kinds of voluntary work. Mrs So received a lot of support from her friends she met in the church. Lai took part in a range of cultural activities held at her supported accommodation. Tina returned to university to continue her studies and some of her classmates supported her to seek help when she experienced a relapse. In the CVSC study we heard examples of people asking their friends and family to translate and interpret for them, of families taking on the main caring responsibilities and of people negotiating complex systems to their advantage, such as one focus groups member who said:

> I've found a good way to get results. You go onto the authority's website and go to adult social care complaints, just click onto that. If you send an email, send a copy of the email to someone and just record everything that you do. (Focus group conducted in English)

We heard from participants in the CVSC study and the Pathways to Mental Health Care Study of the efforts that health and social care professionals had made to find solutions to address their needs. For example, Mrs Lin and Mandy related that:

> The social worker gave us a lot of information. She explained to us about options and arranged someone to look after me so that my husband can go out to do shopping and take a break. We are really pleased with the services. (Mrs Lin, interview conducted in Cantonese)

> My social worker knew that I couldn't speak English, she found me a Chinese chemist in Chinatown. I telephone the chemist and the chemist will contact my GP to organise my prescription. Then I go to the chemist to collect my prescription. (Mandy, interview conducted in Cantonese)

And Mrs So and Fai's Chinese worker praised the psychiatrists thus:

> My consultant psychiatrist is very good. I told him that I saw things, this and that. He advised me to face them, don't be afraid ... he tried to give me the lowest dosage. So now, I am not afraid, I can face them. (Mrs So, interview conducted in Cantonese)

> His consultant is very good. Each time when he sees him (Fai) and also involve his wife in any consultations so that he can find out more about Fai's situation. (Fai's Chinese speaking worker, interview conducted in English)

In the Including People with Learning Disabilities Study service providers talked of the measures that they had taken or plans they had in place to try and break down communication barriers:

> What we need is to sort of almost find another Cantonese-speaking person who could be here. That would be the ideal, because of money issues. I've just spent a couple of grand on training Catherine and she's gone [to another service in the organisation] although she is very useful still. So I can't just get someone else you know cause they say 'ow no you're not' umm, but we know where we are going with that one you know we are on the lookout like students in the holiday, a bit of casual

work. This will give him a little bit of time to talk in his own language and that's a big thing to me to get the opportunity to speak in his first language if he wants to. (Service manager, interview conducted in English)

Chinese welfare organizations

Overwhelmingly, in relation to mental illness and physical disabilities (and to an extent, learning disabilities), it was Chinese welfare organizations that offered the best linguistically and culturally appropriate solutions to Chinese people's obstacles to understanding, accessing and using health and social care services. Chinese welfare organizations tend to be located in or near Chinatown areas and are seen to offer a focal point for Chinese people to meet and develop relationships (Chan et al., 2007). These organizations are found in major cities in the UK with a higher concentration of Chinese population. However, in areas where the Chinese population is smaller there are few, if any, Chinese community centers (Chan et al., 2007).

Participants attested to the benefits of having Chinese-specific services to address their linguistic needs. A strong theme emerging from the data in the CVSC and Pathways to Mental Health Care studies indicated that participants requiring health and social care support felt more at ease and more comforted if care workers could communicate with them in their native language:

> If there is Chinese staff helping me, that's much better. At least we can understand each other. However, there is nothing I can do; I am pleased with the service they (Chinese organization) provide. (Mr Tse, interview conducted in Cantonese)

> Now I go to the Chinese community centre to seek help. In the past, there was nobody' (for linguistic support). (Lai's mother, interview conducted in Cantonese)

These findings concur with the literature surrounding Chinese welfare organizations, which shows that most Chinese people using the services provided by these organizations are Chinese migrants who have limited English language skills and they approach these organizations for translation and interpreting services (Chan, 2004; Chan et al., 2007). Apart from addressing their linguistic needs, many participants reported that they relied on day services provided by Chinese welfare organizations to meet their social and dietary needs:

> I like going to the Chinese community centre for recreational activities such as Tai Chi, Mahjong (a game originally from China and played by four players). (Margaret, interview conducted in Cantonese)

> Our food is different from theirs (the English). At the end of the day, we are not used to what they eat. We like rice porridge, rice, noodles. (Kai-la, interview conducted in Cantonese)

Importantly, the Chinese welfare organizations were shown to have a significant brokering and supportive role. For example, Ann, a fluent English speaker, found that the involvement of the Chinese speaking workers 'was really a big help' in enabling her parents and the mental health workers to understand mental illness from different cultural perspectives. Here, they serve the purpose of shortening the social and cultural distance between participants and western mental health practitioners. Similarly, the literature contends that Chinese welfare organizations serve as a link to mainstream services for Chinese people (Hiew *et al.*, 2008; Ng *et al.*, 2007).

In addition, the Chinese-speaking workers were shown in our studies to be a source of emotional support for people to talk to when they were unable to enlist support from their informal networks:

> The Chinese support worker really cares about her. The support worker is like a friend to her. She likes talking to her about anything ... she is very happy when she meets up with the support worker. (Mandy's husband, interview conducted in Cantonese)

However, the value of the Chinese welfare organizations was less evident in the Including People with Learning Disabilities Study. Partridge (2013) was unable to locate any Chinese-specific organizations that were established to support people with learning disabilities. Consequently, people from Chinese backgrounds with learning disabilities were seeking support from Chinese welfare organizations that were only set up to offer general support. As acknowledged by one manager, this meant that they did not have the skills to deal with people with learning disabilities and therefore may inadvertently have marginalized this vulnerable group of people:

> Unfortunately no [we do not include people with learning disabilities on the staff resident committees] ... I think it's the one thing we need to look into and why they are not ... it's probably because my team are not very, we don't have expertise ... I suppose I need to do a bit more, well there are some support workers that support them quite well but I think they need to be encouraged to get them to help out and take part in the community. (Song-Tao – manager, interview conducted in English)

It seems then that people with learning disabilities are not served well by mainstream or Chinese organizations because these services lack either cultural competence or the necessary appreciation of social inclusion. Similarly, in relation to mental illness, the Chinese support workers of Lai and Mrs So expressed their concerns that:

> we didn't have the skills, we don't have the experiences, we don't have the knowledge to support the people. (Interview conducted in English)

Moreover, some people with physical disabilities or mental health problems expressed a reluctance to work with Chinese organizations. Because most Chinese-speaking workers have strong links with the Chinese community and are based in a local Chinese welfare organization, some participants are concerned that their 'shameful business' will spread across the community and people will 'gossip' about their secret. Mental illness remains stigmatized in Chinese communities, and the fact that people with a label of severe mental illness and their families are considered to have a 'moral defect' (Chang & Horrocks, 2006; Lau & Wong, 2008) has a far reaching impact on Chinese people. It brings shame and embarrassment not only to the individual but also to the whole family (Leung et al., 2012; Yang et al., 2007). Hence, Chinese families are under immense pressure to conceal the labeling of mental illness and therefore can be reluctant to use Chinese services (Lee et al., 2005). Therefore, Susan's father-in-law said that 'the Chinese community worker only knew part of the story' about Susan's (mental health) problem. Peggy's husband initially resisted the input from the Chinese community worker as he was concerned that 'some people really cannot maintain confidentiality' and worried that 'family disgrace' would be broadcast in the community. To a lesser extent, help seeking was also limited amongst people with physical disabilities, because as Alan pointed out:

> It's the habit of Chinese, we like being self-reliant. We seldom ask for help. We are not outspoken, so very often our family helps out as much as they can. However, apart from my daughter, I have no relatives to help me. (Interview conducted in English)

Conclusions

Our studies show that experiences of both health and social care among people from Chinese backgrounds are influenced by individual, professional, structural and cultural factors. For vulnerable individuals with mental illness, physical disabilities or learning disabilities, unending effort is often required to develop understanding, negotiate access and navigate services to meet their health and social care needs. This is especially the case for people who are not proficient in English.

It is evident that many participants are bewildered by the organization of health and social care services and their needs can be overlooked in the system. These services need to develop greater appreciation of the tension between the reluctance to receive support outside the family, the demand of the caring responsibility being placed on the family and the imperative that individuals make their own decisions about the care that they receive.

The role of the family is important for people with Chinese backgrounds who have health and social care needs but their input should not be the only solution. Individuals and their families may welcome the contribution of health and social care services as it provides some relief from the burden of ill health or disability. However, after the initial relief, individuals and their families often found that these services did not fully meet their needs or acknowledge their linguistic or cultural requirements. Moreover, for Chinese people with mental illness and learning disabilities, the stigma attached to their disorders compelled family members to conceal the extent of individual's needs and to take the main responsibility for caring for their relative, and this is not always in the best interests of the individual.

Health and social care services need to address these individual, structural and cultural factors if the needs of people from Chinese backgrounds with mental illness, physical disabilities and learning disabilities are to be met adequately. A clear communication strategy that takes account of the verbal and written languages used by the diverse set of Chinese communities in the UK would provide one solution. This might involve the sharing of resources between culturally specific and mainstream services to better disseminate knowledge that could help improve the care of people from Chinese backgrounds. The diversity of minority cultural groups means that, for services to develop from cultural incapacity to cultural sensitivity, diversity training is needed, which should focus on 'how to find out', rather than outlining the main values and behaviors of single cultures.

Chinese welfare organizations are often in the best place to support and empower people with mental illness, physical disabilities and learning disabilities to help them understand services and assert their rights. They play an important role in meeting the linguistic and cultural needs of Chinese people. To ensure the best outcomes for their service users by facilitating early access and fair and appropriate treatment, health and social care services should develop closer collaboration with Chinese welfare organizations. The development of such collaborations could be mutually beneficial since they would provide a solution to the concerns that disabled people from minority cultural groups often fall between mainstream and culturally specific services (Evans & Banton, 2001; Singh, 2005).

However, Carr (2014) draws attention to the fact that micro providers such as Chinese welfare organizations are vulnerable, particularly in times of austerity. Thus commissioners of health and social care services should consider how they could support these (often) solitary organizations, in terms of mobilizing groups to work collectively and in providing much needed but relatively small financial support to aid stability and sustainability. However, the value of Chinese welfare organizations should not be overestimated, as they are only able to support people who live in high-density Chinese populations and cannot currently meet the needs of all vulnerable groups. Therefore mainstream services must not entirely relinquish their responsibility for providing culturally sensitive, accessible support to Chinese welfare organizations.

References

Bignall, T. and Butt, J. (2000) *Between Ambition and Achievement: Young Black Disabled People: Views and Experiences of Independence and Independent Living.* Bristol: Polity Press and JRF.

Bradbury-Jones, C., Sambrook, S. and Irvine, F. (2009) The phenomenological focus group: An oxymoron? *Journal of Advanced Nursing* 65 (3), 663–671.

Care Quality Commission (2010) *Count Me in 2009: Results of the 2009 National Census of Inpatients and Patients on Supervised Community Treatment in Mental Health and Learning Disability Services in England and Wales.* London: Care Quality Commission.

Carr, S. (2014) *Social Care for Marginalised Communities: Balancing Self-organisation, Microprovision and Mainstream Support.* Policy Paper 18, Health Services Management Centre. University of Birmingham.

Chahal, K. (2004) *Experiencing Ethnicity: Discrimination and Service Provision.* York: Joseph Rowntree Foundation.

Chan C.K. (2004) *A Study of Help-seeking Behaviours among UK Chinese Families.* London: Economic and Social Research Council.

Chan, C.K., Cole, B. and Bowpitt, G. (2007) 'Beyond silent organizations': A reflection of the UK Chinese people and their community organizations. *Critical Social Policy* 27 (4), 509–533.

Chang, K.H. and Horrocks, S. (2006) Lived experiences of family caregivers of mentally ill relatives. *Journal of Advanced Nursing* 53 (4), 435–443.

Chiu, S. and Yu, S. (2001) An excess of culture: the myth of shared care in the Chinese community in Britain. *Ageing and Society* 21 (6), 681–699.

Costa, B. (2013) *Language Support: Challenge and Benefits for Users and Providers of Health and Social Care Services.* London: Race Equality Foundation.

Cross, T.L.C. (2001) Cultural Competence Continuum. *'Focal Point', The Bulletin of the Research and Training Center on Family Support and Children's Mental Health.* See http://www.unc.edu/~wfarrell/SOWO%20874/Readings/cultcompetencecont.htm (accessed 7 August 2015).

Department of Health (2001) *Valuing People: A New Strategy for Learning Disability for the 21st Century.* London: Department of Health.

Department of Health (2012) *The Health and Social Care Act.* London: Department of Health.

Dobbs, J., Green, H. and Zealey, L. (2006) *Focus on Ethnicity and Religion.* London: National Statistics Office/Palgrave Macmillan.

Emerson, E. and Hatton, C. (2004) *Estimating future need/demand for supports for adults with learning disabilities in England.* Institute for Health Research, Lancaster University.

Etherington, K. (2004) *Becoming a Reflexive Researcher: Using Our Selves in Research.* London: Jessica Kingsley.

Evans, R. and Banton, M. (2001) *Involving Black Disabled People in Shaping Services: Findings.* York: Joseph Rowntree Foundation.

Fisher, K. and Glanfield, G. (2009) Services for people with disability from Chinese backgrounds. *Social Policy Research Centre Newsletter* 101 (1), 4–5.

Green, G., Bradby, H., Chan, A. and Lee, M. (2006) 'We are not completely Westernised': Dual medical systems and pathways to health care among Chinese migrant women in England. *Social Science and Medicine* 62 (6), 1498–1509.

Health and Social Care Information Centre (2013) *Community Care Statistics, Social Services Activity, England 2012–2013, Final Release.* Leeds: The Health and Social Care Information Centre.

Hiew, Y., Lok, S., Hollingsbee, C., Man, W. and Yan, C. (2008) *Report of the Community Led Research Tower Hamlets and Hackney in Coping with Mental Health Issues.* London: The National Institute for Mental Health in England.

Hooper, K. and Batalova, J. (2015) *Chinese Immigrants in the United States.* Migration Policy Institute. See http://www.migrationpolicy.org/article/chinese-immigrants-united-states (accessed 7 August 2015).

Irvine, F., Partridge, M., Yeung, E. and Simcock, P. (2015) *Chinese Voices of Social Care: Satisfaction with Social Care for Physical Disabilities Among People from Chinese Backgrounds*. London: NIHR School of Social Care Research. See http://www.sscr.nihr.ac.uk/PDF/Findings/RF27.pdf (accessed 7 August 2015).

Jones, D. (1979) The Chinese in Britain: Origins and development of a community. *New Community* 7 (3), 397–402.

Lau, Y. and Wong, F.K. (2008) Are concern for face and willingness to seek help correlated to early postnatal depressive symptoms among Hong Kong Chinese women? A cross-sectional questionnaire survey. *International Journal of Nursing Studies* 45 (1), 51–64.

Lee, S., Lee, M., Chiu, M. and Kleinman, A. (2005) Experience of social stigma by people with schizophrenia in Hong Kong. *British Journal of Psychiatry* 186 (2), 153–157.

Leung, P., Cheung, M. and Tsui, V. (2012) Help-seeking behaviors among Chinese Americans with depressive symptoms. *Social Work* 57 (1), 61–71.

Liu, Z., Beaver, K. and Speed, S. (2015) Chinese Elders' views on their interactions in general practice: A Grounded Theory study. *Ethnicity and Health* 20 (2), 129–144.

Miltiades, H.B. and Wu, B. (2008) Factors affecting physician visits in Chinese and Chinese immigrant samples. *Social Science and Medicine* 66 (3), 704–714.

Mir, G., Nocon, A., Ahmad, W. and Jones, L. (2001) *Learning Difficulties and Ethnicity*. Leeds: Department of Health.

Ng, A., Hiew, Y., Lok, S. and Tang, R. (2007) *Report of the Community Led Research Project Focussing on the Exploration of the Mental Health Needs and Experiences of the Chinese Community in Barnet*. The National Institute for Mental Health in England.

Office for National Statistics (2012) *Ethnicity and National Identity in England and Wales 2011*. London: Office for National Statistics.

Partridge, M. (2013) including People with learning difficulties from chinese backgrounds: An ethnography of three services. PhD Thesis, Norah Fry Research Centre, University of Bristol.

Poxton, R., Taylor, J., Brenner, D., Cole, A. and Burke, C. (2012) *Reaching Out to People with Learning Disabilities and their Families from Black and Minority Ethnic Communities*. London: Foundation for People with Learning Disabilities.

Rochelle, T.L. and Shardlow, S.M. (2012) Quality of social networks among UK Chinese. *Social Indicators Research* 114 (2), 425–439.

Royal College of Psychiatrists (2011) *Minority Ethnic Communities and Specialist Learning Disability Services*. London: Faculty of the Psychiatry of Learning Disability of the Royal College of Psychiatrists.

Singh, B. (2005) *Improving Support for Black Disabled People: Lessons from Community Organisations on Making Change Happen*. York: Joseph Rowntree Foundation.

Tran, L. (2009) *Evaluation of a Chinese Mental Health Advocacy and Support Project*. London: Kings Fund.

Wong, M.L. (1989) *Chinese Liverpudlians: A History of the Chinese Community in Liverpool*. Liverpool: Liver Press.

Wong, L.Y.M. and Richman, J. (2000b) Chinese mental health. *Mental Health Nursing* 20 (6), 14–18.

Yang, L.H., Kleinman, A., Link, B.G., Phelan, J.C., Lee, S. and Good, B. (2007) Culture and stigma: Adding moral experience to stigma theory. *Social Science & Medicine* 64 (7), 1524–1535.

Yeung, E., Irvine, F., Ng, S. and Tsang, S. (2012) Role of Social Networks in the help seeking experiences among Chinese suffering from severe mental illness in England: A qualitative study. *British Journal of Social Work* 43 (3), 486–503.

Yeung, E., Partridge, M. and Irvine, F. (2015) Satisfaction with social care: The experiences of people from Chinese backgrounds with physical disabilities. *Health and Social Care in the Community*. Published early online. See http://onlinelibrary.wiley.com/doi/10.1111/hsc.12264/epdf (accessed 7 August 2015).

11 A New Zealand Perspective on Providing Health Care for Patients with Limited English Proficiency

Ben Gray, Jo Hilder, Lindsay Macdonald, Rachel Tester, Anthony Dowell and Maria Stubbe

Introduction

New Zealand is a small island nation in the South Pacific with a population of 4.5 million people – about the same size as the state of Colorado. English is the language spoken by the monolingual majority and is one of three official languages alongside te reo Maori, the indigenous language, and more recently, New Zealand Sign Language. Successive waves of migration over the past century have added a large number of other minority languages to a population mix that has become increasingly diverse in the past few decades. The first part of this chapter provides a background to New Zealand's cultural and linguistic diversity, with particular emphasis on the important place of Maori and the more recent influx of migrants from non-English speaking countries. Next, we describe the context of the New Zealand health system (which is predominantly state funded) and the regulatory approach to provision of health care and interpreting services. This is followed by an evaluation of how well the New Zealand health sector has responded to the needs of patients with limited proficiency in English in practice, while attempting to balance cost efficacy, patient safety and patient rights. We then report on our own research looking at the use of interpreters in medical consultations, and discuss how this could inform policy on provision of interpreters for patients with limited English proficiency in New Zealand. The chapter concludes with a brief discussion of what steps could be taken to ensure adequate provision of equitable health services for this vulnerable population.

New Zealand Background

The Maori people and language

New Zealand has a shorter human history than any other country. The indigenous Maori people first arrived in Aotearoa/New Zealand around the 13th century (Wilson, 2015). New Zealand was progressively settled by the British during the first half of the 19th century, and its status as part of the British Empire was cemented by the signing of the Treaty of Waitangi between the Crown and Maori chiefs in 1840. At this time Maori was a spoken language only. Early settlers learned to speak the Maori language, and missionaries devised a writing system and published the first books in Maori. Most migrants during the 19th century originated from Britain and spoke English, although there were localized enclaves of other languages including French, Croatian and Chinese. Until the 1930s the Maori people mostly remained bilingual, speaking Maori in the home and English outside the home. However, at this time government policies advocated a move toward monolingualism, and children were sometimes punished for speaking Maori in school. Everyday use of the Maori language declined between 1920 and 1960 as Maori migrated from rural to urban centers and English became the dominant language in Maori homes (Higgins & Keane, 2014).

Over the last 40 years the Maori people have undergone a cultural renaissance (Taonui, 2013), and this has been reflected in changes in use of the language. The first petition to have Maori taught in schools was presented to government in 1972 (Higgins & Keane, 2014). Since then, the language has become part of the curriculum in all schools and pre-schools. Schools teaching in Maori only (*kura kaupapa*) have been developed. Maori has become an official language and is increasingly used in wider New Zealand society (for example the main radio news program from the public broadcaster greets the audience each morning in Maori, and an annual Maori language week promotes wider use of the language). However, despite a resurgence in the numbers of people fluent in Maori as well as English, there are very few people who speak only Maori (Statistics New Zealand, 2013b) and it is unusual for an interpreter to be essential for health consultations with Maori. Nevertheless, while Maori people rarely face linguistic barriers to health care, there are still significant disparities in health outcomes, even after controlling for socioeconomic differences (Rumball-Smith *et al.*, 2013; Hill *et al.*, 2010; Stevens *et al.*, 2008).

Linguistic and cultural diversity

New Zealand has three official languages: English, Maori and New Zealand Sign Language (NZSL). This means that people have the right to speak in these languages in court and parliament and in other government settings, and that there is a regulatory structure for interpreter competency in Maori and NZSL. However, many other languages are spoken within minority ethnic communities in New Zealand. Among others, New Zealand has a significant number of speakers of Pacific Island languages such as Samoan and Tongan, and increasingly also Asian languages such as Mandarin, Cantonese, Korean and Hindi. As migration patterns have changed in recent years, the New Zealand population has become much more linguistically and ethnically diverse. The proportion of people born overseas has steadily increased from 17% in 1996 to 25.2% in 2013 and, more importantly, the predominant source of new migrants has changed markedly. Between 2001 and 2013, the number of overseas-born migrants from the UK and Ireland dropped from 32 to 26% of all overseas born migrants, whereas overseas-born migrants from Asia increased from 23 to 32%, such that Asia is now the commonest region of birth for the overseas born (Statistics New Zealand, 2013a). There has been a consequential shift in the most commonly spoken 'language in which people could hold a conversation about everyday things' reported in the New Zealand Census (Statistics New Zealand, 2013a). In the most recent Census, conducted in 2013, the top five languages spoken were reported to be English, Maori, Samoan, Hindi and Northern Chinese (which includes Mandarin). In 2006, French was reported as the fourth most common language (although this reflects the fact that French is commonly taught in schools, not that New Zealand has a large number of French-born residents). The New Zealand Census is of limited use, however, in determining how many people need an interpreter for a health consultation, as the question noted above is the only one relating to language proficiency, and this is limited to a self-reported assessment of basic conversational proficiency. The percentage thus lies somewhere between the 2.2% who speak no English and the 18.6% who are multilingual.

This diversity is not evenly spread around the country. New Zealand's largest city, Auckland, has accepted the largest number of new migrants with nearly 40% of its population born overseas, and this demographic reality also has important practical implications for the development and delivery of interpeting services.

The structure of the New Zealand health system

The New Zealand healthcare system has been shaped in part by the need to provide high-quality publicly funded health care for a small population that is unevenly distributed over two narrow main islands approximately 1600 kilometers (1000 miles) in length, comprising a large and often rugged geographic area. As a consequence, New Zealand's health services are quite complex in the way they are structured and also have a number of unique features which are described briefly in this section.

District Health Boards and Primary Health Organisations

New Zealand spends close to the Organisation for Economic Co-operation and Development average per capita on health care, of which 83% comes from government sources (Organisation for Economic Co-operation and Development, 2013). Government funding is distributed by 20 District Health Boards (Ministry of Health, 2014) that together cover all regions of the country. Public hospital services are provided by the District Health Boards and are free of charge to the patient. Primary Care is contracted by the District Health Boards to 32 Primary Health Organizations. Care is provided by primary care services that are members of the Primary Health Organization. These medical services (General Practices) tend to be group practices, owned by the practitioners, by a non-government organization, or, increasingly, by a for-profit organization. Primary Health Organizations are partially funded by government on a capitation basis (a sum of money per patient registered with the practice), with co-payments by the patient making up the balance of the cost. The level of capitation varies according to age (e.g. free care is provided to children under 6) and type of service (e.g. free maternity care), with some weighting for degree of need.

The Accident Compensation Corporation

Health care needed as the result of any accident is funded from a national government-run insurance scheme run by a public organization established for this purpose, the Accident Compensation Corporation. Levies are collected from employers, motor vehicle owners and individuals, and funding is provided on a 'no fault' basis: if the health problem is caused by an accident, then it is covered by the scheme, which provides most of the costs of care and partial income replacement. When the scheme was introduced, the right of individuals to sue other individuals or organizations for damages resulting from accidents was removed. An important consequence of this scheme for the health system is that 'treatment injury' is covered. As a result, in New Zealand there are no lawsuits for medical malpractice, as these episodes are covered by the Accident Compensation Corporation.

Pharmac

New Zealand has a national drug purchasing agency, the Pharmaceutical Management Agency, commonly known as Pharmac. This agency is responsible for purchasing all pharmaceuticals funded by the government in the provision of health care. Pharmac has developed sophisticated processes to maximize the benefit from public money spent on pharmaceuticals, for example by negotiating and coordinating the purchase of pharmaceuticals on behalf of District Health Boards nationwide, or in primary care by subsidising only certain brands (often generic versions) of branded medications prescribed to patients (Pharmac, 2014) This system has gained significant public support, and is also important in that it has resulted in some public acceptance that rationing of care is inevitable and that there needs to be a transparent and fair process for such rationing.

Legal and regulatory framework

There are a number of legal and institutional protections in place for consumers of health services in New Zealand in general, but there are important questions in relation to how well these institutional protections do in fact adequately acknowledge the rights and needs of patients with limited proficiency in English.

Health and Disability Commission

New Zealand has a Health and Disability Commission with jurisdiction over all health and disability service providers: this organization oversees the rights of health consumers and considers formal complaints in relation to health services. This jurisdiction is formalized in the Health and Disability Commissioner's Code of Health and Disability Services Consumers' Rights (Health and Disability Commissioner (Code of Health and Disability Services Consumers' Rights) Regulations, 1996). Right 5, Right to Effective Communication is of particular relevance to the provision of health care to patients with limited English proficiency:

> Every consumer has the right to effective communication in a form, language, and manner that enables the consumer to understand the information provided. Where necessary and reasonably practicable, this includes the right to a competent interpreter. (Health and Disability Commissioner (Code of Health and Disability Services Consumers' Rights) Regulations, 1996)

The limited right to an interpreter is further qualified in:

> Section 3, Provider Compliance:
>
> A provider is not in breach of this Code if the provider has taken reasonable actions in the circumstances to give effect to the rights, and comply with the duties, in this Code. The onus is on the provider to prove it took reasonable actions. For the purposes of this clause, 'the circumstances' means all the relevant circumstances, including the consumer's clinical circumstances and the provider's resource constraints. (Health and Disability Commissioner (Code of Health and Disability Services Consumers' Rights) Regulations, 1996)

This code is administered by an appointed official, the Health and Disability Commissioner. If a person believes that one of their rights under the code has been breached, then they are able to complain to the Commissioner who will, if deemed appropriate, investigate the alleged breach and make findings with recommendations if a breach is found to have occured. Very few complaints are formally investigated however (Health and Disability Commissioner, 2014: 5). The investigation's findings are not legally enforceable themselves, although the commissioner has a significant public profile and adverse findings are usually given prominent coverage in the media. In addition, the commissioner can choose to refer findings to bodies like the New Zealand Medical Council or the Human Rights Tribunal with legal powers to sanction.

Health Practitioners Competence Assurance Act 2003

In 2003 a new law, the Health Practitioners Competence Assurance Act 2003, was passed. This amalgamated the various acts covering the registration of health professionals into one single act ('Health Practitioner's Competence Assurance Act,' New Zealand Government, 2003). The new act covers nearly all practitioners, a total of 16 professions (New Zealand Ministry of Health, 2014), including medicine, nursing, physiotherapy and dentistry. The act states in Section 118 that its purpose is:

> 118(i) 'To set standards of clinical competence, cultural competence, and ethical conduct to be observed by health practitioners of the profession'.

No definition for 'cultural competence' was provided. However the context within which this act was passed was that there was significant pressure from the Maori community to address health outcome inequity. In the early years after the passage of this act much of the focus of cultural competence training related to Maori culture: understanding the history of settlement, the effects of colonization and health outcome disparities for the Maori people. Importantly, as the Maori do not have access issues because of a lack of English, the use of interpreters rarely features in Maori-focused cultural competence training. As a result of the 2003 act, all of the registration authorities have documents on cultural competence, and are responsible for ensuring the competence of health practitioners. They address this by ensuring that undergraduate training adresses the standards of that profession, and that there is a process of ongoing training to maintain competence. Consequently there is an incentive for practitioners to attend training on cultural competence (which could include how to use an interpreter) in order to meet their annual registration requirements. Nine of the 16 cultural competence documents explicitly mention using interpreters currently (Gray, 2014).

Mental Health Compulsory Assessment and Treatment Act 1992

Another law, the Mental Health Compulsory Assessment and Treatment Act 1992 ('Mental Health (Compulsory Assessment and Treatment) Act'; New Zealand Government, 1992) requires in Section 6 that an interpreter must be provided when a person is being assessed under the terms of the act if it is practicable to provide one, and that as far as reasonably practicable competence of the interpreter must be ensured.

Health Quality and Safety Commission

In New Zealand, there is a Health Quality and Safety Commission which aligns with the international standard of the Triple Aim for quality improvement, outlined by the Institute for Health Care Improvement: improved quality, safety and experience of care, improved health and equity for all populations, and better value for public health system resources (Institute for Health Care Improvement, 2015). They have set up a system of reportable events in all public hospitals and are extending the system to include rest homes and primary care. To date they have not done any work specifically relating to communication with limited English proficiency patients. However, in theory at least, the Commission's focus on quality improvement and their use of a systems approach to evaluating adverse events should mean that, as long as the reporting system works well, then issues relating to interpreting will eventually be raised, even if indirectly, and will be addressed where these have impacted on quality performance.

Professional frameworks for interpreters and translators

New Zealand does not yet have a professional structure for interpreters and translators. In 2009, the Office for Ethnic Affairs, which is the government agency responsible for policy and services relating to ethnic communities, said the following in a status report on interpreting services:

> New Zealand has lagged behind in language acquisition as well as provision for language training. We are still in a mono-lingual society – 'everyone speaks English.' There have been some positive developments but unfortunately things have moved at a snail's pace in the provision of language support. Some government agencies have been slow and some reluctant to recognise that there is a legitimate and ongoing need for interpreters and that they have a responsibility to provide equal access to information and services. People with English as a second language are still being asked to bring family members or someone from their community to interpret. More often than not these people are not trained and on some occasions have been children. The deaf community tell of similar experiences. (Clark & McGrath, 2009: 24)

Except for interpreters of Maori and NZSL, New Zealand has no competency or qualifications framework for interpreters or translators, nor is there a registration body. It is possible for any bilingual person to set him- or herself up as an interpreter. Without relying on accreditation from other countries (commonly Australia), a person or organization employing an interpreter can have no idea how competent they are, nor have any meaningful recourse if they do not perform their task well.

Meeting the Needs of Patients with Limited English Proficiency

Health and Disability Commissioner's Code of Health and Disability Services Consumers' Rights

Prior to 1996, there was no expectation in New Zealand that a professional interpreter might be used in a health consultation, nor any mechanism whereby this might be enforced. Unlike the USA, where the case of Ramirez led to a court settlement of $US71 million for failing to use an interpreter (Flores, 2006), people with limited English proficiency in New Zealand do not have similar recourse because of the withdrawal of the right to sue that accompanied the Accident Compensation Act. When the Health and Disability Commissioner's Code of Health and Disability Services Consumers' Rights (Health and Disability Commissioner's Code) was introduced, it initially made little difference to the use of interpreters. The relevant right to effective communication only calls for a 'competent' interpreter and, as discussed above, even this is qualified within the right itself ('where neccessary and reasonably practical') as well as in Section 3 which talks about 'reasonable circumstances' and notes potential 'providers' resource constraints'. Where an interpreter is required but is not provided, over and above issues of patient rights to adequate communication to ensure the safety and quality of the consultation, there are also specific medico-legal issues in relation to ethics and informed consent for procedures. It is not possible to document legally valid informed consent for a major procedure for a patient with limited English proficiency without a registered interpreter (Gray, 2011).

Complaints to the commissioner about breaches of the code are not an immediately effective or guaranteed way of achieving quality improvement. Bismark et al. (2006), in her New Zealand study, documented that, among serious preventable adverse events, only 4% (2/48) resulted in complaints to the Health and Disability Commissioner. Of course any complaint from patients with limited English proficiency about interpreting difficulties or shortcomings is less likely to be made owing to the language barriers inherent in lodging a complaint.

However whilst the complaint process has not had a direct effect on interpreter policy, the Health and Disability Commission's Code requires that health providers must inform consumers of their rights and it is displayed in health service clinics and waiting rooms. As all public hospitals are run by the District Health Boards, they are not only required to give effect to the the Health and Disability Commissioner's Code but are also seen as exemplars for private providers, who may otherwise reason that, if the hospital run by the government does not do it, why should we? As a result, all

District Health Board hospitals have developed individual policies on the use of interpreters, although a review of these policies we conducted in 2011 suggests these are of varying quality with, for example, four of the provincial hospitals still recommending family and friends as the interpreters of first choice. However, the hospitals in the major cities have developed policies more in line with best practice and, as a result, have established a budget to employ interpreters.

Development of interpreting services

Language Line

In 2003, the government established a relationship with Language Line as a publicly funded telephone interpreting service. This was initially aimed at providing services for government departments, but its role soon expanded, initially to all public sector organizations, including in particular all District Health Boards and Primary Healthcare Organizations, and now to all organizations that wish to join. Primary Healthcare Organization and District Health Board users pay a fee for each service episode. As each organization joins Language Line, a trainer visits the organization to train staff on how to use the system and the basics of how to use an interpreter.

This has been a particularly important development because the New Zealand population is spread over a large area. A nationally available telephone interpreting service is the only viable way of ensuring practical access to all health consultations in New Zealand. Language Line currently provides access to 44 languages and has operational links with its sister organization in Australia, the Australian Telephone Interpreting Service for those languages not supported by Language Line interpeters based in New Zealand. Practitioners can ring in and request an interpreter immediately and be connected usually within a minute or two, or they can pre-book an interpreter for a particular appointment. However, unlike the Australian service which is available 24 hours a day, 7 days a week, this subsidised service is still only available in New Zealand for the core business hours of Monday to Friday 9.00 am to 6.00 pm and Saturday 9.00 am to 2.00 pm, owing to government funding constraints

Other interpreting services

Interpreting New Zealand is a not-for-profit organization that provides face to face interpreting in two of the larger cities (Wellington and Christchurch) and also provides telephone interpreting nationally. In Auckand, New Zealand's largest city, the three District Health Boards jointly provide an in-house interpreting service that operates 24 hours a day and covers over 70 languages with both telephone and face-to-face services available. This was set up in 1999, initially providing services to hospital clinicians, and since 2011 has been extended out to primary care. Other District Health Boards around New Zealand contract interpreters on an ad-hoc basis for hospital clinicians. These interpreters may or may not be formally trained.

Interpreter training

The only standard three year undergraduate Bachelors degree course in interpreting is at Auckland University of Technology (AUT), both NZ Sign Language interpreting and foreign language interpreting. There are several, much shorter courses available, for example, a four month intensive course at Unitec Intsitute of Technology in Auckland and an 18 week course through Interpreting New Zealand. All of these courses assume that the student is competent in English and a second language. Owing to the limited amount of interpreting work in New Zealand, most interpreters work across the health, justice, social welfare and commercial fields. Most of the programs provide specific information around health and legal interpreting.

General Practice Standards

As noted above, most primary care in New Zealand is provided by independently owned General Practices. Whilst the model of ownership is changing, historically these practices have been owned by the doctors working within them. Whilst the Health and Disbility Commissioner's Code applies to all these practices, until recently few practices had a policy on the use of interpreters or had ever employed a professional interpreter.

The Royal New Zealand College of General Practitioners (RNZCGP) runs a practice accreditation program. This was first started in 2000. 'Aiming for Excellence' was the publication setting out the collection of standards. Editions 1–3 (Royal New Zealand College General Practitioners, 2000, 2002, 2008) made little explicit mention of the needs of people with limited English proficiency other than citing the Health and Disability Commission code and having a 'desirable' standard (as opposed to an essential standard), which states that the practice 'has identified appropriate local resource people and organizations including interpreters and translators' (Royal New Zealand College General Practitioners, 2002: 15). The fourth edition, published in 2011, makes more mention of the need for interpreters and translators in the commentary of various standards, but the actual criteria are still very weak and still only 'developmental' rather than 'essential', stating that 'The practice team can access interpreters and resources for people with limited English proficiency' (Royal New Zealand College General Practitioners, 2011: 19). There is no standard that requires interpreters to be used for limited English proficiency patients. However, a new standard under patient records requires that the records show (a) primary language; (b) whether or not an interpreter is needed; (c) English proficiency limitations and (d) name of interpreter used, if applicable (Royal New Zealand College General Practitioners, 2011: 43–44). Part of a practice audit is to examine a sample of patient records against these criteria to determine any missing items. As a result, all practices being audited will have had these elements drawn to their attention even if they have not yet implemented them.

The practice standards also refer to staff having cultural competence training, which is a requirement for the individual professionals under their professional registration requirements.

Much of the reluctance to develop stronger standards has been due to the lack of a funding stream to pay for interpreters. Many primary healthcare organizations have a budget for 'Services to improve access' which can be utilized to pay for interpreters, but these are small budgets.

Auckland developments

As the largest city with the most diverse (and growing) community, it is not surprising that Auckland has moved further than the rest of the country in responding to the needs of limited English proficiency patients. There has been a particularly rapid increase in the Asian population in Auckland and, as a result, an Asian health unit was set up at the Waitemata District Health Board. This unit has been influential in developing a comprehensive set of training resources for the staff in the three Auckland District Health Boards, to address cross-cultural care in general and how to use an interpreter in particular (Asian Health Services Waitemata District Health Board, 2010). As noted above, the Auckland District Health Boards have also established an interpreting service that was first made available to the hospital clinicians and since 2011 has provided services to all primary care clinicians in the wider Auckland area. Unlike the rest of the country, this is funded from the District Health Boards budget rather than from the Primary Healthcare Organizations and so is not at the expense of other Primary Healthcare Organization services.

Uptake of interpreter services

There have been two New Zealand studies on uptake of interpreters. A small study in a metropolitan hospital (Gray et al., 2011b) found that, for 22 consultations (mostly in the emergency department) where an interpreter was needed, not a single professional interpreter was used. A study of interpreter usage in General Practices in Christchurch (the largest city in the South Island; Seers et al., 2013) made a calculation based on Census demographic and self-reported language proficiency data to estimate the number of consultations that would have required an interpreter, and compared this with the number of professional interpreters actually employed by the practices over the same time and geographic area. They used the conservative Census figure of those who spoke a language but did not speak English (2.2% of the population). They concluded that a professional interpreter was used in only 75 out of 10,742 (0.7%) of the consultations that might have needed an interpreter according to this criterion. As noted above, the New Zealand Census question does not provide any information on fluency for those who speak some English, and so it is likely that many more than 2.2% of the population in fact require an interpreter for effective consultations. The provision of interpreters in primary care in Christchurch was therefore clearly inadequate.

Bilingual clinicians

Unlike the USA, which has a large preponderance of Spanish speakers in its LEP population, New Zealand has a relatively few speakers of many languages. The commonest languages needing an interpreter (Samoan, Hindi and Mandarin) are rarely learned by people who have English as a first language, unless they are from the relevant ethnic group. As a result most of the bilingual providers will have English as a second language. In primary care a bilingual clinician will attract a language-congruent practice, but because of the relative infrequency of any particular foreign language, hospital clinicians are unlikely to have many patients of their own who speak their native language. They may be called upon by other clinicians to assist, but this is fraught with problems of role definition; are they the clinician responsible or are they an interpreter?

A Research Journey

Bilingual medical students

Our research team began investigation of this topic area with a study on bilingual medical students being asked to use their native languages with limited English proficiency patients in hospital wards (Yang & Gray, 2008). This study was stimulated by some reflective student essays describing episodes of ethical concern. For example, in one case a junior student reported being asked to gain consent for a procedure on a child from the child's father using Mandarin. The main concern in this case was that she was asked to conduct the consultation, not just interpret what the senior doctor wanted to say. In addition the student perceived a possible conflict between the request to interpret and her role as a medical student, exacerbated by her concerns that she had no training or experience as an interpreter, and that her medical training had been entirely in English, which meant that she lacked knowledge of the relevant medical terminology in Mandarin. However, we also suspected that there might on occasion be advantages of students working in this way, both for the student and for the patient. Of the 102 bilingual medical students we identified, half had been asked at some time to interpret and most felt that it had been a good experience, although there were also several examples of difficult episodes. From in-depth interviews, we identified the benefits and risks of students being involved with patients in this way and developed guidance for students and health professionals on how to manage this circumstance safely. We emphasized the importance of the student making a judgment as to whether it would be appropriate for them to interpret in a particular instance taking into account several variables. These included degree of fluency, confusion of the roles of student and interpreter, the availability of a professional interpreter, the degree of urgency of the case and the fact they did not have training in interpreting.

Audits of interpreter use

One of the team (B.G.) is a general practitioner who works in a primary care service with a high number of limited English proficiency patients and a long history of working with interpreters (James & Newtown Union Health Service, 2009). Compared with others in the same city and region, this practice is a very high user of professional interpreter services, including Language Line, a professional interpreting service and several professional interpreters employed part-time at the practice. A simple audit was done of all clinical staff (doctors, nurses and midwives) at the practice to find out how many interpreted consultations they did and whether a professional or ad-hoc interpreter was used (Gray et al., 2011a). Information about language ability of the clinicians was not formally collected, although very few spoke a foreign language spoken by the patients. In this practice, where clinicians were experienced in the use of interpreters, the audit found that 50% of interpreted consultations still involved ad hoc interpreters such as family members, contrary to the general advice that professional interpreters should always be used where practicable. The audit also found that in 75% of these consultations the clinicians reported that they felt that the consultation 'worked well'.

As already noted, our group subsequently did a small prospective study of actual interpreter use and a survey of staff attitudes in our local hospital. We found that, whilst there was some awareness of both the need for interpreters and the clinical risk of not using a professional interpreter, and the hospital did have policy in place and provided access to interpreting services, no professional interpreters were used by the clinicians surveyed for any of the limited English proficiency patient cases we studied (Gray et al., 2011b).

How do we know whether an interpreted consultation 'works'?

During the peer review process of the paper on the audit of interpreters in primary care (Gray et al., 2011a), one reviewer was critical of our asking the clinicians how well their interpreted interactions 'worked' without validating our conclusions on the basis of some other kind of empirical data. We agreed that this was indeed a limitation of the study, but our review of the research literature had also showed that establishing a reliable answer to this question is far from straightforward. Much of the guidance for clinicians on interpreter use uncritically asserts that using professional interpreters is an imperative (Miletic et al., 2006), but this advice is based predominantly on anecdotes of bad outcomes when professional interpreters were not used. Implicit in this assertion also is the presumption that with a professional interpreter all will automatically be well, which fails to take account of other factors that may affect the quality of the interpreting or outcomes.

Whilst there is certainly good research evidence suggesting that quality of care and outcomes are generally better when professional interpreters are used, the literature on the use of interpreters in health care also includes reports that there can be different benefits of using trained interpreters (accuracy, confidentiality, ethical behavior) and untrained interpreters (continuity, trust, mitigating patient resistance to strangers as interpreters). Moreover, there has been relatively little research on the actual patterns of interaction in interpreter-mediated consultations, with most studies focusing on self-reported data from interviews with only one or perhaps two of the parties involved.

Our research team is part of the Applied Research on Communication in Health Group, which has done significant work on the complexity of clinical communication through the close study of authentic video-recorded medical consultations conducted in English (e.g. Dew et al., 2008, 2010; Dowell et al., 2007; Morgan, 2013; Moriarty et al., 2012; Stubbe et al. 2015). This work aligns with a large body of health interaction research internationally, which clearly demonstrates the complexity of interaction in routine health encounters, and that even when both parties are fluent in the same language, issues of understanding arise regularly. That being the case, it is to be expected that adding the complexity of two languages and another party to the interaction will affect the overall complexity of the communication.

We therefore designed our next study to allow us to develop a more robust understanding of the interactional processes that occur in interpreter-mediated consultations, and to gain insight into the perceptions of all participants, not just those of the clinicians (Stubbe et al., 2014; Gray et al., 2016). We video-recorded 18 interpreted general practitioner consultations and interviewed each General Practitioner, patient and interpreter involved immediately afterwards. We had a mix of professional interpreters, family members and bilingual staff in the role of interpreter, and the data set also included some telephone interpreted consultations. The General Practitioners were all experienced in working with interpreters.

Results have yet to be published but the themes that emerged from the study confirmed the complexity of these interactions and highlighted the potential for a lack of role clarity, particularly with family member interpreters, a point that has been widely reported and discussed previously in the literature. The data analysis also revealed much useful detail illustrating effective practice as well as less effective practice, and produced some new findings. For example, we observed many instances where the doctors successfully managed consultations involving family members in a dual role as interpreters, a situation which the parties all considered had added benefits in terms of continuity of care beyond the consulting room. However, it was also clear that, by comparison with having a professional interpreter present, working with a lay interpreter required additional work and a great deal of extra skill on the part of the doctor. We found that patients who have some English, but who still need an interpreter, raise a particular issue that is not often mentioned in the literature. For instance, we had cases where the interpreter interrupted the consultation when it became clear that the patient (and doctor) had thought they understood the doctor's English but in fact had not.

Developing evidence-based guidance for practitioners

How to use interpreters in general practice: A toolkit

In writing the paper on the audit of interpreter use at B.G.'s practice it became very clear that interpreter use in General Practice in New Zealand was very much the exception rather than the rule. Our literature review had similarly shown that low uptake of interpreters was an international problem (e.g. Shuangyu et al., 2010; Huang & Phillips, 2009) and there was no consensus as to why this was happening. At this time there was a significant focus in New Zealand on patient safety and taking a systems approach to improving this (Health Quality and Safety Commission, 2014). In addition, the RNZCGP was developing resources to help practices wanting to improve their service quality. We developed an evidence-based toolkit on best practice in the use of interpreters in General Practice described in Gray et al. (2012) for use by the RNZCGP as a worked example of a quality improvement cycle in a primary care practice to support the College's quality accreditation program, Aiming for Excellence, described above. This is now available as an online module to all General Practices in New Zealand (Gray & Perera, 2012). Our aim was to take a systems approach to the problem of low uptake of interpreters for limited English proficiency patients and attempt to identify the many elements of a practice system that might provide a barrier to the uptake of interpreters. We are currently also designing a set of educational resources based on our research and consultation recordings for New Zealand health professionals to support development of the clinical skill of using an interpreter.

Medical Council ethical and legislative guidelines

The New Zealand Medical Council publishes a guide to Medical Practice in New Zealand which states: 'The book's main purpose is to introduce new entrants to medical practice in New Zealand to the main legislative and ethical standards and guidelines' (New Zealand Medical Council, 2013: 2). As a result of an approach by one of the authors of this chapter, a section on how to use interpreters was added to this guide (Gray, 2013).

Discussion

The New Zealand regulatory structure for providing health care in the context of language barriers is still developing. A major deficit in the current structure is the absence of a regulatory body for interpreters. This makes it hard for clinicians to know how competent an interpreter is. If an interpreter behaves unprofessionally, only those working for an employer (Language Line, Interpreting NZ) are able to be sanctioned and there would be nothing to stop an interpreter fired from one of those organizations from continuing to practice on their own.

The patient code of rights and RNZCGP practice standards are also very weak in relation to provision of interpreting and, given the recent increased availability of interpreters, could reasonably be strengthened. As noted above, while the uptake of interpreters in the health sector is slowly increasing, it is still woefully inadequate. The focus on patient rights in the Health and Disability Commissioner's Code and, in particular, on the importance of informed consent has not resulted in an increased use of interpreters in general. One exception to this is the use of interpreters by psychiatrists when applying the Mental Health Act, which is is anecdotally common in the capital Wellington, but there is no systematic data on how this is being managed. We are hopeful that the focus on fair distribution of resources that is part of the triple aim of the Health Quality and Safety Commission, and the Pharmac model of ensuring best outcome for the dollar spent, will eventually lead to some change in the usage of interpreters. Current access to health services is unfair for limited English proficient patients, and there are examples of resources being wasted as a result of not using interpreters. Both of these problems would be improved with more widespread provision of interpreter services.

Few clinicians in New Zealand have received training on how to use an interpreter. This set of skills is not routinely included in the training of medical students in New Zealand and is unlikely to be included in the training of other health professionals in the absence of policy changes. A consequence of this lack of training is a lack of awareness of the limitations of interpreting aids, particularly computer applications. There is a long history of 'making do'. In addition, we need to teach the clinical skill of how to make the judgment about whether the means of communication that we are using is adequate for the clinical situation we face with limited English proficiency patients (Gray, 2013: 85) An adult family member may be adequate for discussing the care of a minor illness, but discussion of the options for treatment of a cancer would certainly require a professional interpreter. Further research is needed to better understand the clinical circumstances in which family members would be reasonable interpreters.

A complicating factor in considering the care of culturally and linguistically diverse patient groups is the fact that adequate communication is just one, albeit a very significant, ingredient of equitable care. Whitehead defined inequity in health care as referring to: 'differences which are unnecessary and avoidable but, in addition, are also considered unfair and unjust' (Whitehead, 1992: 219). It is indisputable that, if a clinician and patient have no shared language, then there is little possibility of receiving equitable care. However, in the presence of cultural difference (which is inevitably present if language is not shared), providing an interpreter does not ensure equitable care. There is an extensive and growing literature on cultural competence addressing what might be required to improve health outcome inequalities. There is a risk that, in focusing on language barriers, we fail to adequately address the other barriers that minority cultural groups face in accessing equitable health care. It is important that any evaluation of changes in care looks not only at whether interpreting services have been provided, but also at whether health outcomes have been improved as a result.

Conclusion

From our research and understanding of the New Zealand context and the international evidence, we recommend a pragmatic, stepwise, systems-focused approach to improving health care in the context of language barriers. Such an approach could be applied to any jurisdiction and the detail would vary depending on circumstances. For New Zealand the elements that we have identified are as follows.

Governance of the provision of interpreters

(1) Set up a registration body for interpreters.
(2) Seek amendment to the Health and Disability Commissioner's Code to strengthen the requirement for use of interpreters in general, and to introduce wording similar to the Mental Health Act when obtaining informed consent for major procedures.
(3) Lobby government to fund interpreting services centrally rather than from service budgets. Australia has a fully funded telephone interpreter service upon which we could base a New Zealand model.
(4) Continue work to ensure that standards throughout the health sector include the provision of an interpreter where needed.

Service organization

(5) Ensure that all patient records include a field on preferred language and whether an interpreter is required.

(6) Ensure that all health service providers have the ability to contact interpreters when needed and that there is a budget (if not funded centrally) to pay for them.
(7) Ensure that all service providers have policies and practices that address broader issues of cultural competence.

Training

(8) Ensure all health professionals have tuition during their undergraduate training on how to use an interpreter.
(9) Provide access for all postgraduate clinicians to training on how to use an interpreter.
(10) Focus on the clinical judgment of whether the communication mode being used whilst seeing a limited English proficiency patient is adequate for the purposes of that particular consultation or if further help is needed.
(11) Ensure that all clinicians have undergraduate and postgraduate training on cultural competence.

In conclusion, receiving equitable healthcare services is a fundamental right and should not depend on whether patients speak the dominant language, or are part of the dominant culture of the country within which they live. The above recommendations are based on sound evidence, and their implementation would involve a number of simple practical steps that can be introduced progressively. Adopting these policies and practices would demonstrably improve the safety and quality of health service provision to limited English proficiency patients, and would go some way toward enabling better health outcomes for this vulnerable group.

References

Asian Health Services Waitemata District Health Board (2010) CALD Resources. See http://www.caldresources.org.nz/info/CourseLanding.php (accessed 6 January 2014).
Bismark, M.M., Brennan, T.A., Paterson, R.J., Davis, P.B. and Studdert, D.M. (2006) Relationship between complaints and quality of care in New Zealand: A descriptive analysis of complainants and non-complainants following adverse events. *Quality and Safety in Health Care* 15 (1), 17–22; doi: 10.1136/qshc.2005.015743
Clark, D. and McGrath, C. (eds) (2009) *Interpreting in New Zealand the Pathway Forward*. Wellington New Zealand: The Office of Ethnic Affairs.
Dew, K., Dowell, A.C., Stubbe, M., Plumridge, E. and Macdonald, L. (2008) Treating patients differently: A qualitative study of how clinical and social factors shape interactions between doctors and patients. *New Zealand Family Physician* 35, 382–386.
Dew, K., Stubbe, M., Macdonald, L., Dowell, A. and Plumridge, E. (2010) The (non) use of prioritisation protocols by surgeons. *Sociology of Health and Illness* 32 (4), 545–562.
Dowell, A.C., Macdonald, L., Stubbe, M., Plumridge, E. and Dew, K. (2007) Clinicians at work: What can we learn from interactions in the consultation? *New Zealand Family Physician* 34, 345–350.

Flores, G. (2006) Language barriers to health care in the United States. *New England Journal of Medicine* 355 (3), 229–231; doi: 10.1056/NEJMp058316

Gray, B. (2011) Informed consent in patients with limited English proficiency. *New Zealand Health and Hospital* 63 (3), 1.

Gray, B. (2013) The use of interpreters. In I. St George (ed.) *Cole's Medical Practice in New Zealand* (12th edn). Wellington: Medical Council of New Zealand.

Gray, B. (2014) How does the concept of cultural competence affect the practice of bioethics and health law. Centre for Bioethics. Masters of Bioethics and Health Law. See http://hdl.handle.net/10523/5472

Gray, B. and Perera, R. (2012) Improving communication for patients with limited English proficiency. See http://www.rnzcgp.org.nz/assets/documents/Standards—Policy/LimitedEnglishProficiencyModule4web.pdf (accessed 5 January 2015).

Gray, B., Hilder, J. and Donaldson, H. (2011a) Why do we not use trained interpreters for all patients with limited English proficiency? Is there a place for using family members? *Australian Journal of Primary Health* 17 (3), 240–249.

Gray, B., Stanley, J., Stubbe, M. and Hilder, J. (2011b) Communication difficulties with limited English proficiency patients: Clinician perceptions of clinical risk and patterns of use of interpreters. *The New Zealand Medical Journal* 124 (1342), 23.

Gray, B., Hilder, J. and Stubbe, M. (2012) How to use interpreters in general practice: The development of a New Zealand toolkit. *Journal of Primary Health Care* 3, 18.

Gray, B., Hilder, J., Macdonald, L., Tester, R., Dowell, A. and Stubbe, M. (2016) Are research ethics guidelines culturally competent? *Research Ethics* 20, 1–19.

Health and Disability Commissioner (2014) Annual Report 2014. See http://www.hdc.org.nz/publications/other-publications-from-hdc/annual-reports?page=2 (accessed 5 January 2015).

Health and Disability Commissioner (Code of Health and Disability Services Consumers Rights) Regulations (1996). New Zealand Health and Disability Commission. See http://www.hdc.org.nz/the-act--code/the-code-of-rights/the-code-(full) (accessed 16 January 2017).

Health Quality and Safety Commission (2014) About the Commission. See http://www.hqsc.govt.nz/about-the-commission/ (accessed 5 January 2015).

Higgins, R. and Keane, B. (2014) Te reo Māori – the Māori language – Language decline, 1900 to 1970s. *Te Ara – the Encyclopedia of New Zealand*. See http://www.teara.govt.nz/en/te-reo-maori-the-maori-language/ (accessed 23 December 2014).

Hill, S., Sarfati, D., Blakely, T., Robson, B., Purdie, G., Dennett, E., Cormack, D., Dew, K., Ayanian, J.Z. and Kawachi, I. (2010) Ethnicity and management of colon cancer in New Zealand. *Cancer* 116 (13), 3205–3214; doi: 10.1002/cncr.25127

Huang, Y.T. and Phillips, C. (2009) Telephone interpreters in general practice – Bridging the barriers to their use. *Australian Family Physician* 38 (6), 443–446.

Institute for Health Care Improvement (2015) Triple Aim for Populations. See http://www.ihi.org/Topics/TripleAim/Pages/default.aspx (accessed 15 February 2015).

James, K. and Newtown Union Health Service (2009) *Health for the people: Newtown Union Health Service, 20 Years On.* Wellington: Steele Roberts.

Miletic, T., Piu, M., Minas, H., Stankovska, M., Stolk, Y. and Klimidis, S. (2006) *Guidelines for Working Effectively with Interpreters in Mental Health Settings.* Victoria, Australia: Victorian Transcultural Psychiatry Unit.

Ministry of Health (2014) The New Zealand Health and Disability System: Organisations and Responsibilities: Briefing to the Minister of Health. See http://www.health.govt.nz/publication/new-zealand-health-and-disability-system-organisations-and-responsibilities (accessed 23 December 2014).

Morgan, S. (2013) Miscommunication between patients and general practitioners: Implications for clinical practice. *Journal of Primary Health Care* 5 (2), 123–128.

Moriarty, H.J., Stubbe, M.H., Chen, L., Tester, R.M., Macdonald, L.M., Dowell, A.C. and Dew, K.P. (2012) Challenges to alcohol and other drug discussions in the general practice consultation. *Family Practice* 29 (2), 213–222; doi: 10.1093/fampra/cmr082

New Zealand Government (1992) *Mental Health (Compulsory Assessment and Treatment) Act*.

New Zealand Government (2003) *Health Practitioner's Competence Assurance Act*.

New Zealand Medical Council (2013) *Cole's Medical Practice in New Zealand*, I. St George (ed.). See https://www.mcnz.org.nz/news-and-publications/cole-s-medical-practice-in-new-zealand/

New Zealand Ministry of Health (2014) Responsible Authorities under the Act. See http://www.health.govt.nz/our-work/regulation-health-and-disability-system/health-practitioners-competence-assurance-act/responsible-authorities-under-act (accessed 6 January 2015).

Organisation for Economic Co-operation and Development (2013) Health at a glance 2013: OECD indicators. See http://dx.doi.org/10.1787/health_glance-2013-en (accessed 23 December 2014).

PHARMAC (2014) Making funding decisions. See http://www.pharmac.health.nz/about/your-guide-to-pharmac/ (accessed 6 January 2015).

Royal New Zealand College General Practitioners (2000) *Aiming for Excellence*. Wellington: Royal New Zealand College of General Practitioners.

Royal New Zealand College General Practitioners (2002) *Aiming for Excellence*. Wellington: Royal New Zealand College of General Practitioners.

Royal New Zealand College General Practitioners (2008) *Aiming For Excellence: RNZCGP Standard for New Zealand General Practice*. Wellington: Royal New Zealand College of General Practitioners.

Royal New Zealand College General Practitioners (2011) *Aiming for Excellence*. See from https://www.rnzcgp.org.nz/quality-standards/ (accessed 6 January 2015).

Rumball-Smith, J., Sarfati, D., Hider, P. and Blakely, T. (2013) Ethnic disparities in the quality of hospital care in New Zealand, as measured by 30-day rate of unplanned readmission/death. *International Journal for Quality in Health Care* 25 (3), 248–254.

Seers, K., Cook, L., Abel, G., Schluter, P. and Bridgford, P. (June 2013) Is it time to talk? Interpreter services use in general practice within Canterbury. *Jourrnal of Primary Healthcare* 5 (2), 129.

Shuangyu, L., Pearson, D. and Escott, S. (2010) Language barriers within primary care consultations: an increasing challenge needing new solutions. *Education for Primary Care* 21 (6), 385–391.

Statistics New Zealand (2013a) 2013 QuickStats; Cultural diversity. See http://www.statisticsnz.govt.nz/Census/2013-census/profile-and-summary-reports/quickstats-about-national-highlights/cultural-diversity.aspx (accessed 18 December 2014).

Statistics New Zealand (2013b) Census totals by topic official language indicator. See http://www.stats.govt.nz/Census/2013-census/data-tables/total-by-topic.aspx (accessed 23 December 2014).

Stevens, W.M.D., Stevens, G.M.D.F., Kolbe, J.M.F. and Cox, B.M.P.F. (2008) Ethnic differences in the management of lung cancer in New Zealand. *Journal of Thoracic Oncology* 3 (3), 237–244.

Stubbe, M., Macdonald, L., Hilder, J., Tester, R., Gray B. and Dowell, T. (2014) Negotiating role boundaries in interpreter mediated consultations – processes and perceptions. Paper presented at the *European Association of Communication in Health Care International Conference*, Amsterdam. See http://www.each-conference.com/wp-content/uploads/2014/05/EACH2014_abstracts.pdf

Stubbe, M., White, S., Macdonald, L., Dew, K., Dowell, A. and Gardner, R. (2015) Do surgeons want to operate? Negotiating the treatment plan in surgical consultations. In S. White and J. Cartmill (eds) *Communcation in Surgical Practice*. London: Equinox.

Taonui, R. (2013) 'Ngā tuakiri hōu – new Māori identities – Māori renaissance'. *Te Ara – the Encyclopedia of New Zealand.* See http://www.teara.govt.nz/en/nga-tuakiri-hou-new-maori-identities (accessed 3 February 2015).

Whitehead, M. (1992) The concepts and principles of equity and health. *International Journal of Health Services* 22 (3), 429–445.

Wilson, J. (2015) History – Māori arrival and settlement'. *Te Ara – the Encyclopedia of New Zealand.* See http://www.TeAra.govt.nz/en/history/page-1 (accessed 3 February 2015).

Yang, C.-F. and Gray, B. (2008) Bilingual medical students as interpreters – What are the benefits and risks? *New Zealand Medical Journal* 121(1282), 15–28.

12 Toward a New Approach for Culturally and Linguistically Responsive Health Care: A Case Study of Developments in Victoria, Australia

Lidia Horvat

> *Victoria, Australia, has one of the most culturally and linguistically diverse populations in the world and a strong history of policy, programmatic and legislative initiatives in building accessible and equitable health care. Strategic approaches to overcoming language barriers in health care are part and parcel of developing a more coherent healthcare framework for all consumers, patients and communities. This chapter considers key policy initiatives in Victoria, such as the Cultural Responsiveness Framework, which sets standards for culturally and linguistically responsive health care in hospital settings including interpreter provision. It also draws upon insights gained from a recent evaluation of the impact of this policy, and participation in an international pilot of Equity Standards. Considerations for a new framework will be outlined, including equity and cultural responsiveness as key components of quality and safety in health care.*

Introduction

Victoria, Australia, has one of the most culturally and linguistically diverse populations in the world. It has a strong history of policy, programmatic and legislative initiatives in building accessible and equitable health care. Strategic approaches to overcoming language barriers in health care are part and parcel of developing a more coherent healthcare framework for all consumers, patients and communities. Strategies to build a more responsive healthcare system are numerous and diverse in foci. However, identifying what works best, where and for whom, and how to improve care and health outcomes in culturally and linguistically diverse patient groups, remains an ongoing challenge.

This chapter focuses on policy development initiatives in Victoria. It examines how a strategy around standards for culturally responsive care is evolving toward a more coherent framework. The Cultural Responsiveness Framework: Guidelines for Victorian Health Services (CRF) set standards for culturally and linguistically responsive health care in hospital settings including a standard for accredited interpreter provision.

The chapter also considers the inception of the framework and its efforts to embed cultural and linguistic diversity within a quality and safety paradigm. It also draws upon insights gained from a recent review of the impact of this policy, and considers current initiatives including an international pilot of equity standards to focus on key considerations and opportunities for a new framework. Such a framework may bring together key interrelated approaches with common underlying principles. These approaches include equity, person- and family-centered care, health literacy, consumer participation and engagement, human rights, cultural responsiveness and healthcare experience, as key contributors to quality and safety in health care. Considerations and opportunities for a new framework will be posed.

Diversity *is* the Mainstream

Australia is a multicultural and multilingual nation. It has a rich indigenous history spanning at least 50,000 years, and a long history of migration, particularly the mass migration programs commencing after the Second World War, initially predominantly from the UK and Europe. A unique feature of Australia is its successive policy formulations of multiculturalism which began in the early 1970s. Multiculturalism recognized that the Australian population was founded upon successive waves of migration resulting in a broad mix of cultures, languages, identities and experiences. Premised at the outset upon tolerance and acceptance of different cultural identities, multiculturalism became synonymous with people's right to express their languages, cultural identities and practices without discrimination. It focused on shared values, experiences and the benefits that cultural diversity brings, both socially and economically. Not without its challenges, and with supporters and detractors, multiculturalism as a policy continues to evolve as a work in progress.

The claim that Australia is a successful multicultural society is particularly true of the state of Victoria – Australia's most culturally and linguistically diverse state. For Victoria, diversity *is* the mainstream. This is borne out by the most recent Census of 2011, which shows that over 26% of Victorians were born overseas in more than 200 countries. This increases to almost half the Victorian population (over 46%) when you combine Victorians who were either born overseas or have at least one parent born overseas. A large proportion, over 74% of the total overseas born, came from non-mainly English-speaking countries. In addition, 23% of Victorians spoke a language other than English at home and over 67% of Victorians followed one of 135 faiths (Victorian Multicultural Commission, State Government of Victoria, 2011a, 2011b).

This diversity is also increasingly complex. More recent trends in migration and settlement to Victoria have seen an increase in arrivals from North Africa, the Middle East, South-East Asia, North-East Asia and, in particular, Southern and Central Asia. Numbers from these areas have increased in both absolute numbers and as a proportion of the total. Of note, the biggest increase of people settling in Victoria more recently is in those from refugee backgrounds (approximately 4000 people per annum) and asylum seekers (estimated at approximately 10,000 people per annum; Department of Health, 2014). State of Victoria receives around one-third of all refugee and asylum seeker entrants and also receives a high proportion of those who move from their initial location (Department of Health, 2014: 33).

Against this diverse demographic backdrop, the challenges posed to our healthcare system are complex, fluid and ongoing. Increasingly, health professionals and healthcare organizations are required to provide high-quality, safe, culturally and linguistically responsive heath care to very diverse population groups, individuals and communities with varying and complex needs and vulnerabilities.

Policy and Legislation

Although Australia's healthcare system is a mixture of both public and private healthcare providers, predominantly it is known for its universal public healthcare system called Medicare. It also has two other national subsidy schemes: the pharmaceutical benefits scheme, which lists government subsidised medicines to patients with a Medicare card, and a private health insurance rebate, an income-tested private health insurance rebate for people who have private health insurance. National health policies, regulation and funding are developed by the Australian Government. State and Territory Governments are mainly responsible for the delivery and management of public health services as well as the regulation of private hospitals. Health professionals, however, are regulated at a national rather than a state level. Governments at both state and federal levels have developed policy and legislative frameworks for health care which reflect the core principles of multiculturalism and clearly stipulate the requirement for health service systems and health professionals to become more culturally responsive in order to ensure high-quality healthcare provision for the whole population.

Victoria has a strong history of policy, programmatic and legislative initiatives in building accessible and equitable health care. It prides itself in being a national leader in the provision of responsive, integrated and innovative health care (Department of Health, 2014). Despite the different emphases of successive governments, Victoria has maintained a commitment to respecting and responding to diversity as a central feature of state government policies over many decades. Key health policy frameworks such as the Cultural Diversity Guide and the Language Services Policy developed in 2005, both of which articulated strategies for responding to cultural and linguistic diversity considerations in services planning, design and implementation, including the provision of interpreting and translation services, continue to be well utilized today in their new iterations.

The term 'culturally and linguistically diverse' (CALD) is utilized in Australia to commonly refer to people and communities from immigrant and refugee backgrounds. CALD refers to 'the range of different cultures and language groups represented in the population who identify as having particular cultural or linguistic affiliations by virtue of their place of birth, ancestry or ethnic origin, religion, preferred language or language spoken at home' (Department of Health, 2009). Essentially, it distinguishes between communities that may differ from the mainstream dominant culture. It also reflects intergenerational and contextual issues, not only referring to migrant experience. The term does not include Aboriginal or Torres Strait Islander people who are the first peoples of Australia. Separate and distinct policy frameworks address the health, education and participation inequalities experienced by Aboriginal or Torres Strait Islander people.

The term 'CALD' itself is viewed somewhat problematically, with critics suggesting that it continues to marginalize and essentialize difference and that we are *all members of a* culturally and linguistically diverse community. Contributing to this are different conceptualizations and usage of terms to identify and describe patients and communities from diverse population groups which may include different understandings of identity, culture, ethnicity and race. CALD, nevertheless, continues to be widely utilized in policy frameworks even if it may eventually be reconceptualized.

Equity in health care

Equity in health care means that we all have the same and equal right to access and receive high-quality and safe health care, regardless of cultural, linguistic and religious and socioeconomic considerations. This does not mean that everyone receives the same care but rather that all persons have their health care needs equally well met (Department of Health, 2009: 11). It also stipulates that factors that can potentially contribute to differential patient outcomes (e.g. access to accredited interpreters, culturally inclusive care) should be addressed, responded to and minimized (Weinick *et al.*, 2008).

However, access to and utilization of health services and receiving high-quality health care are not the same for everyone. A strong evidence base has emerged (predominantly within the US and Europe) for the provision of culturally competent and responsive health care. Evidence of health inequities and poorer quality health care and outcomes among people from culturally and linguistically diverse backgrounds (Betancourt et al., 2003; Smedley et al., 2003; Flores, 2005; Divi et al., 2007; Task Force on MFCCH, 2010; Ingleby et al., 2012a, 2012b; Mladovsky et al., 2012a, 2012b) has increasingly been utilized by policy-makers and researchers to mount persuasive arguments for the provision of culturally and linguistically responsive health care. In their pilot study of Language Proficiency and Adverse Events in US Hospitals, Divi et al. (2007) confirm that patient–provider communication is a serious patient safety concern and a common root cause of adverse events in healthcare delivery. Their study clearly showed that patients with low English proficiency receive poorer quality health care compared with mainstream patients, and are more likely to experience a 'trajectory of accident opportunity' and/or adverse events in their journey through the health system.

Health inequities and lower quality care are exacerbated when healthcare professionals fail to address ethnicity, culture and language in the provision of health services (Wilson-Stronks et al., 2008). Additional factors such as legal and administrative barriers, lack of familiarity with the health system, socioeconomic determinants and inappropriateness of health services (Mladovsky et al., 2012a, 2012b; Ingleby et al., 2012a, 2012b) can further exacerbate specific and or pre-existing vulnerabilities arising from migration, refugee and asylum seeker experiences, and continue to entrench poorer health status and outcomes. Many of these findings are not only generalizable to the Australian context, but they have also provided a useful evidence base upon which to frame key initiatives in Victoria. Moreover, research within Australia also substantiates the link between culture, language and patient safety outcomes (Heaney & Moreham, 2002; Johnstone & Kanitsaki, 2006; Berner, 2010).

Importantly, to strengthen policy frameworks, Victoria has a legislative base for the support of cultural and linguistic diversity responsiveness. The Racial and Religious Tolerance Act 2001 and the Equal Opportunity Act 2010 are two examples designed to protect Victorians against varied forms of discrimination. Both are underpinned by the Charter of Human Rights and Responsibilities Act 2006, which is designed to protect human rights in Victoria. This Act requires explicit public sector individual and institutional adherence to the promotion and preservation of human rights in decision-making, policy and legislative developments. Significantly, Victoria also has a Multicultural Victoria Act 2011, which recognizes and values the cultural, religious, racial and linguistic diversity of its citizens. The Act outlines a set of principles that promote respect for Victoria's cultural, religious and linguistic diversity.

Three core principles are enshrined within in the Act include:

(1) valuing cultural, religious and linguistic diversity;
(2) recognizing citizenship, expressed as the rights and responsibilities of all people in a multicultural society, as a central tenet of multiculturalism;
(3) ensuring the freedom and opportunity for all Victorians to preserve and express their cultural heritage (Victorian Multicultural Commission, State Government of Victoria, 2011a, 2011b).

A core feature of the Act is the requirement of Government departments to report annually to the Minister for Multicultural Affairs and Citizenship and to Parliament on their achievements in multicultural affairs over the past financial year. Departments are required to report on a range of initiatives and achievements which include the following:

- major improvements (or initiatives developed) to promote multiculturalism and meet the identified needs of Victoria's CALD communities;
- use of interpreting and translating services;
- communications in languages other than English;
- progress under departmental Cultural Diversity Plans to address provision for culturally sensitive service delivery;
- measures to promote human rights in accordance with the Charter for Human Rights and Responsibilities for multicultural communities (Victorian Multicultural Commission, State Government of Victoria 2011a, 2011b).

Attending to Diversity in the Quality and Safety Space

Finding the best ways to respond appropriately to the healthcare inequities experienced by culturally and linguistically diverse communities, including identifying what works best, where, for whom and how, to improve care and health outcomes continues to be a major challenge for healthcare organizations and systems. Despite the value and importance placed on developing effective strategies, policy frameworks have generally provided skeletal frameworks for planning and reporting, lacked intellectual depth and coherence, sufficiently robust performance standards or connected accountability mechanisms. The effect has been to ensure that key initiatives, whilst considered critical, were secondary to clinical imperatives in implementation and corresponding performance measures and standards were not articulated.

In Victoria, an attempt to link cultural and linguistic diversity responsiveness to a quality improvement approach within public hospitals resulted in the Health Service Cultural Diversity Plans (HSCDP) initiative in 2006. For the first time, health services (public hospitals) were required to establish a cultural diversity committee and an HSCDP to respond to its local CALD communities through a strategic coordination and planning process.

Six minimum reporting requirements were established:

(1) understanding clients and their needs;
(2) partnerships with multicultural and ethno-specific agencies;
(3) a culturally diverse workforce;
(4) using language services to best effect;
(5) encouraging participation in decision-making; and
(6) promoting the benefits of a multicultural Victoria.

The purpose of HSCDP was to provide health services with a tool to better plan and respond to the needs of their already defined CALD clients. Identified objectives of the plan were to:

- identify current policy directions and evidence, key result areas and strategies for action to improve health service responsiveness to CALD issues;
- document, evaluate and promote best practice 'multicultural' examples across the health service;
- offer a central coordinating mechanism for responding to and initiating CALD planning at the local health service level;
- support the Victorian Government's whole-of-government reporting framework on responsiveness to cultural diversity;
- integrate CALD issues into the broader planning mainstream of the health service through the quality and safety plan framework, quality reporting requirements and appropriate service delivery plans.

Whilst the intent of HSCDPs was clear, its implementation across all requirements proved to be inconsistent as health services either struggled with identifying and monitoring achievements and tracking progress to improve outcomes for their communities or received insufficient guidance to do this. A review of plans revealed considerable diversity in their scope, content, progress and implementation, identifying a need for greater clarification, support and guidance to health services.

Together with further consultation with health services and a research project, which undertook a review of cultural and linguistic diversity and cultural competence reporting requirements, minimum standards and benchmarks for Victorian health services, the following key constraints for cultural responsiveness were revealed: diverse levels of knowledge and understanding of cultural competence in health service settings; absence of a whole-of-organization approach to delivering culturally responsive services; insufficient alignment between risk management, patient safety, quality improvement initiatives and cultural responsiveness; a lack of integration of cultural diversity knowledge with practical strategies for patient-centered care; challenges in managing the multiple planning and reporting requirements for cultural diversity; and an absence of clearly specified cultural diversity standards, indicators and benchmarks, and effective assessment tools to measure performance (Department of Health, 2009: 5).

The absence of appropriate standards for cultural diversity initiatives within the Australian health system was a key project finding. As a result, a new draft framework was developed and tested with health services through a state-wide workshop and further feedback mechanisms.

Embedding Cultural Responsiveness in Quality and Safety

The CRF grew out of the aforementioned review and was designed to improve and extend the cultural responsiveness performance of Victorian health services. The term *cultural responsiveness* was chosen primarily to ensure consistency and congruence with existing departmental terminology. An additional influencing factor was the lack of agreement about the meaning and interpretation of *cultural competence* and its relatively immature evidence base in relation to improving health outcomes at that time. The often-cited principles and practices of cultural competence include: valuing diversity and similarity; understanding and effectively responding to cultural differences; engaging in cultural self-assessment at individual and organizational levels; adapting service delivery and supports; and institutionalizing cultural knowledge and policies across the organization (Cross, 1989). Of note is that cultural competence, although widely implemented and accepted as a potential strategy to reduce health inequities, still attracts similar criticisms today despite the progress in the field. There is an absence of a commonly agreed definition, content and standardized frameworks (Grant, 2013; Thackrah & Thompson, 2013) and a paucity of evidence to link cultural competence education with patient, professional and organizational outcomes (Horvat *et al.*, 2014; Truong *et al.*, 2014).

The term 'responsiveness' has not always been adequately embedded in the research literature but has enshrined a sense of agency and action with practical merit. Being responsive meant that health services were acting to address issues in a practical way.

Box 12.1: Cultural Responsiveness

'The term *cultural responsiveness* refers to healthcare services that are respectful of, and relevant to, the health beliefs, health practices, culture and linguistic needs of diverse consumer/patient populations and

> communities. That is, communities whose members identify as having particular cultural or linguistic affiliations by virtue of their place of birth, ancestry or ethnic origin, religion, preferred language or language spoken at home. Cultural responsiveness describes the *capacity* to respond to the healthcare issues of diverse communities. It thus requires knowledge and capacity at different levels of intervention: systemic, organizational, professional and individual'. (Department of Health 2009: 12)

The CRF is underpinned by the following principles:

(1) Every person has the right to receive high-quality health care regardless of their cultural, ethnic, linguistic and religious background or beliefs.
(2) Understanding and addressing the links between ethnicity, culture and language will improve health care for culturally and linguistically diverse communities.
(3) Embedding cultural responsiveness in healthcare systems is a viable strategy to reduce disparities in health outcomes which may be exacerbated by cultural, language and religious differences.
(4) CALD consumer, carer and community participation will enhance culturally responsive heathcare delivery.

Significantly, the goal of the CRF was to concretize the links between access, equity, quality and safety and health disparities in culturally and linguistically diverse populations. It sought to firmly embed cultural and linguistic diversity as core domains of quality and safety in health care. Notably, it successfully drew on the aforementioned literature, research and evidence base from the US at the time. It did this in direct response to the aforementioned constraints revealed through the review of the HSCDPs and the research project by ensuring congruence with the Victorian clinical governance policy framework at the time (2009). It also supported and was congruent with the Department's seminal consumer, carer and community participation in the healthcare system policy framework entitled, *Doing it With Us Not For Us*: Strategic Direction 2010–13.

The central premise of the CRF is that health care that is culturally responsive equates to health care that is safe and of high quality. This directly correlates with improved patient satisfaction and experience, equity in health outcomes, cost and error minimization. It applies universally to metropolitan, regional and small rural health services across the state. Based on the four key domains of quality and safety – organizational effectiveness; risk management; consumer participation; and an effective workforce – the framework articulated six standards for culturally responsive practice.

Domain 1: Organizational effectiveness

This domain sought to reposition cultural responsiveness from being 'bolted on' to organizational systems and management practices to being 'built in' as a core activity. It promoted a systemic and whole-of-organization approach in direct contrast with the past tendency to deal with cultural diversity in an ad-hoc way rather than developing high-level strategic governance structures and policies that deeply embed culturally responsive practices across the whole of the health service. This domain set standards for organizational leadership responsibility to strengthen a systems approach including at the highest governance level of the public health service board, in recognition of the key role of executive leadership in 'promoting and sustaining active attention to cultural factors in care' (Chrisman, 2007: 69).

Domain 2: Risk management

Providing health care that is linguistically appropriate and safe is a risk management strategy. Language services provision was strategically located within this domain to concretize the link between culture, language and patient safety outcomes (Johnstone & Kanitsaki, 2006; Garrett, 2009). As the delivery of safe, high-quality care is premised on effective communication between the consumer/patient and the healthcare provider, language barriers between healthcare professionals and patients increase the risks to quality and patient safety (Divi et al., 2007), and increase the opportunity for medical errors and adverse health outcomes. Notably, these risks can be mitigated through the provision of professional interpreters (Flores, 2005; Karliner et al., 2007).

Importantly, failure to provide accredited interpreters also infringes the rights of patients/consumers, carers and communities. The Australian Charter of Healthcare Rights in Victoria specifies the right of communication which includes the right to an accredited interpreter for communication needs within publicly funded healthcare services. The Charter states that interpreters should be provided at important points during a healthcare journey such as when discussing medical history, treatments, test results, diagnoses, during admission and assessment and when people are required to give informed consent (Australian Charter of Healthcare Rights in Victoria, 2007: 12).

The implementation of the Department's language services policy and the provision of accredited interpreters in health settings has been well intentioned and in the main well supported by Victorian health services. Underutilization of accredited interpreters, even when they are made available, commonly referred to as 'getting by', has also been identified as another serious risk management issue (Diamond et al., 2009). The CRF, however, for the first time created a standard for interpreter provision. Moreover, it did this by creating a specific measure with a numerator and a denominator as follows:

- *Numerator* – number of CALD consumers/patients identified as requiring an interpreter and who receive accredited interpreter services.
- *Denominator* – number of CALD consumers/patients presenting at the health service identified as requiring interpreter services.

It specified more systemic and accurate documentation of provision of interpreting services (an accredited interpreter) during the clinical encounter and evidence that those patients who identified as requiring an interpreter in their preferred language were provided with one.

Domain 3: Consumer participation

Engaging consumers and patients as 'safety partners' with health service providers is an effective strategy to identify and help prevent adverse events and improve patient safety outcomes (Johnstone & Kanitsaki, 2009). As consumers, carers and community members from culturally and linguistically backgrounds face a number of specific barriers in accessing health care and optimizing health outcomes, this domain set out to ensure that health services implemented inclusive strategies to work more effectively with diverse consumers to support their participation in informed decision-making about their treatment, care and well-being, that they receive evidence-based, accessible information to support key decision-making along the continuum of care, and that they are active participants in the planning, improvement and evaluation of services and programs on an ongoing basis (Department of Health, 2011). The CRF intersects explicitly with the consumer participation framework *Doing it With Us Not For Us*.

Domain 4: Effective workforce

Developing the cultural responsiveness capabilities of health professionals and healthcare organizations is recognized as a key strategy to improve outcomes for consumers, carers and communities as well as healthcare providers (Cross *et al.*, 1989; Ahmann, 2002; Anderson *et al.*, 2003; Betancourt *et al.*, 2003; Stewart, 2006). Evidence provided through systematic reviews suggests that multifaceted education interventions could lead to improved knowledge, attitudes and skills for health professionals (Beach *et al.*, 2005; van Nuland *et al.*, 2005; Hasnain *et al.*, 2009; Lie *et al.*, 2010; Horvat *et al.*, 2014; Truong *et al.*, 2014) and may lead to improved outcomes for patients/consumers (Harmsen *et al.*, 2006; Horvat *et al.*, 2014).

Cultural responsiveness was clearly stated as everybody's business. Health services were urged to establish more effective systems of workforce development to enhance the cultural responsiveness capabilities of staff across all areas of the organization to develop, implement and evaluate culturally responsive healthcare policy, programs and interventions.

Overall, the CRF specified key performance improvement measures to achieve the standards over time. Each standard specified key measures for achievement. Some were quantitative in nature and include a numerator and a denominator. Others specified clear statements of what is to be achieved. Each standard and measure also identified a series of sub-measures that served as additional guidance for health services in achieving the key measures. The measures ranged along a continuum from a minimal level of activity to more complex and aspirational measure designed to encourage health services to improve.

Box 12.2: Cultural Responsiveness Framework

Domain	Standards
Organizational effectiveness	1. A whole-of-organization approach to cultural responsiveness is demonstrated 2. Leadership for cultural responsiveness is demonstrated by the health service
Risk management	3. Accredited interpreters are provided to patients who require one
Consumer participation	4. Inclusive practice in care planning is demonstrated including but not limited to: dietary; spiritual; family; attitudinal and other cultural practices 5. CALD consumer, carer and community members are involved in the planning, improvement and review of programs and services on an ongoing basis
Effective workforce	6. Staff at all levels are provided with professional development opportunities to enhance their cultural responsiveness

A key tenet of the CRF was its strategic and whole-of-organization approach for health services to work holistically and to strengthen and align planning and documentation with existing policy and reporting frameworks and accreditation processes. A 3–5 year Cultural Responsiveness Plan aligned to the health services strategic plan was sought at the commencement of the implementation of the framework. Thereafter, annual reporting was required on the standards (this was done progressively) in a health services Quality of Care report which was a reporting mechanism to health services communities.

It also sought to both consolidate the multiple cultural diversity reporting requirements for health services and to make explicit the links with other policy frameworks such as the *Doing it With Us Not For Us* consumer participation policy framework and its corresponding Community Participation Plans, Disability Action Plans and Home and Community Care Plans and the Improving Care for Aboriginal and Torres Strait Islander Patients Program. A planning template was provided to assist with this.

Evaluation of the Cultural Responsiveness Framework

There is no doubt that the CRF has promoted a higher standard of awareness and planning for culturally responsive health care among Victorian health services and that the basic requirements of the framework were met. Diversity managers in particular became the CRF champions, arguing that the standards and reporting requirements conferred greater authority to act and respond. In 2014, both the CRF and the consumer participation policy *Doing It With Us Not For Us* policy underwent an independent external summative evaluation. The evaluation process was comprehensive and has provided valuable insights that may inform future policy development. The evaluation found that the both the policy and the framework have been strong influences in Victorian public health services since their introduction and implementation.

A key limitation of this evaluation was the positioning of the CRF as a subset of the broader evaluation ambit. This was primarily concerned with the implementation and evaluation of the consumer policy framework and the state of consumer participation and engagement within Victorian health services. Nonetheless, the evaluation provided a valuable insight into the implementation and the achievements of the CRF thus far.

The standard to provide an accredited interpreter was one of the CRF's major successes. The standard created a high level of commitment and accountability, and was both well understood and promoted within health services as core. The actual provision of interpreter services varied, however, and within different types of health services owing to a number of factors including resourcing constraints. Metropolitan health services had well-developed interpreter provision capabilities, through mechanisms such as on-site interpreter employees or the engagement of external agency interpreters. This varied with regional services that provided a mixture of face-to-face and telephone interpreter services. Rural health services were more likely to engage interpreters in an ad hoc manner. Interpreter expenditure was always a contentious issue for health services, however.

Overall, most health services developed plans and actions directly corresponding to the six standards and measures of the CRF. The evaluation, however, highlighted differences in planning and implementation of the CRF within health services, which were highlighted as follows:

- Metropolitan health services exhibited more mature processes to cultural responsiveness with more comprehensive plans addressing the standards, measures and sub-measures, including better reporting and more measurable outcomes identified. However, there was limited evidence of undertaking some of the more aspirational measures and outcomes beyond what was expected or required.
- Metropolitan health services also reflected better capacity for dedicated workforce and resourcing for cultural responsiveness. They were also more likely to develop stand-alone cultural responsiveness plans than their regional and rural counterparts.
- Regional health services experienced more variation in their planning, implementation and reporting against the standards. They were also more likely to combine congruent planning requirements into one planning process. For example, the development of an Access and Equity Strategy may consolidate key policies into a population planning approach across their catchment area.
- Rural health services were generally less well established in planning, monitoring, and reporting on responsiveness for CALD communities. They were also more likely to combine several congruent plans into one.
- The engagement of CALD communities in health services' planning and participation mechanisms was a general challenge experienced by all three types of health services, although metropolitan health services were more competent in developing diverse strategies to obtain feedback from CALD communities.
- A key limitation of the initial plans was that they outlined health service intent rather than outcomes. Reporting of outcomes and achievements in Quality of Care reports on an annual basis revealed much inconsistency in content and detail. However, this is also a key issue for consideration for the Department in its efforts in supporting health services in performance monitoring and feedback and its ability to provide a coherent framework in which this should occur.
- The CRF had tremendous personal and professional support from key diversity champions (such as Diversity Managers and Language Services Managers and their counterparts with different titles in health services). A limitation, however, was that the CRF, despite its intent to promote a whole-of-organization approach, was not necessarily implemented in this way. This was in part due to the numerous reporting and accountability requirements and pressures that health services faced.

Diversity and equity need to be considered at all levels of the health system: consumer, carer and community, organizational, government and policy. A key finding of the evaluation is that the department and health services should continue to develop, monitor and review effective strategies to engage consumers from CALD backgrounds. This requires not only organizational commitment, but also clearer and more meaningful performance measures that are integrated with other measures. Education interventions are required to build capabilities in cultural competence, person- and family-centered care and intercultural communication for health professionals as well as interventions for consumers. Finally, improved partnerships with consumers and key stakeholders are required. Lessons learned from this evaluation and its key recommendations reinforce the central premise that cultural responsiveness, diversity and equity considerations may need to be better embedded in a comprehensive and coherent framework

Emerging Initiatives – Using an Equity Lens

Three years into the implementation of the CRF and preceding the evaluation, a number of other frameworks and concepts were emerging in the healthcare inequities space. A focus on equity standards was emerging in Europe and the CLAS Standards within the US were being reviewed. Against this backdrop of review and reconceptualization, an impetus for research into new and innovative approaches resulted in an opportunity for the Department to participate in 2012 in an international pilot test. This Equity Standards pilot was viewed as a viable strategy to kick start a new way of thinking about the CRF, its achievements hitherto and what could be a new way forward.

The Equity Standards project was a key initiative in Europe designed to address inequities in health care for ethnic minority and vulnerable populations. Developed by the WHO–Health Promoting Hospitals (HPH) Task Force on Migrant Friendly and Culturally Competent Health Care (the Task Force), it was designed to improve the accessibility, utilization and quality of health care for migrants and ethnic minorities. The Equity Standards have provided an opportunity for healthcare organizations to assess their equity and cultural responsiveness performance. The Task Force grew out of the Migrant Friendly Hospitals project (MFH) in the late 1990s which involved 12 hospitals in 12 European countries. The MFH project aimed to make hospitals more responsive to the needs of migrants and ethnic minorities. It created 12 national best practice models enshrined in the Amsterdam Declaration (LBISM, 2004) and included a series of recommendations. It also established the Task Force on Migrant Friendly and Culturally Competent Health Care in 2005 as part of the international HPH network with a specific mandate to continue the momentum created by the MFH project.

Equity of healthcare access and equity in healthcare provision are important for all individuals and communities. To prevent discriminatory and exclusive practices that result in inequities, health professionals and healthcare organizations are required to respond appropriately to multiple and concurrent aspects of diversity (Chiarenza, 2012) in the consumer and patient groups they serve and work with. This has posed numerous challenges for healthcare organizations, systems and the healthcare workforce.

In Europe, a focus on 'intersectionality' has emerged moving away from hitherto well utilized concepts such as culture and diversity as the central components of developing strategies to address health inequities. A term originally derived from the work by Kimberle Crenshaw (1991) to describe intersecting patterns of racism and sexism, intersectionality may be seen as a way of viewing and understanding both complexity and difference. In positing the intersections or interconnections of all variables that shape and create inequity in health care *as a set of processes* and not as the *possessive characteristics of individuals* (Cattacin et al., 2013), intersectionality, poses a challenge to the 'traditional' focus on ethno-cultural diversity characteristics that may risk stereotyping individuals, groups and communities. In healthcare practice, stereotyping has often occurred and resulted in reductivist recipe 'culture-facts' with 'do's and don'ts' (Kleinman & Benson, 2006) approaches to working with culturally and linguistically diverse communities. A risk for a 'culture facts' approach is that it may both essentialize and homogenize individuals and communities and reduce culture to a static concept. In seeking to generalize, it may dismiss the many differences inherent in individuals, groups and communities.

Equity is seen as a potentially more concrete answer to the challenges posed by pluralism to healthcare organizations today. Using an equity lens means that the focus is not only on single target groups (or variables), but on all factors (or differences) that put vulnerable groups at risk of exclusion and inequities in health or health care. This approach also includes an understanding of the impact of the social determinants of health (Simon & Mosavel, 2008) in health inequities. Equity is inclusive and potentially able to address multiple and concurrent dimensions of diversity and complexity. By focusing on the intersection and interplay of variables that tend to lead to unequal access to healthcare provision, it places the person at the center of concern and not at the periphery as with other approaches. Arguably, some previous approaches, which are seemingly 'equal' on the surface, such as 'treating everyone the same', have resulted in a form of blindness to aspects of difference and sensitivity, resulting in uniformity in health care that can further entrench or exacerbate inequities in health care.

Moreover, equity dovetails readily with co-aligned concepts in health care, such as health literacy, cultural responsiveness, consumer participation and engagement, human rights, and person- and family-centered care. By framing all individuals as having specific and particular needs, it suggests a case-by-case assessment of peoples' healthcare needs by healthcare organizations (Cattacin et al., 2013: 252).

Five Equity Standards

In 2012, the Task Force developed and pilot-tested a framework of five preliminary standards for healthcare organizations to measure performance in equity in health care for migrants and other vulnerable groups.

There are five Equity Standards, focusing on five key interrelated domains which aim to establish the 'creation of equity as a normative orientation in healthcare organisations' (Cattacin et al., 2013: 6). The domains are in the areas of organizational policy development and implementation, access to and utilization of the healthcare service, the quality of care provided and received, consumer participation and engagement in healthcare planning, delivery and evaluation and finally, external stakeholder relationship development and management. Together they contribute to a coherent and systemic organizational approach. The Equity Standards aim at:

(1) *Equity in Policy* – to ensure the development of an equity strategy or plan and to mainstream the implementation of equity in all relevant organizational programs and quality management systems.
(2) *Equitable Access and Utilization* – to assist healthcare organizations to address barriers that prevent people from accessing and benefiting from healthcare services.
(3) *Equitable Quality of Care* – to provide high quality, person-centered care by acknowledging the unique characteristics and needs of the individual in the co-construction of the care process, from diagnosis to discharge.
(4) *Equity in Participation* – to ensure equitable opportunity for service users and community members to participate in service planning, delivery and evaluation.
(5) *Promotion of Equity* – to promote equity activities in partnerships and inter-sectoral collaborations to deliver innovative services to disadvantaged populations (Task Force on MFCCH 2014).

Collectively, the Equity Standards comprise: five main standards (as above), 18 sub-standards and 50 measurable elements. The standards were pilot-tested in 45 healthcare organizations around the world: four in Australia, 10 in Canada and 30 in Europe. Victorian hospitals were the only participants from Australia and the Asia Pacific region. The Victorian Department of Health and Human Services (formerly the Department of Health) became an active member of the Task Force project team in 2012 through its participation in the first pilot phase. It has contributed a Victorian perspective and experience to development of the final standards and the nest phase of the work. The standards were finalized in May 2013 and the Task Force began a new phase of work to aid healthcare organizations to implement the standards.

It received a further three-year mandate to:

- strengthen the evidence base of the standards;
- identify equity-based indicators that complement the five standards;
- develop a self-assessment tool and corresponding manual that healthcare organizations can use to benchmark structures, processes and equity health results;
- undertake a second pilot-test to evaluate how institutions can utilize the standards and self-assessment process, as well as to explore challenges and opportunities for effective uptake in connection with existing policies and practices;
- develop a framework for measuring and monitoring the capacity of healthcare organizations to improve accessibility and quality of care for migrants and other vulnerable groups.

Phase 2 commenced in June 2014, and concluded in March 2015. A Self-Assessment Tool was developed by the project team to provide guidance to organizations to self-assess against the standards. The second phase seeks to establish the practical utility of the standards, and help healthcare organizations evaluate, monitor and improve health equity. A key new component of the standards has been the development of performance indicators for each standard, as well as the opportunity to develop an action plan to address the gaps identified.

Overall, the second phase was implemented in 17 countries including a total of 66 pilot organizations that undertook the self-assessment. Nine Victorian health services have participated in phase 2, doubling our participation rate, and included a mixture of metropolitan regional and rural health services and the Victorian Royal District Nursing Service.

In particular, phase 2 enabled health services to:

- complete a self-assessment process to benchmark organizational performance on each of the standards;
- identify performance indicators that complement the five standards, which measure equity performance and potentially assess progress against the standards;
- analyze and use the results of the self-assessment to identify areas of improvement in each of the standards areas for the inclusion in an action plan to achieve a quantifiable improvement;
- contribute data to strengthen the evidence base of the standards.

The scope and intent of the Equity Standards are consistent with numerous departmental and government policies and legislation. Knowledge and insights from participating in both pilot phases thus far have informed departmental and health services current cultural responsiveness planning and implementation. The second phase of the pilot has been particularly timely as it been concurrent with the aforementioned evaluation of the CRF. Health service participation in the pilot test and insights gained from the policy evaluations may contribute toward a new coherent policy inclusive of equity, cultural responsiveness, person- and family-centered care, consumer participation and health literacy.

How Equity has been Received

The application of an equity lens has resonated with many health services for a number of reasons. Firstly, equity has been embraced as being potentially more inclusive of other co-aligned variables of diversity and wider structural determinants of disadvantage and vulnerability. The significance of the CRF in placing cultural and linguistic issues squarely within a quality and safety framework cannot be underestimated. However, precisely because of this very focus, it was also able to be easily compartmentalized and separated from other co-aligned and congruent initiatives. Health services in Victoria are required to respond appropriately to a broad range of diversities, including CALD communities, Aboriginal and Torres Strait Islander peoples and people from refugee and asylum seeker backgrounds. All are supported by separate, albeit complementary, policy frameworks and initiatives in the main, with corresponding standards and reporting requirements. Each also has different levels of support provided by different areas across the Department. Although the need for specificity is clearly recognized by these policy frameworks, it presents various challenges in implementation and review at health service and departmental levels.

Secondly, equity has allowed health services to focus on a range of issues across their organization. Importantly, whilst it has enabled health services to identify strengths in responding to diverse needs, it has also facilitated a more systemic analysis to identify gaps and areas that were not part of their previous thinking and which may even have precluded equity considerations. Some of the key benefits of participation recently highlighted by health services include:

- congruence with the national accreditation standards with which health services must comply;
- a capacity to apply a population-based approach which is particularly relevant for regional and rural health services;
- alignment with strategic and business plans;
- the identification of gaps in data collection systems that need to be addressed; and
- identification of current strengths and organizational potential.

Using an equity lens has been viewed as a potentially overarching and more inclusive and coherent framework to address all of these issues and some of the constraints revealed by the evaluation of the CRF. Although the CRF was premised on equity in health care, it did not articulate this approach clearly enough. Equity principles formed the foundations of the CRF which clearly stated that all persons have the same right to access and receive high-quality and safe health care, regardless of cultural, linguistic and religious and socioeconomic considerations. This did not mean that everyone receives the same care but rather that all persons have their health care needs equally well met, and that factors that can potentially contribute to differential patient outcomes (e.g. access to accredited interpreters, culturally inclusive care) have been minimized (Weinick et al., 2008). Perhaps by focusing on key cultural and linguistic considerations, the important equity premise was lost. Key lessons learned from the Equity Standards project, including the concept of intersectionality as a basis for reconceptualizing the interconnections between diversity, difference, discrimination and inequity, could be a useful premise for a new framework.

A key challenge, however, in the potential development of a new policy framework will be to not lose sight of the importance of addressing or responding to the specificities that arise from cultural and linguistic considerations in any health care context. Importantly, a new framework may specify aspects of cultural self-awareness and intercultural communication skills as part of more complex and nuanced understandings. These understandings would show deeper analysis of sociocultural barriers to health care at the clinical level (healthcare professional–patient encounter), organizational level (leadership and workforce) and structural level (processes of care) (Horvat et al., 2014).

Reorienting to an equity lens could help develop strategies for a whole-of-organization approach to equity performance and monitoring and bring together complementary and co-aligned concepts and approaches. Although the final results from phase 2 will not be available for some time, valuable learnings and insights from the participation in the Equity Standards self-assessment points to a possible reconceptualization of departmental policy.

Toward a comprehensive policy framework

A comprehensive policy framework may reflect a number of emergent initiatives and approaches, key policy drivers and existing frameworks, both nationally and within Victoria. One of the major changes that has taken place in Australia in recent years has been the introduction of the National Safety and Quality Health Service Standards under the Australian Health Service Accreditation Scheme. Standard 2 of these national accreditation standards is entitled *'Partnering with Consumers'*. This specific standard has one of the most significant drivers for consumer participation strategies and outcomes and the provision of person- and family-centered care within public health services across Australia.

The reconceptualization of the care relationship and the role of consumers as equal and active partners seeking engagement and empowerment in their healthcare experience and journey has also been a significant contributor to this. The growing body of evidence of improved clinical outcomes when consumers are involved in decision-making (Australian Commission on Safety and Quality in Health Care, 2011) has also had a significant impact. Similarly, research into health literacy interventions as an enabler of communication and participation in health care (Department of Health, 2013) has focused on the appropriateness of health information systems in the care continuum. In addition, a new approach in measuring health experience, which is a deliberate move away from measuring patient satisfaction, is resulting in a sharpened focus on improved measures, data and outcomes of health care as a core quality improvement strategy for health services.

A process of co-locating and aligning key concepts has already commenced in Victoria in order to synthesize core common underlying principles and approaches. A skeletal framework is emerging from this process that may evolve to a new level. At its core, however, is locating equity as a key component of the broader quality and safety agenda, which enshrines three fundamental principles for high-quality and safe care: that 'care is consumer centred, driven by information, and organised for safety' (Australian Commission on Safety and Quality in Health Care, 2010: 1). Other co-located concepts and approaches include cultural responsiveness, consumer participation and person- and family-centered care, and addressing health literacy and information considerations at consumer, community, healthcare workforce and healthcare systems levels. The congruence between these co-aligned concepts and approaches to address healthcare inequities are increasingly apparent (Beach *et al.*, 2006; Like, 2011; Australian Commission on Safety and Quality in Health Care, 2011; Department of Health, 2013).

It is clear that policies that aim to address health inequities require better alignment between core concepts, core underlying principles, theories and approaches. These must be communicated in such a way that their mutually reinforcing components are made explicit. The aforementioned core concepts and approaches together with the recommendations arising from the evaluation of the CRF and the *'Doing it With Us Not For Us'* and the insights from the Equity Standards will be extremely useful in informing future policy. A new integrated and coherent policy may articulate a strong focus on equity and participation and include the alignment of the aforementioned concepts and approaches within a quality and safety framework.

Disclaimer

The views expressed in this chapter are those of the author and do not necessarily represent the views of the Department of Health and Human Services, State Government of Victoria, Melbourne.

References

Ahmann, E. (2002) Developing cultural competence in health care settings: National Center for Cultural Competence. *Pediatric Nursing* 28 (2), 133–137.

Anderson, L., Scrimshaw, S., Fullilove, M., Fielding, J.E. and Normand, J. (2003) Culturally competent healthcare systems, a systematic review. *American Journal of Preventative Medicine* 24 (3S), 68–79.

Australian Charter on Healthcare Rights in Victoria (2015) See http://docs.health.vic.gov.au/docs/doc/A828F4D7161E1D77CA2578AA007DDA38/$FILE/1105029_ACHCR_A5_FA_web.pdf (accessed 7 March 2015).

Australian Commission on Safety and Quality in Health Care (2010) Australian Safety and Quality Framework for Health Care. See http://www.safetyandquality.gov.au/wp-content/uploads/2012/01/32296-Australian-SandQ-Framework1.pdf (accessed 7 March 2015).

Australian Commission on Safety and Quality in Health Care (2011) Patient centred care: Improving quality and safety through partnerships with patients and consumers, ACSQHC, Sydney. See http://www.safetyandquality.gov.au/wpcontent/uploads/2012/03/PCC_Paper_August.pdf (accessed 1 March 2015).

Beach, M.C., Price, E.G., Gary, T.L., Robinson, K.A., Gozu, A., Palacio, A., Jenckes, M.W., Feuerstein, C., Bass, E.B., Powe, N.R. and Cooper, L.A. (2005) Cultural competence: A systematic review of healthcare provider education interventions. *Medical Care* 43 (4), 356–373.

Beach, M.C., Saha S. and Cooper, L.A. (2006) *The Role and Relationship of Cultural Competence and Patient-centeredness in Health Care Quality*, Vol. 36. Commonwealth Fund, 2006.

Berner, S. (2010) Health care interpreters – vital partners in client care. Diversity Health Institute. Diversity (pp. 2, 7).

Betancourt, J.R., Green, A.R., Carillo, J.E. and Ananeh-Firempong, O. (2003) Defining cultural competence: A practical framework for addressing racial/ethnic disparities in health and health care. *Public Health Reports* 118 (4), 293–302.

Cattacin, S., Chiarenza, A. and Domenig, D. (2013) Equity standards for health care organisations: A theoretical framework. *Diversity and Equality in Health and Care* 10 (4), 249–258.

Chiarenza, A. (2012) Developments in the concept of cultural competence. In: D. Ingleby, A. Chiarenza, W. Devillé and I. Kotsioni (eds) *Inequalities in Health Care for Migrants and Ethnic Minorities* (pp. 66–81). Antwerp: Grant.

Chrisman, N.J. (2007) 'Extending cultural competence through systems change': Academic, hospital and community partnerships. See http://tcn.sagepub.com/cgi/content/abstract/18/1_suppl/68S

Crenshaw, K. (1991) Mapping the margins: intersectionality, identity politics, and violence against women of colour. *Stanford Law Review* 43, 1241–1299.

Cross, T.L., Bazron, B.J., Dennis, K.W. and Isaacs, M.R. (1989) *Towards a Culturally Competent System of Care, Volume I*. Washington, DC: Georgetown University Child Development Center, CASSP Technical Assistance Center.

Department of Health (2009) *Cultural Responsiveness Framework: Guidelines for Victorian Health Services*. Melbourne: Victorian Department of Health. See https://www2.health.vic.gov.au/getfile/?sc_itemid=%7b1DD19A35-BBF8-4B36-80B3-63BA2E1F5F7C%7d&title=Cultural%20responsiveness%20framework%20-%20Guidelines%20for%20Victorian%20health%20services (accessed 6 August 2015).

Department of Health (2011) *Doing it With us Not For Us: Strategic Direction 2010–13*. Melbourne: Victorian Department of Health. See http://health.vic.gov.au/consumer/policy.htm (accessed 6 August 2015).

Department of Health (2013) *Health Literacy: Enabling Communication and Participation in Health*. Department of Health Background Paper. Melbourne: Victorian Department of Health. See http://health.vic.gov.au/consumer/health-literacy.htm (accessed 6 August 2015).

Department of Health (2014) *The Victorian Refugee and Asylum Seeker Health Action Plan 2014–2018*. Melbourne: Victorian Department of Health.

Department of Human Services (2006) Health service cultural diversity plans. Victorian Department of Human Services.

Diamond, L., Schenker, Y., Curry, L., Bradley, E. and Fernandez, A. (2009) Getting by: Underuse of interpreters by resident physicians. *Journal of General Internal Medicine* 2, 256–262.

Divi, C., Koss, R.G., Schmaltz, S.P. and Loeb, J.M. (2007) Language proficiency and adverse events in US hospitals: A pilot study. *International Journal for Quality in Health Care* 19 (2), 60–67.

Flores, G. (2005) The impact of medical interpreter services on the quality of health care: a systematic review. *Medical Care Research and Review* 62 (3), 255–299.

Garrett, P. (2009) Healthcare interpreter policy: Policy determinants and current issues in the Australian context. *Interpreting and Translations* 1 (2), 44.

Grant, J., Parry, Y. and Guerin, P. (2013) An investigation of culturally competent terminology in health care policy finds ambiguity and lack of definition. *Australian and New Zealand Journal of Public Health* 37 (3), 250–256.

Harmsen, J.A.M., Bernsen, R.M.D., Meeuwesen, L., Pinto, D. and Bruijnzeels, M.A. (2006) Cultural dissimilarities in general practice: development and validation of a patient's cultural background scale. *Journal of Immigrant and Minority Health* 8 (2), 115–124.

Hasnain, R., Kondratowicz, D.M., Portillo, N., Balcazar, F., Johnson, T., Gould, R. *et al.* (2009) The use of culturally adapted competency interventions to improve rehabilitation service outcomes for culturally and linguistically diverse individuals with disabilities (Review). The Campbell Library.

Heaney, C. and Moreham, S. (2002) Use of interpreter services in a metropolitan healthcare system. *Australian Health Review* 25 (3), 38.

Horvat, L., Horey, D., Romios, P. and Kis-Rigo, J. (2014) Cultural competence education for health professionals. *Cochrane Database of Systematic Reviews* 5, article no. CD009405.

Ingleby, A., Krasnik, A., Lorant, V. and Razum, O. (eds) (2012a) *Volume 1: Health Inequalities and Risk Factors Among Migrants and Ethnic Minorities*. COST Series on Health and Diversity. Antwerp–Apeldoorn: Garant.

Ingleby, D., Chiarenza, A., Devillé, W. and Kotsioni, I. (eds) (2012b) *Volume 2: Inequalities in Health Care for Migrants and Ethnic Minorities*. COST Series on Health and Diversity. Antwerp–Apeldoorn: Garant.

Johnstone, M.J. and Kanitsaki, O. (2006) Culture, language, and patient safety: Making the link. *International Journal for Quality in Health care* 18 (5), 383–388.

Johnstone, M.J. and Kanitsaki, O. (2009) Engaging patients as safety partners: Some considerations for ensuring a culturally and linguistically appropriate approach. *Health Policy* 90, 1–7.

Karliner, L., Jacobs, E., Chen, A. and Mutha, S. (2007) Do professional interpreters improve clinical care for clients with limited English proficiency? A systematic review of the literature. *Health Services Research* 42 (2), 743.

Kleinman, A. and Benson, P. (2006) Anthropology in the clinic: The problem of cultural competency and how to fix it. *PLoS Medicine* 3 (10), e294.

LBISM (2004) The Amsterdam Declaration: Towards migrant-friendly hospitals in an ethno-culturally diverse Europe. Ludwig Boltzmann Institute for the Sociology of Health and Medicine (LBISHM) at the University of Vienna, Faculty of the Social Sciences. Vienna/WHO Collaborating Centre for Health Promotion in Hospitals and Health Care. See http://www.mfheu.net/conf/downloads/AmsterdamDeclaration2004.pdf

Lie, D.A., Lee-Ray, E., Gomez, A., Bereknyei, S. and Braddock, C.H. (2010) Does cultural competency training of health professionals improve patient outcomes? A systematic review and proposed algorithm for future research. *Journal of General Internal Medicine* 26 (3), 317–325.

Like, R.C. (2011) Educating clinicians about cultural competence and disparities in health and health care. *Journal of Continuing Education in the Health Professions* 31 (3), 196–206.

Mladovsky, P., Ingleby, D., McKee, M. and Bernd, R. (2012a) Good practices in migrant health: The European experience. *Clinical Medicine* 12 (3), 248–252.

Mladovsky, P., Rechel, B., Ingleby, D. and McKee, M. (2012b) Responding to diversity: An exploratory study of migrant health policies in Europe. *Health Policy* 105 (1), 1–9.

Simon, C. and Mosavel, M. (2008) Key ethical and conceptual issues in the forging of 'culturally competent' community health initiatives: A South African example. *Cambridge Quarterly of Healthcare Ethics* 17 (2), 195.

Smedley, B.D., Stith, A.Y. and Nelson, A.R. (2003) *Unequal Treatment. Confronting Racial and Ethnic Disparities in Health Care*. Washington, DC: The National Academies Press.

Stewart, S. (2006) Cultural competence in health care. Diversity Health Institute Position Paper.

Task Force on MFCCH (2014) WHO-HPH Task Force on Migrant Friendly and Culturally Competent Health Care. See http://wwwold.ausl.re.it/HPH/FrontEnd/Home/Default.aspx?channel_id=38 (accessed 20 March 2015).

Thackrah, R.D. and Thompson, S.C. (2013) Refining the concept of cultural competence: Building on decades of progress.*Medical Journal of Australia* 199 (1), 35–38.

Truong, M., Paradies, Y. and Priest, N. (2014) Interventions to improve cultural competency in healthcare: A systematic review of reviews. *BMC Health Services Research* 3 (14), 99.

van Nuland, M., Hannes, K., Aertgeerts, B. and Goedhuys, J. (2005) Educational interventions for improving the communication skills of general practice trainees in the clinical consultation. *Cochrane Database of Systematic Reviews* 4.

Victorian Multicultural Commission, State Government of Victoria (2011a) 2011 Census: A snapshot of our diversity. See http://www.multicultural.vic.gov.au/population-and-migration/victorias-diversity/2011-census-a-snapshot-of-our-diversity (accessed 14 February 2015).

Victorian Multicultural Commission, State Government of Victoria (2011b) Multicultural Victoria Act 2011. See http://www.multicultural.vic.gov.au/about-us/legislation/multicultural-victoria-act-2011(accessed 14 February 2015).

Weinick, R.M., Flaherty, K. and Bristol, S.J (2008) Creating equity reports: A guide for hospitals. The Disparities Solutions Centre, Massachusetts General Hospital

Wilson-Stronks et al. (2008) *One Size Does Not Fit All: Meeting the Health Care Needs of Diverse Populations*. Oakbrook Terrace, IL: The Joint Commission.

Epilogue

This edited volume provides an excellent overview of the global challenge healthcare providers and linguistically diverse patients face when patients seek health care in settings where it is delivered in a language other than their own. The contributing authors provide a diverse set of insights into these challenges and means for overcoming them and highlight how the likely best solutions to the problem of language barriers in health care vary depending on where you are in the world, what means of overcoming them are available, how policy shapes or does not shape these solutions, and the culture, language and language abilities of the patients being served. They also provide a number of practical ideas and recommendations as to how to address these challenges, from how to work effectively with informal interpreters to developing means for measuring physician language proficiency. These recommendations sometimes conflict, indicating that, while the challenge is consistent and global, the means for addressing language barriers in healthcare settings are varied and context dependent. This book serves as evidence for that diversity and as a resource for understanding this increasing global challenge and for considering different means for addressing it and issues that must be addressed when developing solutions.

Glossary

Bilingual health communication: Health communication that has to occur in two languages.

Bilingual speakers: Individuals who speak two languages relatively fluently.

Bilingualism: The existence of more than one language in an individual or community.[1]

Census: An official count or survey of a population. The US conducts an official survey of its population every 10 years. It was last conducted in 2010. Data from the US Census is frequently used to characterize the population in the US who are Limited English Proficient (LEP; see definition below).

Community health needs assessment: An evaluation of the needs of community members, which may include health-related needs, transportation needs, legal concerns, access to subsidized public assistance programs, and other needs.[2]

Community interpreter: Interpreting takes place in the course of communication in the local community among speakers of non-dominant languages. The community interpreter may or may not be a trained interpreter. Community settings include schools, social service agencies, clinics, legal services, and businesses that serve a diverse clientele.[3]

Culturally and Linguistically Diverse: A term used in Australia and New Zealand to describe those individuals who identify as having a specific cultural or linguistic affiliation by virtue of their place of birth, ancestry, ethnic origin, religion, preferred language or language(s) spoken at home, or because of their parents' identification on a similar basis.[4]

Informal interpreters: Individuals who act as interpreters but who have not been formally trained or paid to provide interpretation. Also referred to as ad-hoc interpreters.

Language concordance: When a clinician is truly fluent in the language of his/her limited English proficient patient.

Languages of Lesser Diffusion: A language 'that has relatively few speakers in one specific location or geographical area in relation to the population as a whole'.[5]

Limited English proficiency: A legal concept used in the US referring to a level of English proficiency that is insufficient to ensure equal access to public services provided in English without an interpreter.

Medicaid: Federal Health Insurance in the US that provides health insurance for families and individuals with limited financial resources.

Medicare: Federal health Insurance in the US that provides health insurance to Americans aged 65 years of age or older who have paid into the service, through their paychecks, over time. It also provides insurance to younger people with disabilities and for people with certain conditions, like end-stage renal disease.

Professional interpreter: Individuals who have been assessed for professional skills, demonstrate a high level of proficiency in at least two languages and have the appropriate training and experience to interpret with skill and accuracy.[6]

Role conflict: When the expectations about the role an interpreter should play in an encounter diverge or are in conflict between the interpreter, provider, patient/client, family and/or health system.

Title VI of the Civil Rights Act: Title VI, 42 USC. §2000d et seq., was enacted in the US as part of the landmark Civil Rights Act of 1964. It prohibits discrimination on the basis of race, color and national origin in programs and activities receiving federal financial assistance. If a recipient of federal assistance is found to have discriminated and voluntary compliance cannot be achieved, the federal agency providing the assistance should either initiate fund termination proceedings or refer the matter to the Department of Justice for appropriate legal action.[7] National origin includes primary language, so that discrimination based on language is prohibited in the US under this Act.

Translation: The conversion of a written text into a corresponding written text in a different language. Within the language professions, *translation* is distinguished from *interpreting* according to whether the message is produced orally (or manually) or in writing. In popular usage, the terms 'translator' and 'translation' are frequently used for conversion of either oral or written communications.[8]

Translator: A person who translates written texts, especially one who does so professionally.[8]

Notes

(1) https://en.wikipedia.org/wiki/Bilingualism
(2) https://www.cdc.gov/stltpublichealth/cha/plan.html
(3) Pöchhacker, F. (1999) 'Getting organized': The evolution of community interpreting. *Interpreting* 4 (1), 125–140.
(4) http://www.dhi.health.nsw.gov.au/Transcultural-Mental-Health-Centre/Information-for-Consumers-Carers-and-Community/Community/FAQs/FAQs/default.aspx
(5) Giambruno, C. (2014) Dealing with languages of lesser diffusion. In C. Giambruno (ed.) *Assessing Legal Interpreting Quality through Testing and Certification: The Qualitas Project* (pp. 93–107). Sant Vicent del Raspeig: University of Alicante Publications.
(6) http://www.ncihc.org/assets/documents/NCIHC%20Terms%20Final080408.pdf
(7) https://www.justice.gov/crt/fcs/TitleVI-Overview
(8) National Council on Interpreting in Health Care (October 2001) *The Terminology of Health Care Interpreting: A Glossary of Terms*.

Index

Note: Page numbers in **bold** refer to the Glossary.

Adelson, N. 151–152, 163
AILIA (Language Industry Association of Canada) 59, 67n3
Aitchison, J. 136
Altarriba, J. 132, 133
Amsterdam Declaration (2004) 225
Appave, G. 1
Applied Research on Communication in Health Group 203
Arendt, H. 82
Arksey, H. 121
Asociación Mayab 152, 157–158, 162–163
asylum seekers 4
Auer, P. 121
Australia
   Health Service Accreditation Scheme 230–231
   Telephone Interpreting Service 198
   see also Victoria, Australia

Baker, C. 120
Baker, D.W. *et al.* 105
Bandura, A. 80
Baraldi, C. 58
Bath, P.A. 46
Beaufort Research 122, 123*t*, 125, 127, 132, 135, 139–140
Begay, M.-G. 160
Benson, P. 226
Betancourt, J. *et al.* 141
Bhatia, T. 121
bilingual health communication xvi, 35–36, 93, 95, 96, 97, 98–99, **236**
   bilingual health care staff 78, 79, 201–202
   see also bilingual speakers in Wales
Bilingual Health Communication Model (BHC Model) 39

communicative goals 39–40
individual agency 40–42
individual-level constructs 39–47, 39*f*
interpersonal-level constructs 47–51
propositions 51
quality and equality of care 44–47
system norms 42–44
temporal dimension 49–51
Trust–Control–Power 47–49
conclusion 52
bilingual speakers **236**
bilingual speakers in Wales xvii, 116–118
   bilingual context 118–120
   bilingualism 120–121, 120*t*
   methodology 121–122
   findings and discussion 122–140
      (acknowledging significance of bilingualism 124–126
      bilingualism and cultural identity 136–140
      bilingualism and emotion 132–136
      bilingualism and expression 128–132
      perceived models of bilingualism 126–128
      research studies in scoping review 122, 123*t*)
   study limitations 140–141
   conclusions and recommendations 141–143
   realist synthesis framework 142–143, 143*f*
bilingualism 120–121, **236**
   complementarity principle 127
   key dimensions 120*t*
   see also bilingual speakers in Wales
Bischoff, A. *et al.* 97–98
Bismark, M.M. *et al.* 197
Bond, M. 133
Bourhis, R. *et al.* 129–130

Brisset, C. et al. 58, 75
Browne, A. 139, 140
Bruno, R. 153

CALD *see* culturally and linguistically diverse
Canada
 AILIA (Language Industry Association) 59, 67n3
 see also community interpreters
Carr, S. 187
Carter, H. 136
CAT (Communication Accommodation Theory) 129
Cattacin, S. et al. 226, 227
CBDIO *see* Centro Binacional para el Desarrollo Indígena Oaxaqueño
censuses **236**
 New Zealand 192, 200–201
 United Kingdom 170, 172
 United States 7, 24, 150t, 165
 Victoria, Australia 212–213
Centro Binacional para el Desarrollo Indígena Oaxaqueño (CBDIO) 149, 152, 157, 161
Chan, C.K. et al. 184
Chang, K.H. 186
Chen, J. et al. 106
Chen Wu, A. et al. 63
Chiarenza, A. 226
Chinese culture 45, 46, 48, 50, 172–173, 178, 186
Chinese population of the UK xvii–xviii, 170
 background 170–173
 methodology 173–174
 challenges 174
  (accessing services 176–178
  understanding services 174–175
  using services 178–182)
 Chinese welfare organizations 184–186, 187
 learning disability services 172, 174, 175, 177–178, 180–181, 182, 183–184, 185
 mental health services 171, 175, 176, 179–180, 181, 182, 183, 184, 185–186
 social care services 172, 173–174, 175, 176–177, 180, 181, 182–183, 184
 solutions 182–184
 conclusions 186–187
Chrisman, N.J. 220

Circos, Krzywinski, M. et al. 2f
Clark, D. 196
CLAS standards *see* Culturally and Linguistically Appropriate Services
code-switching 128, 130, 133
Communication Accommodation Theory (CAT) 129
communication modalities 93
 bilingual providers 93, 95, 96, 97, 98–99
 and clinical outcomes 95–96
 in-person interpretation 26, 94, 96
 internet-based applications 28
 and interpreter accuracy 94–95
 interpreters 5–6
 of languages of lesser diffusion 154
 online translation tools 28, 94
 and patient satisfaction 96–97
 and patients' willingness to disclose 97–98
 relay interpreting 154
 remote modalities 26–28, 94, 96–97, 154
 telephonic interpretation 27, 41, 96
 videoconferencing 27–28, 154
 conclusions 98–99
communicative competence 137
communicative goals 39–40
community health needs assessment **236**
community interpreters 7–8, 57, **236**
 assessment of patients 66
 ethnic minorities 56–57
 interpreting in public institutions in Canada 58–59
 mental health care interpreting 60–64
 research in healthcare interpreting 59–60, 66–67
 role 57–58
 training 59, 61, 63–64, 65, 66
 working with community interpreters in mental health 64–67
competence
 communicative competence 137
 of interpreters 84, 85
 see also cultural competence in health care
conference interpreting 57
confidentiality 84, 85
control 37, 42, 43, 47–49, 72, 73, 79–83, 84
convergence 129–130
Cooper, R.J. 8
Crenshaw, K. 226

CRF *see* Cultural Responsiveness
Framework
cross-cultural care 45–47, 48, 50, 63–64, 86–87
Cross, T.L. *et al.* 138, 218
Cross, T.L.C. 182
cultural competence in health care 137–138, 141, 182, 195, 206, 218, 225
see also intersectionality
cultural identity and bilingualism 136–140
Cultural Responsiveness Framework (CRF) 212, 218
cultural responsiveness defined 218–219
principles 219
1: organizational effectiveness 220
2: risk management 220–221
3: consumer participation 221
4: effective workforce 221–223
evaluation 223–225
see also Equity Standards initiative
Culturally and Linguistically Appropriate Services (CLAS standards; US) 21–22, 103, 104, 122, 138
culturally and linguistically diverse (CALD) 213, 217, **236**
culture shock 3
Culyer, A.J. 46

Damschroder, L. *et al.* 142
Davidson, B. 43
Davies, D. 134
DeCamp, L.R. *et al.* 104
dialogue interpreters *see* community interpreters
Diamond, L. *et al.* 220
Diamond, L.C. *et al.* 104, 107, 108, 109, 111–112
divergence 130
Divi, C. *et al.* 215, 220
Drennan, G. 78
Durazo-Arvizu, R. 134

Eamranond, P.P. *et al.* 105–106
Elman, S. 137
emotion and bilingualism 132–136
equality of care 44, 46–47, 103, 206, 207, 214–216
Equity Standards initiative 225–226
five Equity Standards 227–229
reception of 229–232
toward a comprehensive policy framework 230–232

ethics 45, 57, 58, 59, 64, 81–82, 155–156
ethnolinguistic vitality 124
'Ethnologue: Languages of the World' 152
Etyan, A. *et al.* 97–98
European Union 73
expression and bilingualism 128–132

Fagan, M.J. 97
Fernandez, A. *et al.* 105, 106, 108, 110
fidelity 84, 85
Fishman, J. 119
Flores, G. 197, 220
Ford, L.L. *et al.* 163, 164
Free, C. *et al.* 83
French, J.R.P. 82, 88n3

Gany, F. *et al.* 97, 158, 166
Gavioli, L. 58
Giles, H. *et al.* 124, 129
global trust 84, 85
globalization xv, 1–3
Goldsmith, D.J. 36, 37
González, J. 158, 166
Gray, B. *et al.* 197, 200, 201, 202–203, 204, 205
Green, A.R. *et al.* 105, 109
Greenhalgh, T. *et al.* 82
Gregg, J. 117–118
Grosjean, F. 126–127, 128
Gubrium, J.F. 40
Gumperz, J. 137

Hall, M.A. *et al.* 84–86
Hardin, D.M. 111
Hardin, K.J. 111
Hasnain-Wynia, R. *et al.* 152, 153
health im/migrant effect 56
health worker experience 7
Heikkila, K. *et al.* 137
Hernandez, R.G. *et al.* 111
Hiew, Y. *et al.* 185
Holstein, J.A. 40
honesty 84
Horrocks, S. 186
Horvat, L. *et al.* 230
Hsieh, E. 5–6, 107

'I Speak' language identification cards 152
Iaith 117, 122, 123t, 124, 126, 131, 135–136, 139
ILR (Interagency Language Roundtable) scale 109, 111–112

IMIA (International Medical Interpreters Association) 151
in-person interpretation 26, 94, 96
Indigenous Interpreting + 158, 163–165
individual agency 40–42
informal interpreters xvi, 41, 71–73, 103, 155, **236**
   bilingual healthcare staff 78, 79
   control and power in health encounters 72–73, 79–86
   family members 5, 24, 41, 48, 61, 72, 78, 79, 81, 83, 85–86, 103, 155
   need for research 73–79
   and role conflict 75–79
   trust and distrust 72, 84–85
   types of 78, 87n1
   conclusion 85–87
Institute for Healthcare Improvement Quadruple Aim 6–7
International Medical Interpreters Association (IMIA) 151
internet-based applications 28
interpretation type and clinical outcomes 95–96
interprète en milieu social see community interpreters
interpreter accuracy 94–95
interpreter-mediated medical encounters 35–38
   see also Bilingual Health Communication Model (BHC Model)
interpreter training 42
   and clinical outcomes 95–96
   community interpreters 59, 61, 63–64, 65, 66
   and interpreter accuracy 94
   in New Zealand 199, 205, 207
   and patient satisfaction 96, 98–99
   in US 155–157, 158–160
interpreters 5–6
   financial costs 62
   standard for provision 220–221
   see also communication modalities; community interpreters; informal interpreters; professional interpreters
intersectionality 226, 230
Irvine, F. et al. 173, 175, 176, 180, 181, 182–183, 184

Jacobs, E. et al. 132
Jacobs, E.A. et al. 112

James, K. 202
Johnstone, M. 130–131
Johnstone, M.J. 221
Jones, S. 120, 137

Kanitsaki, O. 130–131, 221
Karliner, L. et al. 152, 220
Karliner, L.S. et al. 22
Kaufert, J. 59–60
Kehayia, E. 142
Kleinman, A. 226
Korean Americans 45
Kuo, D. 97

Labun, E. 63
Laczko, F. 1
Lai, T. 133
language access services in the US xv–xvi, 20–22
   CLAS standards 20–22, 103, 104, 122, 138
   communication modalities 26–28
   human communication 28–29
   identification of patients 22–24
   importance of professional interpreters 21, 24–25
   limited English proficiency 20–21
   REAL data collection 23–24
   see also language concordance between LEP patients and clinicians
language awareness 137
language barriers in health care xv, 102
   see also communication modalities
language concordance 24, **237**
language concordance between LEP patients and clinicians xvii, 102–103
   and better quality of care and outcomes 95, 96, 105–106
   clinician awareness of own limitations 41, 110–112
   language services in practice 106–108
   measure/regulation of clinician language proficiency 108–110
   needs of patients 103–105
   conclusions 112
language dominance 8
language interpretation 24
language planning initiatives (LPI) 8
language planning theory (LPT) 8
language services 5–6
   in acute care 7

community-based services 7–8
defined 5
in home care 7–8, 9
implementation 6–9
interpreters 5–6
long-term care 9
in nursing 10
outcomes 9–11
in primary care 7
in rehabilitation services 9–10
conclusion 11
see also language access services in the US
languages of lesser diffusion (LLD) **237**
languages of lesser diffusion in US xvii, 149–151, 150*t*
interpretation services resources 155–156
medical interpreting training programs and initiatives 156–165
modalities of interpretation 154
predicting and assessing language access needs 151–154
discussion 165–166
Lau, Y. 186
Leanza, Y. *et al.* 58, 64
learning disability services *see* Chinese population of the UK
Lee, S. *et al.* 186
Leininger, M. 137–138
LEP *see* limited English proficiency
Levac, D. *et al.* 121–122
Lewin, K. 87
Lewis, J. 124
Lewis, M.P. *et al.* 152
limited English proficiency (LEP) xvii, 5, 20–21, 151, **237**
see also language concordance between LEP patients and clinicians; New Zealand: meeting the needs of LEP patients
linguistic access xv–xvi
Lion, K.C. *et al.* 108
LLD (languages of lesser diffusion) **237**
see also languages of lesser diffusion in US
LPI (language planning initiatives) 8
LPT (language planning theory) 8

McGrath, C. 196
Madoc-Jones, I. 122, 123*t*, 125, 128, 131, 135, 139, 140
Manson, A. 105, 109
Matiasek, J. 141
Mazor, S.S. *et al.* 107
Medical Interpreting Training Program 156–157, 158–160
mental health care xvi, 56–57
Chinese population of the UK 171, 175, 176, 179–180, 181, 182, 183, 184, 185–186
community interpreters 60–67
New Zealand 195, 205
professional interpreters 78
see also community interpreters
Mexican Americans 45
Migrant Friendly and Culturally Competent Health Care Task Force 225, 227
Migrant Friendly Hospitals (MFH) project 225
migration xv, 1–2, 2*f*, 56
asylum seekers 4
documented individuals 3–4
and health 2–3, 56
and healthcare systems xvi, 3
identity and health 3–4
language 4–5
refugees 4
undocumented individuals 4
see also language services
Miletic, T. *et al.* 203
Miller, K. 46
minority languages *see* languages of lesser diffusion (LLD)
Misell, A. 117, 122, 125, 127, 137
Moreno, M.R. *et al.* 111
Morier, R. 132, 133
Mosavel, M. 226
Murphy, J. 130

Natividad Medical Center (NMC) 163–164
Natividad Medical Foundation (NMF) 163, 164
Navajo Nation Community Health Representatives Program 157, 160
Nelson, M. 111
Nerenz, D.R. *et al.* 104, 105
Netherlands
informal interpreters 74–75
Law on Medical Treatment (1995) 74
migrants 73–74
professional interpreters 74, 75

New Zealand xviii, 190
    cultural safety 138
    linguistic and cultural diversity 191–192
    Maori people and language 191, 195
    professional frameworks for
        interpreters and translators 196
New Zealand health system 192
    Accident Compensation Corporation
        193, 197
    District Health Boards 193, 197–199
    Medical Council ethical & legislative
        guidelines 204–205
    Pharmac 193–194, 205
    Primary Health Organisations 193, 198
    Royal New Zealand College of General
        Practitioners (RNZCGP) 199,
        204, 205
New Zealand legal and regulatory
        framework 194
    Health and Disability Commissioner's
        Code 194–195, 197–198, 199, 205
    Health Practitioners Competence
        Assurance Act (2003) 195
    Health Quality and Safety
        Commission 196, 204, 205
    Mental Health Compulsory
        Assessment and Treatment Act
        (1992) 195, 205
    Office for Ethnic Affairs 196
New Zealand: meeting the needs of LEP
        patients
    Auckland developments 200
    bilingual clinicians 201
    development of interpreting services
        198–199, 205–206
    general practice standards 199–200,
        206–207
    Health and Disability Commissioner's
        Code 197–198, 199
    interpreter training 199, 205, 207
    Interpreting New Zealand 198, 205
    Language Line 198, 202, 205
    uptake of interpreter services 200–201
New Zealand research
    audits of interpreter use 202
    bilingual medical students 201–202
    does interpreted consultation 'work'?
        202–204
    evidence-based guidance for
        practitioners 204–205
    discussion 205–206
    conclusion 206–207
Newtown Union Health Service 202

Ng, A. et al. 185
Ngo-Metzger, Q. et al. 105–106, 109
NMC (Natividad Medical Center)
    163–164
NMF (Natividad Medical Foundation)
    163, 164
non-verbal communication 86
normative theory 36, 37–38

Ó Riagáin, D. 136
Office of the French Language
    Commissioner 117, 121, 127
O'Hagan, K. 136, 137
O'Malley, L. 121
O'Neil, J. 60
online translation tools 28, 94
Organization Maya K'iche 157, 162

Parsons, J.A.B. et al. 107–108
Partridge, M. 174, 175, 177–178, 180–181,
    182, 183–184, 185
patients' willingness to disclose 97–99
Pavlenko, A. 133, 134
Pawson, R. 142–143
Pelto, D. 152, 163, 164
Perera, R. 204
Pérez, A. 163
Perez-Stable, E.J. et al. 105
Pinto, D. 87
Pöchhacker, F. 57, 58
power 37, 43, 47–48, 72, 73, 79, 82–83,
        87n2–3, 106
    expert power 48, 82, 84
    institutional power 41
    and language 130, 138
    legitimate power 48, 82, 84
    social power 48, 82
Prince, D. 111
professional interpreters 21, 24–25, 42,
        84–86, **237**
    in-person interpretation 26
    in mental health care 78
    Netherlands 74, 75
Program for Medical Interpreting
    Services and Education
    (PROMISE) 158
Prys, C. 122, 123t, 125, 131, 132
public service interpreters see community
    interpreters

Quadruple Aim 6–7
quality of care 44–47

racial discrimination 182
Ramsden, I. 138
Raven, B. 82, 88n3
Reddy, M.J. 64
Rees, C.E. 46
refugees 4
Regenstein, M. et al. 110
relational contexts 47
Reuland, D.S. et al. 109, 110, 111
Ritchie, J. 124
Ritchie, W. 121
Roberts, G. et al. 122, 123t, 125, 126, 127–128, 131, 135, 139
role conflict **237**
Rosenberg, E. et al. 81
Royal New Zealand College of General Practitioners (RNZCGP) 199, 204, 205

Sachdev, I. 129
Saha, S. 117–118
Samson, A. 133, 137
Santiago-Rivera, A. 133
Schenker, Y. et al. 106–107
Schrauf, R. 134
Schwartz, L. 78
Schwei, R. et al. 130
Seale, C. et al. 43
Seers, K. et al. 200–201
Segalowitz, N. 142
self-efficacy 80
Shin, H.B. 153
sign languages 150t, 191–192, 199
Simon, C. 226
Smye, V. 139, 140
social care services 7–8, 9
 see also Chinese population of the UK
Social Cognitive Theory 80
Sosa, V. 152
Spector, N. 133, 137
speech accommodation 129
Stubbe, M. et al. 203
system norms 42–44, 75, 76–78

telephonic interpretation 27, 41, 96
Theory of Planned Behavior 80
time 49–51
Tracy, K. 37
trans-cultural nursing theory 137–138
translation **237**
translators **237**
trust 47–49, 63, 64, 72, 73, 84–85

truth-telling 45
Turkish migrant patients 82, 83

United Kingdom
 Health and Social Care Act (2012) 172
 interpretation services 172, 179
 Valuing People 177
 see also bilingual speakers in Wales; Chinese population of the UK
United Nations (UN) 4
United Nations Development Programme (UNDP) 56
United States
 Agency for Health Care Research and Quality 9
 American Community Survey 7, 20
 American Hospital Association (AHA) 23
 Chinese population 171
 Culturally and Linguistically Appropriate Services (CLAS standards) 21–22, 103, 104, 122, 138
 Institute for Diversity in Health Management 23, 104–105
 Institute of Medicine 23, 24, 104, 153
 Interagency Language Roundtable (ILR) 109, 111–112
 International Medical Interpreters Association (IMIA) 151
 The Joint Commission 24, 103
 Language Proficiency and Adverse Events 215
 Medicaid 21, 104, **237**
 Medicare 21, 104, **237**
 National Council on Interpreting in Healthcare (NCIHC) 25, 151, 158
 Title VI of the Civil Rights Act 21, **237**
 see also language access services in the US; language concordance between LEP patients and clinicians; languages of lesser diffusion (LLD) in US

Van Lier, L. 137
Vásquez Santos, L. 149, 154, 161
Victoria, Australia xviii, 211–212
 Australian Charter of Healthcare Rights in Victoria (2007) 220
 Charter of Human Rights and Responsibilities Act (2006) 215

Victoria, Australia (*Continued*)
    Cultural Responsiveness Framework (CRF) 212, 218–225
    culturally and linguistically diverse (CALD) 213, 217
    diversity *is* the mainstream 212–213
    Doing It With Us Not For Us 219, 221, 223, 231
    Equal Opportunity Act (2010) 215
    equity in health care 214–216
    Equity Standards initiative 225–232
    Health Service Cultural Diversity Plans (HSCDP) 216–218, 219
    Multicultural Victoria Act (2011) 215–216
    policy and legislation 213–216
    Racial and Religious Tolerance Act (2001) 215
videoconferencing (VMI/VRI) 27–28, 154
Virtual Interpreting Training and Learning (VITAL) Program 158, 166

Wadensjö, C. 58
Wagstaff, A. 46
Wales *see* bilingual speakers in Wales
Wei, L. 121
Wepa, D. 138–139
Westermeyer, J. 60
Whitehead, M. 206
WHO–Health Promoting Hospitals (HPH) Task Force 225
Wilson-Stronks, A. *et al.* 215
Wong, F.K. 186
Wright, C. 64
Wynia, M. 141

Yac, E. 162
Yang, C.-F. 201
Yeung, E. *et al.* 173, 175, 176, 179–180, 181, 182, 183, 184, 185–186

Zook, E.G. 46